Suddenly Silenced

Forty Years as an Associate Evangelist with Billy Graham

John Wesley White (D.Phil [Oxon])

SUDDENLY SILENCED

Forty Years as an Associate Evangelist with Billy Graham

JOHN WESLEY WHITE, D.PHIL, OXON

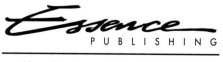

Belleville, Ontario, Canada

SUDDENLY SILENCED
Second Edition
Copyright © 2010, John Wesley White

First printing: June 2010
Second Printing: November 2010

All Rights Reserved. No part of this publication may be reproduced, stored in a retrieval system or transmitted in any form or by any means—electronic, mechanical, photocopy, recording or any other—except for brief quotations in printed reviews, without the prior permission of the author.

All Scripture quotations, unless otherwise specified, are taken from the New King James Version. Copyright © 1979, 1980, 1982. Thomas Nelson Inc., Publishers. • Scripture quotations marked KJV are taken from *The Holy Bible, King James Version*. Copyright © 1977, 1984, Thomas Nelson Inc., Publishers. • Scriptures marked ASV are taken from *The Holy Bible, American Standard Version*. Public domain.

ISBN: 978-1-55452-470-9

To order additional copies, visit:
www.essencebookstore.com

For more information, please contact:
Join the Family Christian Ministries
Dr. John Wesley White
P.O. Box 120
Markham, ON L3P 7R5
www.johnwesleywhite.ca

Essence Publishing is a Christian Book Publisher dedicated to furthering the work of Christ through the written word.
For more information, contact:

20 Hanna Court, Belleville, Ontario, Canada K8P 5J2.
Phone: 1-800-238-6376. Fax: (613) 962-3055.
E-mail: info@essence-publishing.com
Web site: www.essence-publishing.com

First edition by Advantage Publishing
Library of Congress Control Number: 2007943062

Table of Contents

Letter to Billy Graham 7
Introduction by David Mainse 11
Chapter 1   At the Stroke 13
Chapter 2   The Early Years 19
Chapter 3   My Spiritual Roots 27
Chapter 4   The Moody, Wheaton Years 33
Chapter 5   Launching Out 43
Chapter 6   Marriage—A Beautiful Romance 51
Chapter 7   The Left Side of the Road 65
Chapter 8   The Oxford Years 77
Chapter 9   The Green Monster 91
Chapter 10 The Right Side of the Road 103
Chapter 11 International Evangelism: 7 Continents,
            100 Countries, in 5 Years 121
Chapter 12 George W. Bush 135
Chapter 13 Agape 171
Chapter 14 Richmond College 191
Chapter 15 Near Death 215
Chapter 16 Phoenix: Rising Up from the Ashes 251
Chapter 17 Y2K and 9/11 291

Chapter 18   Lessons from a Stroke 303
Acknowledgments 311
Definition of a Stroke 317
Stephen Edward Trelford Bio 319
Index of Names: By Chapter in Order of Appearance 321
Index of Names: By Alphabetic Order 327

Letter to Billy Graham

June 14, 2007

Dear Billy:

On Friday your close friend George Beverly Shea telephoned us twice, and we spoke at some length. We know, don't we, that heavenly baritone voice Bev possesses. How are we to offer condolences to you, when Ruth, perhaps the greatest spiritual woman of the 20th century and your beloved wife, has gone to heaven? Billy, Bev said that Ruth had died at 5:05 p.m. on June 14, 2007. Then, on Sunday afternoon June 24, I had another telephone conversation with Bev and Karlene. We weep with you. We assume that Gigi, Anne and Bunny are worshipping with Pastor Richard White at your home Presbyterian church.

On June 14 I was praying and meditating on Ruth, now in heaven. In my hands lay open the book of Ezekiel. As you know, grief and mourning are the topics of the first half of the book of Ezekiel. A passage of Scripture came boldly to me. With great clarity of mind and spirit, *"The heavens were opened and I saw visions of God"* (Ezekiel 1:1). Having the gift of spiritual sight I knew *"[The Lord] sought for a man [you, Billy] among them, that should make up the hedge, and stand in the gap before me for the land"* (Ezekiel 22:30). I saw that you had traveled among the children of Israel, who were gathered on the bands of the river Chebar. As I came to chapter 3 a great outpouring of revelation cascaded upon me. The Lord proclaimed, *"Son of man [Billy], I have made thee a watchman unto the house of Israel: therefore*

Suddenly Silenced

hear the word at my mouth, and give them warning from me" (Ezekiel 3:17). Billy, you have been that good and faithful servant.

Then in dazzling shards of light the vision concluded with the fulfillment of the Word:

> *Son of man [Billy], behold, I take away from thee the desire of thine eyes with a stroke [I know this well]: yet neither shalt thou mourn nor weep, neither shall thy tears run down. Forbear to cry, make no mourning for the dead...and cover not thy lips, and eat not the bread of men. So [you] spake unto the people in the morning: and at even [your] wife died; and [you] did in the morning as [you were] commanded* (Ezekiel 24:15–18).

Indeed, a stalwart servant staying the course until for yourself...heaven! But perhaps there will be another decade, until you are 100 like George Beverly Shea—or the rapture.

In my opinion the greatest man in the first half of the 20th century was Winston Churchill. By God and his own oratorical skill Winston motivated the free world to rid itself of the atrocities of the Second World War. When living in England in the 1960s, the White family resided in Tralee House, just three miles from Blenheim Palace, Churchill's home.

To me, you, Billy, are the greatest man in the second half of the 20th century. Throughout your tenure as the world's best recognized preacher and statesman you have counseled kings and queens, presidents and the leaders of the world with unfailing integrity. You have always displayed God-given wisdom in spiritual matters concerning your lifelong commitment to Jesus Christ. You were glorified in Him and have become a household name around the world. I thank the Lord for the forty years I've spent with you.

Genesis informs us concerning creation, *"Adam called his wife's name Eve, because she was the mother of all living"* (Genesis 3:20). In the book of Proverbs we read, *"Who can find a virtuous woman? for her price is far above rubies"* (Proverbs 31:10). To the world Ruth is that woman far above rubies.

Ruth and Calvin were close friends. He was the pastor to two generations of your family. Billy, you'll remember that many times I joined Calvin at "Little Piney Cove."

Letter to Billy Graham

On June 14, 2007, Ruth went to heaven. The news media, in a worldwide tribute, transmitted Ruth's story. She was a saint to people on every continent. *The National Post* quoted your words from Ruth's funeral: "She was a vital and integral part of our ministry…These last few years we've had in the mountains together, we've rekindled the romance of our youth, and my love for her continued to grow deeper every day. I will miss her terribly and look forward even more to the day I can join her in heaven" (*National Post,* June 18, 2007). Your words were touching and loving for the woman who meant so much to you and to the world. She dedicated her life to helping you spread the gospel of Jesus Christ. Indeed, the world mourns.

Transformation. Then I prayed and ultimately envisaged my role as a servant to the Lord Jesus Christ as the words of Paul became clear: *"We preach not ourselves, but Christ Jesus the Lord; and ourselves your servants for Jesus' sake"* (2 Corinthians 4:5).

Your Servants For Jesus' Sake,

John and Kathleen

Introduction by David Mainse

Pictures flash before my mind as I focus on the extraordinary life of John Wesley White. I see him as an associate evangelist with the premier evangelist of our time, Billy Graham. Dr. White is addressing great throngs of people all over the world, and at his invitation thousands are coming forward to receive Christ as Savior and Lord of their lives.

I see this son of the Saskatchewan Prairies leaving the farm to follow the call of God to ministry, preparing his heart and mind in experience and education, studying at various colleges—culminating in a doctor of philosophy degree from Oxford University in England—before joining the Graham organization.

An enduring image for me is one of this preacher-scholar traveling from north Toronto by subway to make his frequent guest appearances on Canada's daily TV show *100 Huntley Street*. He's dressed for the occasion, and there's a ready smile and greeting for other passengers. The morning newspaper is before him as he prepares to share the Scriptures in light of the headlines on network television and later on send his comments on the news to Dr. Graham. He walks briskly into the studio, newspaper tightly tucked under his arm.

These are not just "still shots"; they are "moving pictures." I see John pouring his life into the life of Franklin Graham, while mentoring this future leader of the Billy Graham Evangelistic Association. I see a grieving father at the funeral of his pilot son, Wesley, whose life was lost due to a plane crash in the far north.

This montage of images shift to Mt. Sinai Hospital in Toronto, where I visited John for the first time following his stroke. He initially speaks only one word, "Jesus." Next time I visit, he speaks three words, "Jesus is Lord." Never have I witnessed more dogged determination to regain speech. I see him again with me on *100 Huntley Street*; his determination to once again communicate the gospel is evident to all. He is a powerful example to others, including other victims of strokes and their loved ones. His appearance shouts across the continent, "Never give up!"

This book is proof that, with God's help and a stubborn refusal to give up, his brilliant mind and great heart need not continue to be trapped inside a prison of a body that refuses to co-operate. I'm amazed and challenged by this publication of yet another of the many wonderful books authored by such a great man, Dr. John Wesley White.

David Mainse
Founder of Crossroads Christian Communications, *100 Huntley Street*

CHAPTER I

At the Stroke

The three best-selling works in the English language have been the King James Version of the Holy Bible, the writings of William Shakespeare and the works of Stephen Hawking. Stephen Hawking was one of my contemporaries at Oxford University from 1959 to 1963. He became a world-renowned physicist. At Oxford Stephen was healthy, academic and athletic. He was the coxswain on his boat and frequently rowed on the Thames River. Stephen would later be afflicted with Hodgkin's disease, and he would one day rise from the ashes to become like the phoenix.

I was among a privileged class of students to spend four years at ground zero of the academic world, Oxford University. In my time at Oxford I, like Stephen Hawking, spent countless hours at the Bodlean Library in research. Like Stephen Hawking, who rowed, I was athletic. I played for the Oxford Blues hockey team. Later I would know the strange world of speechlessness and like Stephen Hawking would rise like the phoenix.

Three internationally recognized leaders graduated from Oxford University in the twentieth century: former prime minister Winston Churchill, former prime minister Tony Blair and former president Bill Clinton.

I had been an Oxford scholar and a fervent evangelist. I knew nothing about strokes. Then, at 11:30 p.m. on April 28, 1996, the bell tolled; my wife, Kathleen, with her sky-blue azure eyes, stopped dead in her tracks when she saw me staring into space, transfixed on the void. When she questioned me, I just smiled a crooked smile, and she knew I had suffered some kind of a stroke. Through her panic she managed to call for an ambulance.

I had fallen to a severe and paralyzing stroke. Jesus said to Peter concerning the post-resurrection, *"Most assuredly, I say to you, when you were younger, you girded yourself and walked where you wished; but when you are old, you will stretch out your hands, and another will gird you and carry you where you do not wish"* (John 21:18). I had been preaching around the world for half a century. My life had been busy. Actually, I had never given any consideration to writing my personal story. But I was silenced by a devastating stroke.

For nine months there was nothing for me to do but to think and pray. Hour after hour in lonely hospital wards I lay numbed. The smell of the antiseptic, the sounds of the people in pain, the icy darkness when the lights went out. That first incredible Monday in hospital, friends and loved ones swarmed me. I trembled and laughed a weak, nervous laugh, but through a strange mist I heard the crying. Words of prayer and hope fell upon me—well-wishes and speculation and meaningless answers, reasons and causes.

In remote isolation that first morning in the Greeneville, Tennessee, hospital, I could not reply. I remember squinting hazily as through a revolving kaleidoscope; I detected the mass of bodies. I could see the outline of a person somewhere beside me. I recognized that it was Ted Cornell—my friend, a pianist from New York. Yes, it was Ted whom I first saw when I came out of the coma.

There, looming in the fog, was another, a giant figure of a man; it was Perry Ellis, a six foot nine inch Texan, who towered in the foreboding shadows. He had been a friend of mine for thirty-five years. Perry had been our chairman since that first crusade with the Billy Graham Evangelistic Association in Maryland.

But mostly, I listened through the mysterious mist. I could hear the talking, some of which I could not understand. I did understand the sounds. The sounds of Calvin Thielman, the pastor to two generations of Grahams and one of my closest friends, could be heard; Calvin stood by. He knew, firsthand, the trauma of a stroke. He suffered his stroke more than a quarter of a century ago. I sensed the presence also of John Dillon, Tom Bledsoe, and myriad other friends scattered throughout the room. What could they be thinking? I could not say.

At the Stroke

That first night I fell to a place that we evangelists sometimes refer to—a place where confusion reigns—a cold, hopeless place where loneliness pervades everything, where the soul burns. I was in hell. I was inundated with an ominous new reality full of physical pain and mental torment. It was Blue Monday.

In the beginning I could see no hope for the future. My preaching was surely at an end. So, heaven awaited, just one small step ahead. For weeks, in the daytime I lay flat on my back. My friends and family buzzed at my bedside. I felt invisible, yet strangely hidden behind a thick wall of secrecy. I knew. But how could they know? How could anyone know? I was in the company of many loved ones, yet I was totally alone. Later, in the dark night, I was abandoned, to lie in lonely isolation.

My son Paul, a professor at Purdue University, drove over 600 miles from Indiana to Greeneville, Tennessee, to be with me. He hurried to the hospital not knowing what condition his beloved father was in. What would he find when he arrived?

I can only imagine that trip. When he arrived at my bedside, he broke down in tears. My son, shocked, wept as a toddler weeps when his parents depart from him in his walled crib in the dark night.

Franklin Graham, another welcome visitor to my room, had preached that Monday night and then traveled to join the worried. In a moment of relative quietness, I could hear him mention that the last sermon I had delivered was the most powerful and effective of my fifty-two years of preaching. Franklin was a friend.

I remained at the Greeneville General Hospital until Wednesday morning, when Billy Graham provided a jet for Kathleen and me to fly to the Mayo Clinic in Minnesota. As a survival mechanism I began to savor the reflections of my whole life. I remembered those sweet days of youth, the exciting days of my salvation, the call I heard from God and my answer to Him. Then there were the days of my ministry. I drifted for hours at a time in quiet thought.

I was speechless. I had no means of communicating anything, except that I had one outstretched and trembling left hand. My right hand—the one I write with—had been paralyzed. After twenty-three books, the writing stopped. Further, I had that very frightening impression that other people in the room were hidden behind an invisible veil

Suddenly Silenced

and they could not or would not penetrate it to find me. I knew loneliness such as few people know. I came to a profound understanding of 1 Corinthians 13:12: *"For now we see in a mirror, dimly, but then face to face. Now I know in part, but then I shall know just as I also am known."*

As I slowly drifted out of the coma, the icy realization invaded. The extent of what had happened to me blindsided me again, like a train screaming down the tracks on a midnight run. I was struck with one incredible thought. Once I had been driven and focused, diligent concerning microscopic detail that some refer to as too small to mention, but now I was lying frigid, semi-paralyzed—in deep space.

Although I was articulate to a large degree throughout my adult life, my vocabulary now contained one word—for nine months—scribbled on a scrap of paper: *Jesus*! That single word was etched deeply into my being.

My sense of hearing remained sharp. A din of noise and a cacophony that sounded like 1,000 people screeching into my ears prevented even a semblance of serenity. Kathleen brought me scores of spiritual tapes. I crowded out the pain with the Word of God.

My evangelistic preaching had taken me to 100 countries through 1,000 crusades: from Moscow to Melbourne; from Sydney, Nova Scotia, to Sydney, Australia; from Belfast to Brisbane; from Tokyo to Toronto. For twenty-five years I had reached television viewers across North America and into Russia each week.

Time passes. It inexorably passes. In hospital, I lay quietly, allowing those personal thoughts to penetrate the silence. There were thoughts of half a lifetime with Billy Graham. I had been one of the chosen few who have had the opportunity of addressing, well, millions of people, in hundreds of cities, from hundreds of platforms. In 1995, in Minneapolis, I preached at the Promise Keepers' rally—to 61,000 men. They came to the rally in cars, on bikes, and on foot to hear the Word. A record 9,000 came forward on one night to receive Jesus as their Savior. President Randy Phillips told Brent Smith later that this was the largest number of decisions recorded in Promise Keepers' history! Lying there, I could very clearly see the technicolor images of the cover of *Time* magazine in my mind. Billy Graham and Franklin, his son, appeared; their busts, like the busts of Mount Rushmore, filled the

At the Stroke

cover. T*ime* wrote three paragraphs about me in this issue. The words I had spoken had been heard!

I had spoken words, words and more words. A torrent of terminology, from Christology to doxology. Then, I was silenced. My mouth was still, but my brain—oh, my brain!—was active and alive. This is the devastation of an aphasic stroke victim.

With respect to precursors, I wish to relay the story of the 1990s—my decade of affliction. In 1991, our son Wesley was killed when his twin-prop plane crashed in northern Quebec. In 1992 my heart stopped one hour before I was due to preach at The People's Church service that was to be televised across Canada. In 1996, I suffered a severe stroke on the left side of my brain. Ultimately, like an old oak tree in the still forest, I fell down.

I spent time in four hospitals: the Greeneville General Hospital, for two days; the Mayo Clinic in Minnesota, for five weeks; the Queen Elizabeth Hospital in Toronto, for seven weeks, and the North York General Hospital, for seven months as an outpatient.

In November following my stroke, I suffered a toxic gallbladder attack. The attack was so explosive that it nearly killed me! Franklin Graham phoned me that Christmas, comparing my condition to the biblical account of Zacharias in the book of Luke. Both Zacharias and I fell silent: for nine months—not one word! The therapists had voices. They were clamoring that I would never speak again.

I felt like a modern-day Job: *"The LORD gave, and the LORD has taken away; Blessed be the name of the LORD"* (Job 1:21).

CHAPTER II

The Early Years

I was born John Wesley White, on September 15, 1928, on a farm four miles south of Pangman, in Saskatchewan, Canada. Although bearing the name of the great eighteenth-century evangelist and founder of Methodism, I was actually named after another John Wesley: a preacher from Manitou, Manitoba, of whom my mother was particularly fond. I was named John also after John Kirk, an uncle on my father's side. I am proud to say that his son, principal Gordon Kirk, made his decision for Christ during my crusade in Dresden, Ontario, on April 2, 1993.

My parents were Martha Jean and Charles Earle White. The Whites immigrated to Canada in the nineteenth century. Fifty years ago, I learned something about my family ancestry while preaching in a Presbyterian church in the Scottish Highlands, researching my doctorate thesis at Oxford. Following my message I was entertained in the home of the church's elderly minister who, on showing me his family tree, quipped, "your name is White. I believe you're related to the campbell clam." Now I further want to let you know that the Whites were a rotten bunch of that family. They were rebels and they disgraced the family name. It was so bad that they had to change their name from Campbell to White. Paradoxically, it seems to trace a curious historical footpath to royalty, the King. My father was born on April 15, 1889. He came from a farm in Berkeley, which is south of Owen Sound, Ontario. This is located close to the birthplace of Nellie McClung, the nationally recognized feminist and social reformer of the 1930s and 1940s who is referred to as the "Great Manitoba Suffragette" (*Toronto*

Star, June 4, 2006) and whose face appears on the Canadian fifty-dollar bill. Dad was one of seven children: four boys and three girls. He was one of those pioneers who ventured by rail to a southern Saskatchewan town, where he homesteaded in 1905. As a reeve, he presided over the local council.

It was 1912 and the days of the sinking of the *Titanic* and the opening of the Black Oak School, which was situated on our White property. Responsible and hard working, from an early age throughout his entire life, my father could be seen working our large fields at harvest time. His rugged hands were swollen with the passage of years and the grip of the wrench. He was the third youngest of the four boys in his family, but he was clearly the leader. My father, a Presbyterian by persuasion, purchased the Halliday homestead the year he married my Anglican mother, in 1916.

My mother, Martha Jean McCaffrey, was a westerner by birth. She was born on July 9, 1888, in Manitou, Manitoba. She had grown up there and was one of nine children: five boys and four girls. She was a young pupil of Nellie (McClung) Mooney's in secondary school, in rural Manitoba. Nellie was my mother's teenage teacher and also her mentor and friend for fifty years. Nellie Mooney boarded at the McCaffrey home while she taught at Hazel School, a one-room schoolhouse that offered a curriculum for grades through 10. Such a powerful model was Nellie to my mother that my mother became a teacher herself a couple of years after she had been Nellie's pupil. Mom began her career at Kinghorn School, an elementary school southeast of Pangman.

In 1913 settlers from Eastern Canada and the United States were putting down roots in southern Saskatchewan. During the winter of 1913 in the brutal cold, a score of men spent time in the loft of our barn praying for revival. Then, in the Black Oak district, two women evangelists, Sisters Peden and Andrews, came from Winnipeg to hold tent meetings. A townswoman, Mrs. Charles Clews of Pangman, is recorded as having written in her diary on April 25, 1913, "The boys have gone to hear the 'Holy Roaring Rollers' at the school south of town." And on June 20, 1913, Mrs. Clews wrote, "Went to the Holy Rollers. A cyclone." These were likewise historic meetings. These meetings were held across the road from Harry Sheppard's land near our farm. A tidal

The Early Years

wave of salvation swept across the district. Dr. Strand was moderator of the Presbyterian Church, from Scotland, and was involved in the historic evangelistic meetings in the Black Oak district in the teens of the twentieth century.

Brothers Fred and Harold Hollands emigrated from England to the Pangman area during this period, and they knew the Lord. They took an active part in the meetings. My mother's sister Emma married Harold Hollands. They were Brethren.

Most significant to me was the fact that two other brothers moved from Ontario to Pangman. They were Frank and Charles White. Charles, my father, was the chairman of Trossachs Camp during the 1930s and 1940s. Uncle Harold Hollands sparked the Full Gospel Bible College. Out of those meetings came the foundation for the long-term blessings of Trossachs Camp meetings, the Full Gospel Bible Institute, renamed Full Gospel Bible College (1946-2007), and the Full Gospel Missions, later known as the Evangelical Churches of Pentecost (ECP) (*Streams of Grace*, Linda Wagner). I was ordained in the Evangelical Churches of Pentecost in 1948.

Yes, in 1913 there spread a fire of authentic revival in a barn in the Black Oak district. In the 1990s a Vineyard revival reminiscent of those Black Oak meetings took place near Pearson International Airport in Toronto. This charismatic bonfire saw our son Randy's wife, Lorraine, who was a nominal Christian at the time, swept up into the flame of the Holy Spirit. She lifted her arms and wept tears of joy as she was really and truly born again. Additionally, Kathleen's brother Billy Calderwood, a PhD and a Congregational minister, reveled in this revival. He received a second blessing.

In April 2007 the Canadian Broadcasting Corporation announced that there were then 600 million charismatic Christians in the world. They were quoting the Harvard University historian Harvey Cox, who pointed out that charismatic Christianity was only one century old.

After my father and mother married in 1916, they went to a local revival held by two women in a tent. They were converted to Christ there. My wife, Kathleen's, parents had a similar experience. They were born again at a revival held by two women in Belfast.

After marrying, my parents built a house, a barn, and some granaries. They settled into a life of farming. My father began farming as the birth of new technology transformed the agricultural industry in the early decades of the century. A threshing machine was a prime example of this. My father's first threshing machine was so enormous that it took a dozen strapping men to haul the wheat bundles from it. This was part of the great wheat harvest.

The automobile was at the time still a marvelous mechanical machine and rare enough on the prairies. My father's first car was purchased in 1914, the first year of the "Great War." The years of the Great War and teen decade ended with the most devastating flu epidemic of the century. My brothers Roy and Elmore died. For three years Roy's little red wagon rode inside our big wagon that hauled the wheat. My parents were understandably heartbroken.

The roaring 20s stormed in, leaving in their wake great prosperity for my mother and father. History reveals that this was a record decade of affluence. We living children were all born in the 1920s. From the heights of fantastic wealth followed the blight of hardship during the Great Depression. A barren wasteland grew like a giant tumor, replacing the green and golden lands. A period of severe drought on the prairies ensued, which the author John Steinbeck referred to as "The Grapes of Wrath." Previously flourishing wheat fields were sunburned into whirling dust fields. And a sea of wheat leaned into a crusty and parched earth.

In one of those years, my father's magnificent wheat crop was entirely spoiled, and his great combine was left to rust. The corrosion also diminished our hopes as people looked to their dreams with tears in their eyes. History has recorded that the summer of 1937 produced the hottest days ever in Canada in southern Saskatchewan.

Hugh was my oldest brother. He enlisted in the Royal Canadian Air Force in Regina in 1942. During the remainder of the war, he was stationed in Montreal and at other Canadian postings, including the Pacific coast in British Columbia. He married Aileen Milligan. After completing a bachelor's degree in science at the University of Saskatchewan, he taught school at Briercrest High School, which became the leading Bible institute in Canada.

In the 1950s, Hugh and Aileen moved to Victoria, B.C. Hugh took a job as a seismologist with the Canadian government. He continued his studies during those years and earned his PhD in physics from the

The Early Years

University of British Columbia. Hugh and Aileen had two boys and two girls. Both boys earned doctoral degrees: one, a physician, and the other, a physicist. Hugh's family moved to the Toronto area in the 1960s, where Hugh was instrumental in founding Richmond College.

Lewis was my second oldest living brother. Lewis' wife, Clara, was the cousin of Doctor Earle Cairns, a history professor at Wheaton College, who was of tremendous support to me. Dr. Cairns recommended that I study at Oxford University in England. Lewis and Clara raised their five children, four daughters and one son, on the farm outside Pangman. Lewis continued the family business. Lewis also spent much of his life on evangelical and secular boards. Their oldest daughter received her PhD at McGill University. Her husband is a neurologist in San Antonio, Texas.

Betty, my sister, became a teacher in Saskatchewan. Prior to my attending Moody Bible Institute, Betty attended that formidable school in Chicago. She married Elmer McVety, my earliest best friend. Betty and Elmer had four children and then adopted another boy. Their son Charles obtained his PhD at the University of St. Petersburg in Russia and is now the president of Canada Christian College in Toronto.

These were some of the hardest and happiest days of my life. Among other significant events, the decade of the 1930s featured hockey. I was a hockey fanatic. NHL stars Syl Apps, Gordon Drillon and Nick Metz were my idols. Metz came from the Milestone district. I still recall the excitement as I would sit by the radio on Saturday nights, listening to the shrill voice of Foster Hewitt, which was broadcast all the way from Toronto. He delivered the play-by-play action of the game. I sat spellbound with my ear pressed to the radio.

I have been hooked on hockey throughout my whole life. I practiced my hockey skills every chance that I could—on the sloughs. I dreamed that one day I would become a Toronto Maple Leaf. I would be a star! I fancied myself a star hockey player, known everywhere—within ten miles of my home! For two years I was a rushing defenseman for the Pangman team, and one of my greatest thrills was scoring five goals against Parry before my hometown on our local open-air rink.

I played baseball, too. I remember one night I wanted to show the Ogema crowd that I was as great at this game as I was at hockey. I

Suddenly Silenced

recall standing in the batter's box. I glared at the pitcher. I braced myself, feeling the energy surging through my sinewy arms. I stared the pitcher down. The pitcher wound up and hurled a fastball—right down the pipe. With fantastic power, I lashed a liner down the first base line. I streaked down the line and made a head-first slide into the base. The dust rose into a mushrooming cloud. I was safe—by half a step. I'd silenced the Ogema fans.

Again, feeling the excitement surge through my body, I took a step toward second. I would attempt to steal a base. The crowd was silent, still. I glanced over to see the pitcher hurl the ball to home plate—to the hitter. With my head down, I began sprinting toward second.

I heard the voices of the crowd come up. I thought they were cheering in amazement at my daring steal. But I quickly shot a glance back to first, to see the enormous first baseman standing on his base, with the ball in his glove. I was stranded in no-man's land!

I scampered to get my feet, moving back to first. The first baseman was laughing at me. He simply reached down and tagged my hand. My ears stung with the sounds of the jeering crowd and the umpire's incredible cry: "*Yer out!*" The pitcher had faked a fastball to the batter at home plate and fooled me with one of the oldest tricks in the book.

I left the field sheepishly. I slunk off to the bench, with my eyes to the ground. This moment immortalized my illustrious career as a ball player. For a young boy on the prairies, this was thrilling!

Before any of us could catch our breath, it was June 1939, and the world was about to decay into the madness of World War II. Hitler was mesmerizing his troops in readiness for their terrible march through Europe. Few on the prairies believed that such a thing could happen or would happen. The pleasantries of pre-World War II were about to be dashed to dust. The dreams of millions would be reduced to rubble, and a new world was about to emerge. We, to varying degrees, blinded ourselves to the awesome change that loomed before us.

That June 1939, the White family climbed into the "Hupmobile" with all the bubbling enthusiasm of a summer day and wheeled sixty miles north, bumper-to-bumper, to Regina, which derives its name from Latin, meaning "Queen City." In those days Regina was a city of 58,000, which exploded to become a city of half a million people who made their pilgrimages from Montana, the Dakotas and the prairies to

The Early Years

see King George VI and Queen Elizabeth, the late Queen Mother. The vast lawns along the route of the travelcade were sprawling with spectators who had come in droves to crane their necks, breathlessly awaiting even a glimpse of the royals. Even the back alleys and side streets were flooded with those too tired or unable to elbow their way to the front of the crowd for fear of causing a stampede. Regina was a beehive of activity, and the queen was about to deliver the honey. The dizzying mass of bodies managed to picnic in gleeful anticipation of the impending splendorous event. London, England, with its attendant pageantry was coming to town! Even as a youthful juvenile of ten, I could feel the radiant beauty emanating from Queen Elizabeth. It was here that I was awakened to romance.

I still vividly recall scrambling to gather myself together as my heart beat like a tribal drum in my young chest. I sped to the fence and was able to get within six feet of Her Royal Highness in her Rolls Royce. I think I saw the royal white-gloved hand wave at me. This was blue-blooded infatuation for sure. Queen Elizabeth had sky-blue azure eyes.

Exactly fifty years later, in 1989, I once again beheld Her Majesty. I was jogging down Leslie Street near a mansion in Toronto when I suddenly glanced up. I froze in my tracks. There, only a few feet away, through the window of a Rolls Royce that was stopped directly beside me, shone the same sky-blue azure eyes that had enchanted my youth. It was the queen! And she telegraphed eye contact with me. Although it was for but a fleeting moment, time stood still. Notably, Kathleen's mother, of Scottish derivation, was a dead ringer for the Scottish Queen Mother. Those eyes! The two women were born the same year and demonstrated the same kind of dignity and elegance. In the millennial year 2000, the Queen Mother turned 100. In 2002 and at the dignified age of 101, the Queen Mother died. Headlines around the world bled red ink immortalizing the favorite royal in print. The world mourned.

Another romantic event fastened itself to memory when I was at the inquisitive age of fourteen. Another pair of sky-blue azure eyes made their way into my life. After a year or two of my continual badgering, my father reluctantly agreed to bring home a Royal Enfield English motorcycle. He had purchased it in Regina—for $100. My mother grew several new gray hairs, I recall. The war was on, but I felt a new freedom. The thrill of the kick-start, the chilling sensation of thundering pipes, the invincibility of acceleration! As a lad, I cruised up and down the main street of Pangman. The other boys lined the sidewalks of the small town and turned green with envy.

It was not long before I had impressed my school sweetheart, Glenna Graham. She had the eyes of the queen. They were sky-blue azure eyes. It would be years until I married the sky-blue azure eyes of my wife, Kathleen. Glenna was the daughter of an Irish pharmacy owner from Belfast. I was as big as a house, with Glenna riding shotgun on the back of my bike as I rumbled down Main Street. Eat your heart out, fellas!

My cruising continued for a while. No one could have been more proud than I was in those days of my two-wheeled chariot. I paraded and waved to my friends and others.

Then, as if the black curtain fell on the final act of a tragic play, on one bright and shining day there was a clinking, a clunking and a puff of smoke. My bike ground to a halt. Glenna's face turned tomato red as she fled into her father's drugstore. I snuck past the store, dragging my broken bike through the back alley. I could hear the painful reverberations of the jeering onlookers. I made a fool of myself!

CHAPTER III

My Spiritual Roots

It was a brutally cold winter day in 1935. The White family crested the snow in a closed-in sleigh, referred to as a "cutter," from our farm near Ceylon to the home of the Merriths. The Merriths were neighbors who lived some eight miles away from our farm. There was in progress an evangelistic meeting featuring evangelist Howard Cantalon. He was an itinerant preacher in the area. Howard caused a wave of revival that year across the prairies. When we entered the Merriths' house, the Reverend Cantalon was there. He took us directly to the family's dining room table, where he began ministering to us. He was strong and preached Christ and the cross. My ears filled with the booming authority of his words. I was born again.

When I was still just nine years old, I listened daily to the sermons on salvation that aired from CKCK radio. Evangelist Oscar Lowry of Moody Bible Institute in Chicago was the radio evangelist. I was indelibly impressed with this series of programs, and I soon obtained Lowry's book, which was filled with Scripture. His book provided cards that presented biblical reference on the fronts and text on the backs. I spent countless hours memorizing them. This was undoubtedly the genesis of my biblical education.

There were other books of sermons and devotions that were part of my personal religious education and spiritual development. At the age of twelve, I was rummaging through an abandoned old caboose in our backyard when I came across a musty book entitled *Anecdotes and Illustrations*. This edifying book was written by Dr. Reuben A. Torrey, a graduate of Yale University and a most effective evangelist. Torrey followed in the footsteps of Dwight L. Moody. From 1901 to 1907, like Moody and Sankey before them, the team of Torrey and Alexander traveled the world, from Australia to New Zealand, South Africa, England, Scotland, Ireland, Wales, Canada, and to the big cities in the USA. They campaigned to millions. O.J. Smith, the founder of The Peoples Church, was converted to Christ in 1906 as a teenager at Massey Hall in downtown Toronto, along with thousands of others.

R.A. Torrey pastored the Moody Church in Chicago in 1908. Then he founded the Open Door Church, which was the largest church in Los Angeles. The Open Door Church expanded to include a Bible college, which has evolved into the highly respected Biola University. Two other relevant names were connected with the Open Door Church. The tennis pro and evangelist Percy Crawford, who hailed from Manitou in southwestern Manitoba, was converted at the Open Door Church. Crawford established himself in Philadelphia. In the 1940s and 1950s, he was the very first to bring evangelism to television. His program was syndicated across North America. J. Vernon McGee pastored the Open Door Church for a generation. McGee died in the 1980s, but his radio series built around Genesis to Revelation still airs around the world.

Interestingly, at Wheaton College Torrey's daughter was a favorite professor of Ruth Graham's. A generation later, Torrey's granddaughter's husband, Tom Landry, was the coach of the Dallas Cowboys football team in Texas. He led the Dallas Cowboys to a record that made them the winningest football team in NFL history. In 1971 Tom became the chairman of a Billy Graham crusade. Tom and I discussed many pertinent issues on the platform.

R.A. Torrey underwent a dramatic baptism of the Holy Spirit. My call to evangelism at least partly resulted from my scouring his book *The Personality of the Holy Spirit*. In 1928 Torrey died and was buried in Montreal. That same year I was born. For sixty-five years, I have adopted the theology of R.A. Torrey.

The theme of the team of Torrey and Alexander, like Trossachs Camp theme, comes from that song "O That Will Be Glory":

O that will be glory for me,
Glory for me, glory for me,

My Spiritual Roots

*When by His grace I shall look on His face,
That will be glory, be glory for me.*
(Charles H. Gabriel, 1900)

However greatly these early experiences ignited my youthful mind, the spiritual zenith of my youth was the glorious two weeks I spent each summer at Trossachs campground. Upon entering Trossachs Camp in the valley, located about an hour's drive from the farm in Pangman, we were confronted by an enormous sign that boldly read "Grace and Glory" (Psalm 84:11). It was Shekinah! Trossachs was a collection of charming wood cabins, and the area was dotted with tents. At Trossachs I was privileged to have Hugh McVety, Glen MacLean and Lorne Pritchard instruct me in the Word of God. The words of Doctor Luke kept flashing through my mind, *"When the day of Pentecost was fully come"* (Acts 2:1).

At a camp meeting at Trossachs, my spiritual life underwent the unforgettable and immutable infusion of being baptized in the Holy Spirit. I found myself on my knees in prayer, vigilantly seeking the answer to my life and to the existence of God, when Jesus' words were revealed to me in a *"still small voice"* (1 Kings 19:11–13). Jesus prophesied, "You *shall be baptized with the Holy Spirit...and began to speak with other tongues, as the Spirit gave them utterance"* (Acts 1:5;2:4). Then the spiritual fire came upon me.

The flame of the Holy Spirit swept through me like a furnace force. It happened in an instant, so short that there is no word to identify it. I was filled with a sense of joy and power that was clearly beyond this world. A love so radiant, a love so profound, swept over me that I knelt as the thunderclap struck. The love of Christ shone in and through me so that I could not contain it. The Spirit of the Living Christ was complete, and there appeared at that time nothing else.

Amazingly, His *"grace and glory"* had prepared me. It was Shekinah! I was filled with total understanding. I wept tears of joy. In that moment, the entire spectrum of time, the Alpha and Omega was encompassed. In a nanosecond I beheld all eternity. The bright light had perforated me. The inner illumination had set me aglow. All was revealed in the love that can only be received from the One. "I am He," He said. And, it was all for me. Where I had been asking, I was

Suddenly Silenced

answered. All things had become new. I was a new creation in Christ! The full force of the Holy Spirit was upon me.

I cite my thesis from Oxford, quoting D.L. Moody:

> I really felt that I did not want to live if I could not have this power...I was crying all the time that God would fill me with His Spirit. Well, one day, in the city of New York—oh, what a day!—I cannot describe it, I seldom refer to it; it is almost too sacred an experience to name. Paul had an experience of which he never spoke for fourteen years. I can only say that God revealed Himself to me, and I had such an experience of His love that I had to ask Him to stay His hand. I went to preaching again. The sermons were not different; I did not present any new truths; and yet hundreds were converted. I would not now be placed back where I was before that blessed experience if you should give me all the world—it would be as the small dust of the balance.

As Moses cried out to the Lord 3,000 years ago from Mount Sinai, *"Please, show me Your glory"* (Exodus 33:18).

Trossachs Camp produced four of the most significant Canadian evangelists who were born in 1928: Elmer McVety, Arthur Sheppard, Jimmy Pattison and myself. We all underwent the baptism of the Holy Spirit before becoming evangelists. It was white heat. Arthur Sheppard has been an evangelist to the world for sixty years. Jimmy Pattison was referred to as "The Boy Evangelist from Vancouver" in the April 2004 issue of "Report on Business" in the *Globe and Mail*. In 1999, the report stated that Jimmy was the third wealthiest man in Canada. Today, according to the *Globe and Mail*, he is listed in *Forbes Fortune 500* magazine as the 93rd wealthiest man in the world.

That momentous spiritual experience stirred in me a passion to win souls. I still recall my first convert, Jerry Carpenter. He went to high school with me in Pangman.

Jerry was a party animal. When his father was killed in a tragic Wheat Pool elevator accident, his entire community went into mourning. His mother and sister wept for a long time. Jerry became lost in a tunnel of darkness. My chance came. I was anointed and led Jerry to Jesus—in the night. In the morning I could see that Jerry had made a

My Spiritual Roots

180-degree turnaround. Jerry had a mission. He went out witnessing to the grieving, first to his mother and sister, then to his friends and then to his community. Jerry was born again. I was winning souls.

My career in preaching began at the tender age of fifteen. The arrangement was that Elmer McVety and I would take turns preaching. Sunday evening, Elmer preached beneath that little packed tent. He was superb. Monday night in 1944 in Southey, north of Regina, it was my turn. Very few people were in attendance. I was disappointed. I recall delivering my first sermon and bungling it. I had prayed throughout the day for power and clarity. I was full of the Holy Spirit, but I was nervous.

At once a gargantuan man named Gilbert Dynna gazed down at me. He had a hand the size of a ham. He squeezed my fledgling hand, and he barked, "The other boy will preach for the rest of this week." I collapsed inside. I felt like going back to the farm! That was 1944.

In later years I learned of the fruits of that first year in evangelism. In 1974, George Beverly Shea and I held at a television rally in Red Deer, Alberta, for my weekly program *Agape*. It was here that I was greeted by Lillian, a pastor's wife, who had just spent twenty-five years as a devoted missionary in Africa. She moved toward me and with an air of gentle conviction declared, "It was my father, Gilbert Dynna, who shook your hand in that tent the first Monday night you preached. I was a teenager then and was saved that night. I went to Bible School in Saskatoon, married and was called to Africa." This news helped to bolster my own confidence and assurance of Romans 8:28.

At a Franklin Graham–John Wesley White crusade in the hockey arena in Moose Jaw, Saskatchewan, in 1989, I met Pastor Harold Dynna, the son of Gilbert Dynna. He was Lillian's brother. As I approached Reverend Dynna I was awestruck with his powerful countenance. He strode directly up to me and recalled a Wednesday night in 1944 when he was converted at one of my meetings. Harold's ministry has been a faithful one on the prairies ever since. Harold's son, Dole Dynna, is part of an evangelistic music trio that travels throughout western Canada and the western United States. In 2006, they released a record of an evangelistic song. Dole returned to Trossachs Camp, which after three generations is still in the business of training evangelist souls.

For a brief time during my late teens, I was sidetracked into the teaching profession. There was a great shortage of teachers during World War

II. On account of this I was persuaded to enroll in "normal school" (teachers college) in Moose Jaw. My mother was a teacher. Five hundred budding young teachers were training at the college when I was there.

During the first six weeks of my teacher training I was sent around practice teaching. I had preached for two years but had not yet taught. In a rural school fifteen miles south of Moose Jaw, while I was teaching a class, the superintendent of schools saw me at it. He approached me and tried to convert me from my preaching career to a teaching career. Although I had given careful consideration to his offer, day and night I was beset with a burning desire to be an evangelistic preacher!

While I struggled with my internal conflict I continued to teach for a while. Notably, the teacher shortage crisis was critical in Preeceville, sixty miles north of Yorkton, where the student body was split between students of Norwegian and Ukrainian descent. These northern Europeans made great hockey players. The Ukrainians were particularly passionate about the game. I thought I loved hockey, but for these students it was an all-consuming pastime. You can well imagine that the circumstances in which I found myself were not ideal in the building of one's self-confidence as a teacher. Surely God did not want me to spend my life barking out the three Rs, only to fall on the deaf ears of would-be NHL-ers. Respectfully, my students referred to me not as "Mr. White" but as "Johnnie." In the entire high school, only a few of them studied. They fooled around and played hockey, and their extra-curricular activities amounted to chasing after the girls and partying with the boys. There are, I suppose, compensations for almost all of life's hardships. What made the Preeceville experience most memorable was winning the provincial high school hockey championship that year.

Many years later I had the opportunity to meet my Preeceville students again. During the 1970s George Beverly Shea and I were holding an Agape rally in Yorkton, sixty miles north of Preeceville. Of the 1,000 people who attended, many of those Preeceville students showed up. After the rally, many of my ex-students came to shake the hand of Dr. John Wesley White, the Oxford graduate and TV celebrity. To them I was no longer "Johnnie"!

CHAPTER IV

The Moody, Wheaton Years

When September 1948 arrived, I was enrolled in the Moody Bible Institute in Chicago. I had been hungry to preach, but I realized that I needed to continue studying the Scriptures. Something brand new, however, was added to the mix. I was being introduced to the world of skyscrapers and city pavement. The opportunity to preach formally evaporated. After a period of deep reflection, I tucked my Bible under my arm, picked myself up, and descended into the depths of the inner city to take the Word of God to the blistering streets. It was here that I took my stand as a street-corner preacher. The crowds that I attracted consisted mainly of the poor, the vagrant and the skid row alcoholic.

Kathleen comes from a Brethren background. At seventeen years of age she and her sister Mina, just nineteen, attended the Billy Graham and Cliff Barrow Youth For Christ meeting at the 1,200-seater auditorium Wellington Hall. It was the winter of 1946–47. The teenage girls made their way to the meeting through the rubble of a bombed-out Belfast in the wake of World War II. Brethren preachers of that time were rather dull and plain. To the girls, when Billy and Cliff took the platform it looked like glitzy and glamorous Hollywood had come to town. America the Big had come to Belfast. The two men were flamboyant, handsome and fiery, with flashy suits, loud ties and cowboy hats. Billy would hold the Bible way up high and wave it, proclaiming the truth. Later, I discovered that Billy's mother, Morrow Graham, was Presbyterian, but much influenced by the Brethren, just as Kathleen was. She was steeped in Scripture. She always preached, "The Bible says…The Bible says…" In retrospect this event foreshadowed the life-changing events of one personally historic night in November 1948 at the Paul Rader Tabernacle in North Chicago.

My roommate introduced me to the Bob Jones Evangelistic Soul Winning Conference. Serendipitously, it was here that I saw Billy Graham for the first time. He was as yet unknown to me. Looking back, my attendance at the conference had been divinely ordained. That night, it all changed for me. When the statuesque and anointed Billy Graham took the platform, I was entirely overcome. The tabernacle was just a third full, though he possessed the fiery oratory skills of a Winston Churchill. I found myself sitting in the front row and eye-to-eye with the piercing blue eagle-eyes of Billy Graham, who had pointed that evangelistic index finger, maybe at me. I was mesmerized—completely taken back.

He delivered a dynamic message on "Crises in the World: Philosophic Crisis, Economic Crisis, Social Crisis, Moral Crisis and Spiritual Crisis; Revival in the World." Cliff Barrows, Billy Graham's fellow evangelist and music director, played his gleaming trombone. I remember the air was ignited with the electricity of an almost ethereal sound. I was again filled with the Spirit. I was overcome with excitement. My blood surged. I was flooded with energy. My spiritual enthusiasm flowed from Billy's message.

I returned to my room at Moody realizing that I had had an epiphany. I reflected night and day on the words of Ezekiel. *"The heavens were opened and I saw visions of God"* (Ezekiel 1:1). Other words of Ezekiel flooded into my mind: *"I sought for a man among them, that should make up the hedge, and stand in the gap"* (Ezekiel 22:30). That was Billy Graham. And I knew the apostle Paul's words to be true: *"We all, with unveiled face, beholding as in a mirror the glory of the Lord, are being transformed into the same image from glory to glory, just as by the Spirit of the Lord"* (2 Corinthians 3:18). Then I prayed, and I ultimately envisaged my role as servant to the Lord Jesus Christ as the words of Paul became clear: *"We preach not ourselves, but Christ Jesus the Lord; and ourselves your servants for Jesus' sake"* (2 Corinthians 4:5). In my vision, Billy was the leader. I was the servant. So, for the next fourteen years I prayed night and day for the ministry of Billy Graham,

The Moody, Wheaton Years

and that torch was aflame to evangelize. And I have carried that torch for the rest of my life.

During the Christmas vacation of December 1948, I accepted an opportunity to preach an evangelistic campaign at a packed little Methodist church in a village three miles from Bloomington, Wisconsin, where Reverend Arlo Twist was the pastor. Following this campaign we held a week of meetings in a medium-sized church in a town five miles from Bloomington. To my delight, and perhaps even to my surprise, many came forward to receive Christ.

We moved into a larger church, in the city, for three weeks of meetings. It was here that floods of people made decisions for Christ. By any yardstick, this was revival—and something new for me. Like the blast from a shotgun, the reverberations of the revival resounded. I was on fire. I might seek some small place as His servant.

Ed Janecek was singularly the most important pillar of the Bloomington area. He was a real character. He came from an affluent farming family, and as a teenager, he was voted the most popular student at Richland Center High School. Among other things, Ed was a partyer. I recall that he majored in jokes on stuttering. He bought his own red roadster, his own Hog (Harley Davidson motorcycle) and his own airplane! He displayed the wiles of a man possessed of a witty, yet dramatic, personality. Ed was among those convicted at the campaign and came forward the last night as the crowd fled to the altar. Ed knelt in a state of profound humility before that mourner's altar.

Ed's life changed in an instant. He was a new man. At the time, Ed had been married for three months to Janine, whose first cousin was the Hollywood actor Lou Ayers. I was the best man in Ed's bridal party.

Ed pursued the dream of his new life with Christ and was trained and ordained as an evangelical minister. Years later he wrote me a letter about the 1995 Promise Keeper's rally in Minneapolis, notifying me that his son Phil had attended that rally. In 1998 Phil wrote me a letter stating that his father had passed away from cancer. The Janecek family had been touched by the fire.

In January 1949 I arrived at Moody Bible Institute, late for my first year. I had returned from the revival. I was spiritually uplifted by the terrific response. But in terms of being a major name in evangelical circles, I was still relatively unknown; I was still a "rookie." Dr. Harrison,

Suddenly Silenced

the field ministry leader of the Moody Bible Institute, invited me to give a forty-five minute address to the student body about the revival. I was anointed and Christ-centered. It was one of the most moving addresses I had ever delivered. Both the faculty and the entire student body gave me encouraging feedback.

Dr. Harrison reported my success to Dr. Robert Cook, the president of Youth for Christ, and Dr. Don Hustad, the head of the music department at Moody. They were delighted. It was then that we formed an evangelistic team. Our team was comprised of tenors Ron Kendall and Lester DeBoer, Arthur Nunn, a baritone and song leader from Texas, and pianist Dwayne Benjamin, who stood a towering six feet six inches tall. I sang bass, preached and was the leader of the team. We worked on weekends. During the holidays we ventured throughout Iowa, Wisconsin, Illinois, Indiana, Michigan and Ohio spreading God's Word.

This evangelistic team was greatly blessed. It was customary for our team to meet with some friends five days a week for spiritual fellowship and prayer. Our team also rehearsed our performances for one hour a day. Monday to Friday each week, I was busy with my studies. On Saturdays I traveled to our evening Youth for Christ rallies. Sunday mornings and evenings the team sang and I preached at church services.

In the 1960s, Don Hustad had "become professor of church music at Southern Baptist Seminary in Louisville, where he...trained a whole generation of church musicians" (Billy Graham, *Just As I Am*). In 1949 Don was the organist and head of music at the Moody Bible Institute. At Moody, one day during a frigid winter, Don turned to me and said, "You've got a great preaching voice, John, but it's not for singing."

My head was still swollen from the accolades accruing from the revival. However, the bubble now burst. In an instant I went from being a Horatio to being a loud but nasal and mediocre singer. Yes, I had spent five years performing what I considered good singing, only to be informed by Dr. Hustad that I was a mediocre singer.

I couldn't understand it. My mother was a music teacher. My brother Hugh had held a degree from the Royal Conservatory of Music from the age of sixteen. My sister Betty was a well-respected church pianist. But now it seemed I was born with a voice, although loud, that was perceptively nasal and "not for singing"!

The Moody, Wheaton Years

During the winter of 1949, I had an opportunity that was rivaled by few experiences in my life. Our team was thrilled and honored to perform in the Orchestra Hall in Chicago, one of the world's premier music houses. George Beverly Shea, a close friend of Don Hustad's, was featured. It was Bev who wrote the music to that amazing song "I'd Rather Have Jesus":

> I'd rather have Jesus than silver or gold;
> I'd rather be His than have riches untold;
> I'd rather have Jesus than houses or lands;
> I'd rather be led by His nail-pierced hand.
> Than to be the king of a vast domain,
> Or be held in sin's dread sway;
> I'd rather have Jesus than anything
> This world affords today.
> (Rhea F. Miller, 1922)

In 1943, I had attended a meeting in Regina held by a native evangelist, in full headdress, by the name of Chief Whitefeather. In London, before King George VI and Queen Elizabeth, he sang Bev's "I'd Rather Have Jesus." As an evangelist, I selected this song to be my theme, and for over five years I sang it as a solo many times before I preached. But, in the Orchestra Hall, and in light of Don's echoing sentiments concerning my voice, I retired from singing solo.

In 1949 we finally met the emerging leaders of the Youth for Christ movement: Billy Graham, Cliff Barrows, Charles Templeton, Paul Smith, T.W. and Grady Wilson, Jack Shuler, Merv Rosell, Torrey Johnson—the founder of Youth for Christ, Bob Cook—the president of Youth for Christ in the 1950s, and Bob Pierce, the founder of World Vision and Samaritan's Purse. It should be noted here that Samaritan's Purse has been headed by Franklin Graham for the last thirty years.

That September, my second and senior year at Moody, our evangelistic team resumed our road trips. On weekends we carried the Word of God to those in the breadbasket in the Midwest. I was making new friends at the institute. I joined Moody prayer meetings with Al Christiansen. Al, who became a strong influence and close friend of mine, had grown up in an affluent New England family. Who could have seen that he would later become a well-known and powerful evangelist? I may not have been able to foresee the exact details of Al's future, but I came to see that Al possessed enormous potential to reach people with the Bible. Al was my good friend. He has enjoyed a distinguished career and was a chaplain at Billy Graham's training centre "The Cove" in North Carolina throughout the 1990s.

In September 1950, I was enrolled at Wheaton College, west of Chicago. In the mid-western evangelical circles we were the cream of the crop, and Earle Cairns was the best professor I had at Wheaton. He was both a historian and a mentor to me. In 1963 he was named "Teacher of the Year" at Wheaton College.

Another important figure appeared from the wings and onto the stage of my life. It was Jean Graham. Jean came from Charlotte, North Carolina, to study at Wheaton; she was Billy Graham's sister.

Soon after her arrival Jean and I struck up a vigorous friendship. We talked about evangelism every chance we could get. We would talk about the evangelism of Jean's brother, his dedication, his calling, and his future. The year before, Jean and I had attended a founder's day conference for 2,000 evangelicals at the Moody Bible Institute at Wheaton College. I had accompanied Jean to many events.

A tall and exceedingly bright young man became my best friend at Wheaton. Leighton Ford was one of those men gifted with senatorial good looks. I was only slightly surprised when upon graduation Leighton Ford achieved the highest marks in philosophy of any Wheaton College student. Leighton was a distinguished Canadian from Ontario. On weekends, he was a dynamic preacher in the Youth for Christ movement who rose in prominence in the 1940s and the 1950s.

On the Ides of March, March 15, 1951, Leighton approached me and told me that he had found a date. This would set the stage for a lifelong and loving relationship, but not with his date. Jean Graham, who was then unacquainted with him, and Leighton's date and I took off to Chicago in Leighton's luxurious new Buick.

We were on our way to the grand Chicago Stadium. This night, I had boyish entertainment in mind. I had a chance to see the Black Hawks play the Boston Bruins. So I was excited about going with them to the game. On the road, Leighton drove, and his date sat in the passenger seat in the front of the car. Jean joined me in the back seat.

The Moody, Wheaton Years

When we arrived at the stadium, I was in anxious anticipation. My heart was palpitating. I was about to see my first live National Hockey League game. When we entered the gargantuan building, we were confronted with row upon row of brightly colored seats. Eventually we found ours.

It happened quickly. Leighton and Jean got a face-to-face glance at each other, and that was it. They were smitten with each other. Through the entire game, the only play they saw was the activity going on in each other's eyes. I couldn't get a word in edgewise. Leighton's would-be date vied for my attention.

I was interested in the game. I was especially delighted to see the amazing play of one of my true hockey heroes, Bill Mosienko. Bill was the Black Hawk's center. His stick handling reminded me of a magician waving his magic wand. He could make it do many tricks, including scoring hat tricks! I was mesmerized. I had heard Foster Hewitt on the radio praising Bill's dazzling play. But no complimentary commentary could do Mosienko justice when I actually witnessed his spectacular ability live. My eyes followed the gleam of his skates all night long.

During the drive home to Wheaton my mind was filled with colorful snapshots of Bill Mosienko. Leighton and Jean were filled with each other.

In May 2006 I sat in awe in the front row of Toronto's Queensway Cathedral, taking in the dynamic spectacle of Leighton Ford holding sway. Before a large congregation of those about to graduate from Tyndale University College and Seminary, Leighton's oratory and message were spellbinding and edifying. Following the ceremony, Leighton briskly took me aside. He told me the story of another hockey game in Chicago on the Ides of March.

Leighton and his now wife Jean Graham Ford were high in the stands, as was the case in 1951. They were straining to see the game. Suddenly, they were distracted by an old man who, above them somewhere and all at once, became frantic. Craning their necks to see what was the matter, Leighton and Jean decided that the man was desperately searching around for his false teeth. The man made such a scene over such a protracted time that Leighton and Jean could no longer concentrate on the game. Finally, the man gave up, deciding that there was nothing more he could do, now that his ivories were gone. So, disgruntled and toothless, the man plummeted into his seat. Then, quite unexpectedly, the old geezer, with his neck lurching forward and his mouth wide open, let out a terrific screech. The man's false teeth were parachuting down. They landed on Leighton's lap! Leighton and Jean broke into hysterics.

These were the good old days. Frank Nelsen—a sparkling Christian and close friend of mine from Boston—Leighton, Jean and I spent what seemed like forever in joyous and meaningful conversation. Leighton, Jean, Frank and I shared precious camaraderie. We had formed a union of wonderful friends.

We were off to that classic and majestic ball park Wrigley Field. Off to watch the Chicago Cubs play. It was here on one of those unforgettable fresh spring days that I got to see Stan "The Man" Musial and his St. Louis Cardinals play. When Musial stepped out of the dugout we were riveted to our seats. With the shining sun, the clear blue sky, the green grass and the smell of popcorn wafting through the air, I could hardly believe that I was actually getting to see that great Cardinal, Musial, at bat.

As he approached the plate from the on-deck circle I could feel my spine tingle with the thrill of anticipation. I leaned forward, straining to see the cut of his jaw and the tilt of his head. As he stood in, he assumed his own trademark batter's stance, the one most boys try to emulate at some time in their lives. He looked the pitcher down. The southpaw hurled the rotating cutter right down the pipe, but Stan saw it coming. It was as if the ball was frozen in time. Stan "The Man" calculated both velocity and trajectory and put his body, then his bat, into it. The crack of the bat and the ball screamed airborne past a lunging first baseman; in there, for a clean single. Silenced were the Chicago faithful as Stan "The Man" Musial strode confidently to stand on first base and to his leadoff.

Yes, Leighton, Jean, Frank and I went out to the ballparks, Wrigley Field on the north side for the Chicago Cubs of the National League and Comiskey Park on the economically challenged south side to watch the American League Chicago White Sox play. In 2005, the Chicago White Sox won it all. They were the World Series champions. The previous year, 2004, the Boston Red Sox did what most of the baseball world thought impossible. They broke the "Curse of the Bambino."

The Moody, Wheaton Years

They won the World Series for the first time since 1918. They did it in four straight games.

Some would say that what Stan "The Man" Musial was to the National League, Boston's Ted Williams was to the American League. To this day I hold a memory that is as clear as day. On an otherwise nondescript day in the 1980s in a rural New Hampshire restaurant, I had the opportunity of meeting arguably the greatest baseball player of all time, "Teddy Ballgame"—Ted Williams. He was a towering six feet six inches of athletic excellence. His presence even at his table loomed over the otherwise sedate restaurant. It was written of Ted "The Kid" that only one in 10,000 men have eyes with the visual acuity and depth perception that he was blessed with. Amazingly, it has often been said that the Red Sox "Splendid Splinter" visually picked up the seams of the baseball as it was leaving the pitcher's hand. The engineered mastery of his level swing was a marvel for all to witness. In the game's most traditional park, Fenway Park, Ted Williams repeatedly belted "frozen ropes" the distance of the park only to ricochet them off the "Green Monster" in left field that he knew like the back of his hand.

In 1941, the Boston Red Sox "Great" accomplished what others had previously laughed off as impossible. On the last day of the season he finished the year with a whopping .406 batting average. This was a new high-water mark in the annuls of baseball history. Indeed, this mark has never again been achieved. Most contend that it never will. Following a meal, a backward glance at the patrons, a quick hello and a turn to the door, he was gone. His memory remains.

Those were precious days. Leighton, Frank and I all had evangelistic teams. We would travel independently on weekends, preaching at our Saturday evening Youth for Christ meetings and in churches on Sundays throughout the Midwest. It was noted that I held the record number for meetings in a single day. I held seven one Sunday in Hammond, Indiana. This was all-out evangelism.

During the ten-day Easter holiday of 1951, I took my team to preach in Galt, Ontario. The team included my sister Betty, the pianist, and singer Don Holliday; I was the preacher. At the Galt meeting, hundreds of teenagers made decisions for Jesus Christ. This number included another Don—Don Newman, who was a rebellious teenager.

Suddenly Silenced

Don later became the pianist and choir leader at the People's Church in Toronto.

Yes, the music ministry since the Peoples Church began has been magnificent. The founding pastor, O.J. Smith, was heralded for his memorable hymns. Smith wrote in excess of 600 poems. Many of them have become hymns. The worship leaders, too, have been most capable: Eldon Layman, Don Newman, and, for over thirty-one years, David Williams, who introduced The Living Christmas Tree to Canada. For the past five years, Russell Wells' son-in-law Jared Erhardt has picked up the baton and continues the superb musical ministry at The Peoples Church.

One memorable teenage girl made up her mind for Jesus at the Galt meetings. She went on to marry the successful developer Bill McClintock. In the 1980s Bill's family purchased the land on which Tyndale University College resides. Tyndale is just beyond my backyard in North York, Ontario. In an act of compassion, the board of Tyndale dedicated one of its rooms to the memory of our late son Wesley, who was killed when his twin-prop plane suddenly crashed in northern Quebec in 1991.

CHAPTER V

Launching Out

In February 1952, I rode the rails to the Billy Graham crusade in Washington, D.C. I felt like a square peg in a round hole. I was living in a seedy hotel room that I used as a prayer station as much as anything else. Before the crusade prayer meetings I would pray alone to boost my spiritual strength. At the crusade prayer meetings I would be fired up for the crusade and Billy's message. I studied Billy Graham's preaching style and was overwhelmed by his charisma and the mighty power with which he delivered the Word of God. Billy Graham's messages were powerful, hard-hitting exclamations of the love of Christ. I was inspired.

Following the crusade each night, I continued my routine. I grabbed my Bible and descended into Washington's inner city. There were more alcoholics, prostitutes and illiterate ethnics to reach with the unchanging Word of God. I was both discovering my mission and making my mission a complete dedication to Jesus Christ, whom, for many years, had lived in my heart.

I returned to Chicago from Washington by train. When I arrived in the windy city I met my friend Clarence Carter, an affluent layman who resided in Florida.

There were two preachers of notoriety at that time who were particularly well known for dynamic preaching. They were pastors W.A. Criswell from the Baptist Church of Dallas and Robert Lee from Memphis. Responding to invitations, these giants would preach at the Moody Bible Institute's founder's conference. For four key years of my life, I was enthralled with the scriptural preaching of these men. They were strong influences on my oratory and delivery style. My preaching was taking shape.

I was a close friend of Robert Lee's. Dr. Lee presided over the Bellevue Baptist Church in Memphis, Tennessee. When I beheld the largest church in the South, I knew immediately that it was by far the largest that I had ever seen. The membership roll of this church was an astounding 17,000. Of relevance when considering the numbers at Bellevue Baptist, one must understand that there were 12 million members in the parent Southern Baptist Association.

Pastor Lee was a most eminent preacher. He was captivating. A brilliant spectacle kneeling on one knee in a white suit gazing up into heaven, Dr. Lee always found the spotlight before the huge congregation. Further enhancing his charisma, he projected his beautifully modulated voice in mesmerizing waves.

I escorted Clarence Carter to the altar at the invitation. The Bethel Mission in Pangman had no members. So he enrolled at Bellevue. He has been a member there for over a half a century.

Following the death of Pastor Lee, another voice was ushered forth from this pulpit. It was the baritone voice of the inimitable pastor Adrian Rogers. For an entire generation there were but three pastors who presided over the enormous congregation at Bellevue Baptist Church. Pastor Rogers was the third.

In February 1976, Adrian Rogers attended a Billy Graham Crusade. I happened to be sitting behind Billy and Adrian on the platform. I tapped Dr. Rogers on the shoulder. I wished to congratulate him on his appointment as president of the Southern Baptist Association with its, by then, 15 million members and on his article in the religion section in *Time* magazine. I managed to inform him that I had been a member of his church for twenty-five years. Before I could congratulate him, Dr. Rogers turned around and declared, "John Wesley White, a member of Bellevue Baptist Church for twenty-five years?" He paused and then spoke again—"Are you tithing?"

Sadly, in 2006 Adrian Rogers passed away as a result of contracting cancer. Happily, reruns of his program air around the world. I watch them regularly from 11:00 to 11:30 on Sunday mornings.

That August in 1952, I joined the World Congress of the Youth for Christ movement. Bob Cook was the president of Youth for Christ. Al

Launching Out

Christensen, Bob Cook and I departed from Chicago. We headed east to the edge of North America. We found ourselves in Newfoundland, and from there we winged our way to Ireland. Al, Bob and I were entirely jubilant. We were on our way to Belfast, for our first intercontinental campaign! We knew that there were many souls in Belfast in need of the Word of God.

Upon arriving in Ireland we were overcome with the fact that we were among hundreds of preachers there. They must have felt the same way about those hungry souls. They represented scores of cities from Europe, Africa, Asia, South America and North America. What had been billed as a campaign emerged as a great evangelistic congress and a powerful spiritual revival.

Yes, there were preachers on every street corner in Belfast. There were enormous assemblies of Protestants and Catholics congregating in the streets of this city of 500,000. This was a festival of preachers, lay ministers and common folk. The sounds of music wafting down the narrow lanes of Belfast added persuasive overtones to our message. At Windsor Park on the outskirts of Belfast, on the last day of our campaign, a round-up of 42,000 people gathered at the invitation. People literally spilled out of the park waiting for their turn to answer the call to Christ.

Following the completion of the congress, Al Christensen and I went 100 miles west to the predominantly Roman Catholic county of Donegal. The town's Catholicity meant that we preached before sparse crowds, often of fifty or less. Those who attended had heard the echoes of Belfast. At the end of a long day's night, we were discouraged about the small numbers that attended our meetings in Donegal. After an entire week of preaching, there were absolutely no converts! The result was that the many assembled preachers went home at the end of August. We were discouraged.

Then it dawned on me, one Monday beneath a tent, that the apostle Paul had declared, *"By occupation they were tentmakers"* (Acts 18:3). Our tent in southern Saskatchewan sat perhaps 100 people. Our tent in Belfast sat perhaps 2,000 people. In 1995 in the Minneapolis Metrodome (a very big tent) I preached to 61,000 men. So I guess that you could call me a "tentmaker".

For four weeks Al and I would take turns preaching. In the wake of the congress campaign there was a spiritual turnaround. Our unplanned meetings resulted in hundreds of souls coming forward. Al and I rejoiced beneath the big top tent!

On our first Thursday of preaching, in September 1952, two-thirds of our giant tent was filled to overflowing with those seeking the Word of God. Al and I prayed fervently for these Irish people. The Reverend Ian Paisley took over in the tent from 10 p.m. to 3 a.m. As soup and tea were being served he would shout out the Word of God to the prostitute, the homeless and the drunkard who stumbled into the Big Top. Paisley is a Free Presbyterian minister who has always been known for his outspokenness. He was a "fundamentalist." In 1952, he was known throughout Ireland as a highly assertive and effective preacher, who, for his opinionated views, was loved and feared. For a generation Ian Paisley has been famous and infamous around the globe. He is still preaching. His bellowing voice resounds down the alleyways and into the crannies of the world.

Ian Paisley has lived his life as a vocal fundamentalist, but now at eighty-three years old, he is a moderate. *The London Times, The New York Times, USA Today,* the leading newspapers of the world, CNN, CBC, BBC and the leading television stations of the world herald Ian Paisley as a moderate peacemaker. In May 2007, Ian Paisley became the prime minister of Ulster.

On the first Sunday night in Belfast, Al and I were faced with up to 3,000 people packing the inside and outside of our tent. Hundreds more world-weary souls fled to the front at the invitation. It seemed that all Northern Ireland attended those meetings.

There was no question about it—we were in a spiritual heat wave! For forty-five years ministers and missionaries have retold tales of the awesome events of God's work in Belfast. These were crucial days for me in Europe.

In Belfast, in September 1952, a fifteen-year-old girl named Lynda made a decision for Jesus Christ and was born again beneath our tent. Prior to that time, she had been a nominal Christian. Following her college education, she became a teacher. Later, she was called to become a missionary in Pakistan, a country that is 95 percent Muslim. She met her husband, Norman Lynas, a missionary, there before they returned to Belfast, where they have three grown sons and several grandchildren.

Lynda is a leader of evangelicals in Irish society. In April 2008, she attended Franklin Graham's highly successful festival in Belfast. Norman was the chairman of the festival.

The June 2008 edition of *Decision* magazine featured a two-page article about Lynda and her experience in 1952. The article contained a beautiful picture taken of her over half a century ago in Belfast.

Trevor Harris is a pastor of a megachurch in Seattle, Washington. As a young orphan, he was converted to Jesus Christ beneath the tent as I preached in Belfast in September 1952. Trevor immigrated to Saskatchewan to attend Full Gospel Bible Institute in Eston, three years after the tent. He then immigrated to the United States to found a little church in the late 1950s. Today, that little church has swollen its congregation to become that megachurch. Trevor is now an anointed pastor and evangelist. In 2006, the last time that I spoke to Trevor, he was a powerful preacher at Trossachs Camp.

One story of God at work in Belfast is that of an Irish police sergeant from Belfast. Sam Baird was built like the Rock of Gibraltar. His wife and three sons all made decisions for Jesus Christ at our meetings. The topic one Sunday night was a favorite of mine: "The Signs of the Times: The Second Coming of Christ." When the Baird family was returning home on a double-decker bus, Sergeant Baird apparently was sure that he was witnessing the prophetic signs of the end times. In the spirit of conviction, Baird suddenly inquired of his sons, "If Jesus Christ were to come tonight, would you go?"

His son Trevor shocked his father and confessed that "No! At this time I would not go with Jesus." But the power of conviction was laid upon young Trevor, and the change began. In a remarkable revolution, and with unreserved conviction, the youth exclaimed, "Yes! I want to go with my Lord Jesus Christ—I am a sinner and I want to be saved—for Christ's sake." Trevor's moment had come. He was transformed, turned inside out. He had now entered into a personal relationship with the living Christ.

Sergeant Baird had two other, younger, sons, Neville, a Christian business entrepreneur, and Clifford, a psychologist. They both found Jesus Christ at our crusade, just three weeks after Trevor had been reborn.

The Baird family immigrated to Guelph, Ontario, in the late 1950s. Trevor enrolled in the Moody Bible Institute in Chicago. After he graduated from Moody he moved to Texas, where he then graduated from the Dallas Seminary in the 1960s. He was training and ordaining in the Baptist ministry. Once ordained, Trevor relocated to Canada. He was elevated to the position of senior minister at Calvary Baptist Church in Oakville, Ontario. The topic again was "The Second Coming of Jesus Christ."

In 1978 our son Wesley and I were using our revolutionary media system at Pastor Baird's church when, seemingly emerging from a meltdown, stepped forward Sergeant Baird's grandson Stephen. His father, Trevor, broke down in a pool of tears. I spoke to him years later, and he informed me that Stephen's son came to the Lord during a church service in Ontario. Stephen was married and had three children. They were converted. An amazing four generations coming to Christ!

Trevor's wife was the sister of Dr. Reverend Gordon Freeland, who in the '90s was the president of the Fellowship Baptist churches across Canada and the chairman of the board of Tyndale University College in North York, Ontario. Tyndale University, for the sum of 40 million dollars, acquired St. Joseph's Morrow Park with its attendant buildings, making it a sprawling university campus. In 2006, the president of Tyndale was Dr. Brian Stiller, and the chancellor was Dr. William McCrae. They are both friends of mine.

There was another who found his way beneath our big top tent. He was Sam Sherrard. Later he immigrated to Canada and organized the *Rex Humbard Program*, which aired nationally in the '60s and the '70s.

Kathleen's brother Billy took up a career in soccer. Then he immigrated to Saskatchewan to attend Full Gospel Bible Institute in Eston. He earned three degrees, including a PhD in London. He married a woman named Maidra. Billy took up preaching. He pastored a church in Lethbridge. He switched from the United Church of Canada to the Congregational church in Lethbridge. He founded a Bible school connected with his church, and he pastored a large and vigorous church there.

Of the scores of people who were called to the ministry in Ulster, there was one special young man in our tent—Jim Wetheral, the son of a dentist. He was a teenager when he heard the Lord calling him to evangelism. Jim has served throughout the world as an effective evangelist and pastor. He specialized in church history en route to his doctoral degree in theology. He earned his doctorate in theology in Switzerland. It was in this spectacular country that he married Evelyn, a direct descendent of Napoleon Bonaparte.

John Abraham was an affluent youth who came to the tent and declared that he was called to be an evangelistic preacher. This Abraham was a descendant of the Old Testament Abraham. He drove a Jaguar and owned a linen factory in Lurgan, Ulster. In the 1950s and 1960s he was one of my associate evangelists throughout Great Britain. He held hundreds of meetings throughout England, Scotland, Ireland and Wales. He immigrated to Canada and for a long twenty-five years spent his life evangelizing back and forth across the two great oceans, the Atlantic and the Pacific. He wound up living in Vancouver, British Columbia. In India, Indonesia, and Southeast Asia, he made thousands of converts.

My cousin Louis Peskett was born on March 9, 1931, making him two and a half years my junior. When he was a little boy in the late '30s, his mother bought him a Shetland pony, on which he picked me up for school. I rode bareback to Black Oak School with Louis. He grew up to reach a height of six feet three inches. At Trossachs Camp Louis underwent the Baptism of the Holy Spirit. He later went on to Full Gospel Bible Institute in Eston. Prior to preaching at fifty Youth For Christ rallies he became an ordained minister. Louis advanced to head the Youth For Christ in Alberta. In his adult life he became close friends with Premier Ernest Manning.

In 1966 I flew to North Carolina to join the Billy Graham team following the news that Louis had been tragically killed while climbing in the Rocky Mountains of Alberta. A stone had broken lose from the mountain, killing Louis. As Elisha did, Louis may have cried, "*My father, my father, the chariot [of heaven]!*" (2 Kings 2:12). A gravesite was erected at the place of his death. The epitaph on his headstone simply read "Climbing."

In memoriam of Louis, scores of Youth for Christ rallies were held. Premier Manning named that particular mountain where Louis met the end of his earthly journey Peskett Mountain. Interestingly, John Abraham married Louis Peskett's widow, Shirley. Recently, on the worldwide television program *It Is Written,* Louis Peskett's headstone was mentioned, as was the apt inscription "Climbing." Louis' Aunt Pearl White revealed Louis' memorization of Scripture as a child and, most poignantly, his recitation of his life's verse: *"The path of the just is like the shining sun, That shines ever brighter unto the perfect day"* (Proverbs 4:18).

CHAPTER VI

Marriage— A Beautiful Romance

During our third week in Belfast in 1952, I met the most beautiful woman in the world. I fell in love. It was perhaps fitting that her name happened to be Kathleen. Soon I would be singing the Irish song "I'll Take You Home Again, Kathleen." I had spent my entire life answering the call of the Lord. But I had been lonely for the kind of companionship only a wife could offer. I had never been seriously involved with a woman, and I had never been truly in love.

It was during the third week of our campaign, and I was preaching up a storm. I found myself gazing down into the crowd. All at once I found myself suspended in rarified air. All I could see were the most sky-blue azure eyes I had ever seen.

Kathleen was standing there like a vision before me, and only eighteen months before she had stood there before Billy Graham. The vast crowd disappeared in a gray fog. I could see only the one with those sky-blue azure eyes. I was distracted. I found it hard to continue my sermon. I fumbled on the platform. I spoke as though I had marbles in my mouth; she was so lovely.

Out of the fog I could see that Kathleen was standing beside another beautiful woman, a brunette. Later I discovered that this Irish beauty was Kathleen's cousin. Her name was Jean Sargent. The pair of them were illuminating. I can't remember how the sermon ended, but I somehow got through it.

A little errant thought whisked across my mind as I stood drifting away in a dreamlike state. It was staggering to realize that I'd faced countless crowds and delivered hundreds of sermons to strangers, in cities I had never before set foot in, yet I had never known the excitement, the sheer exhilaration, of being so completely swept away by a person as I was in that instant. We—all of us—could feel the electricity in the air.

God provided me the opportunity to walk Kathleen home after the sermon the following night. *At last, a chance to be alone*, I thought. But her father joined us. My heart temporarily sank; I thought that I could feel it in my stomach. Yet just to be with her, regardless of the conditions or the company, set my heart pounding and my mind reeling. I more floated than walked down those winding streets of Belfast. I thought that I detected just a hint of jasmine in the air.

To my delight, I had a second wonderful discovery. Kathleen's father was the most scriptural man that I had ever met. Walking between Kathleen and her father was an overwhelming experience for me. I was sure that I was levitating.

Our winding course took us three blocks up High Street, then down Royal Avenue to the train station, then onto Antrim Road. I cannot remember how long it took us to get to our destination, for time lost all meaning for me. However, when we finally reached the Calderwood home, I met Kathleen's family. As I entered the obviously Irish house, subtle lighting and fragrances met my senses. In this exotic state I beheld Kathleen's sisters assembled around the living room as one arranges beautiful bouquets of wildflowers on a wedding table. Entranced, I felt like I had entered a harem of mysterious beauties in the ancient days of Moses. I was engulfed in a spirit of romance.

I averted my eyes, only to cast a glance over to Kathleen's father's extensive library of expositories and commentaries of the Bible. Kathleen's father was a layman, but I found him to be both spiritually extroverted and intellectually learned. And as time went on I was privileged to hear him speak. His oratory skills were decidedly advanced. He was magnetic. But that evening I spent two hours captivated by four pairs of blue eyes and two pairs of brown eyes. As I have alluded to, I had to persevere with the greatest discipline to muster the conviction to leave that house that night. When I did, I again noticed the fullest of moons spying down on me and graciously lighting my way back to my lodgings.

Kathleen hailed from a family of six girls and one boy. One piece of information that emerged from the voluminous communication that transferred between Kathleen and me in the following days was that

Marriage—A Beautiful Romance

Kathleen's first cousin was the reigning flyweight boxing champion, John Joseph (Rinty) Monaghan. He was known throughout the entire sporting world. Rinty had defeated the champion of the Philippines at King's Hall in Belfast, the largest coliseum in the country. The *London Times* stated that Rinty was rated 32nd in the top 100 all-time greatest boxers who have found their way into the ring. Rinty and the Philippine boxer fought before enormous crowds until the Philippine boxer received the thundering knockout blow and fell unconscious to the mat. And Rinty led all of Ireland in a resounding rendition of "When Irish Eyes Are Smiling." Rinty wasn't renowned for his coarse vocal tones, but Ireland roared their love to him anyway.

For the next seven nights I held Kathleen's hand on our journey home to her father's house. I floated on air, and now the whole world sustained the fragrance of the resplendent rose of summer. Upon reaching her father's house we all talked about many things and discussed the Scriptures. We chatted about the marvelous passages and parables and about the glory of Christ. We shared conversation well into the night.

By way of introduction to Kathleen's family it must be stated that the matriarch of the family was Kathleen's mother, Wihelmina Calderwood. She was a gracious woman and prided herself in the knowledge that she was a relative of the American president Woodrow Wilson. Kathleen's oldest sister, Dorothy, was married, and her other sisters were not. Dorothy and her husband, Albert Sommerville, were married in 1948. The next year they gave birth to Kenneth, Kathleen's favorite nephew. He lived close to the Calderwood home in the north section of Belfast. In 1966 he moved in with us in Toronto. He stayed for two years. Later, Kenneth spent years as a successful and affluent engineer in Albany, New York, then Florida, 2006-2010.

Jean, Kathleen's second oldest sister, immigrated to Canada in the 1950s and was married to Bruce Bullock. Mina, the third oldest sister, named after Kathleen's mother, married Billy Matier in Belfast, also in the 1950s. The fifth oldest sister, Mary, attended Bible school in Saskatchewan, then married James Briggs from Ontario. Kathleen's youngest sister, Ruth, has remained single.

It took no time at all to learn that Kathleen's family was strict Plymouth Brethren. They met six times a week at the Brethren's Hebron Hall.

Suddenly Silenced

Before I had really noticed, it was time for Al Christensen and me to uproot. The pain of disentrenching was almost unbearable for me, as I was by then in love.

Al Christensen and I made our way from Ireland to England and on to southern France by train. Southern France is highly secular, as evidenced by the small crowds we preached to. However, we held ten days of meetings there. From every city, town, village and hamlet there flows an interesting story. From one of France's southern cities comes such a story.

Al and I somehow came across a motorcycle-straddling Protestant pastor in the south of France. One day we found him preaching in the park. Al came up with the ingenious idea of placing his cowboy hat on the seat of the preacher's motorcycle. Al placed his Bible under the hat and began loudly proclaiming, "The hat that you see before you is a powerful hat. Under it is something as explosive as the atomic bomb." The gathering had not noticed the huge cowboy hat at first, and they approached it cautiously. Al would again point an index finger to the hat and deliver a verse of Scripture. Then, I would deliver another verse of Scripture. This twinning system continued. The crowd, at first small, eventually swelled.

The message was called "The Seven Points of Life." This message was based on possibly the best-known Scripture in the Bible: *"For God so loved the world that He gave His only begotten Son, that whoever believes in Him should not perish but have everlasting life"* (John 3:16). This was the first point, and it took Al three or four minutes to explain the verse. Then, there was "Life" under the hat.

It was my turn. So, I delivered the second point, which was that there was "Power" under the hat, like the atomic bomb. *"I am not ashamed of the gospel of Christ, for it is the power of God to salvation for everyone who believes"* (Romans 1:16).

Then came Al's turn for the third point, that there was "Talking" under the hat. *"God, who at various times and in various ways spoke in time past to the fathers by the prophets, has in these last days spoken to us by His Son, whom He has appointed heir of all things, through whom also He made the worlds"* (Hebrews 1:1–2).

It was my turn again. There were "Answers" under the hat. *"Jesus said to [Thomas], 'I am the way, the truth, and the life. No one comes to the Father except through Me'"* (John 14:6).

Marriage—A Beautiful Romance

Al was up again. There was "Joy" under the hat. *The Revelation of Jesus Christ, "whom having not seen you love. Though now you do not see Him, yet believing, you rejoice with joy inexpressible and full of glory"* (1 Peter 1:7–8).

I got up again. There was "Peace" under the hat. Jesus declared, *"These things I have spoken to you, that in Me you may have peace"* (John 16:33).

Al returned to speak. There was "Eternity" under the hat. Jesus said, *"In My Father's house are many mansions; if it were not so, I would have told you. I go to prepare a place for you. And if I go and prepare a place for you, I will come again and receive you to Myself; that where I am, there you may be also"* (John 14:2–3).

The crowd that had gathered wanted to see what was under the hat. But we held our position. Al had a climactic conclusion to this unusual approach.

At the invitation, in a breathtaking moment he finally lifted the hat, and the Bible was exposed. Al then hefted the Bible and began waving it vigorously. He testified, "This is the Bible, the Living Word of God. Come forward to receive a new life, for man must be born again." The mass of people swarmed around us and took the invitation. What a joyous celebration of salvation God had engineered through us! This strategy kept people coming to hear the Word.

It was on to Rome. We held meetings for a week in the ancient coliseum. Al and I had an interpreter. Those who stopped to listen could hear the Scripture in Italian. They were but a *"little flock"* (Luke 12:32), yet they stayed to hear the Word.

Al and I then found ourselves in Madrid, Spain. They were persecuting Protestants. After considerable reflection, Al and I decided to return to Belfast.

After a short rest and a long ride we disembarked in Northern Ireland. In the Crossgar Presbyterian Church, fifteen miles outside of Belfast, I met John Robb, the son of an Irish clergyman. In the early 1950s John was a teenage Irish rebel with a motorcycle. The broken muffler rattled windows all over the neighborhood. While John disturbed the peace, I was conducting a series of crusade meetings at the church.

One of the influential members of the church was a factory owner who had a tale to tell. A few weeks before the crusade, John Robb had gone to the factory owner looking for work. On Monday, the second day of the crusade, the factory owner invited him to come to the evening meeting to hear me preach. John was a hostile young rebel and left halfway through the sermon.

On Tuesday afternoon, the owner of the factory threatened John Robb, shouting, "It is a free country, but jobs are scarce. Make sure tonight you sit all the way through the meeting, or you're fired!" That night John Robb returned to the church, slinking into a pew. This was the night that he listened and upon hearing was convicted, then converted. Like Saul on the Damascus Road, his life was forever changed.

After graduating from university and seminary and being ordained into the ministry, the one-time Irish rebel biker immigrated to Canada. John Robb's spiteful energy had been transformed into sparkling Christian enthusiasm. He planted Alliance churches in Oshawa, London, and Brandon. Further, he built a large church of 800, the Alliance Foothills Church, in Calgary. Ten years ago, John Robb was appointed the senior pastor of a large church in Regina.

It was a glorious fact—I was in love. So it was natural that Kathleen and I decided to get married. We knew that we couldn't get married in the Hebron Hall, because the policy of the Closed Brethren stated that there should be no marriage outside the Brethren. So we made arrangements to have the legal ceremony performed in Scotland. Al and I met a doctor, Gordon Hendry, while Al and I preached at a Baptist church in Bathgate, Scotland. Gordon made arrangements for Kathleen and I to be married legally in the morning in Scotland. Then Mary, Al, Kathleen and I journeyed to London to Westminster Abbey, and beneath the arch, in front of the big door, we rang in the new year. It was 1953.

Following the thrown bouquets, the confetti and the well-wishes was the most romantic time in our lives. Though we traveled extensively on our honeymoon, we could barely keep our eyes from each other. Each day we walked the garden of bliss. We were lost in each other.

This was not the case for Mary Calderwood and Al Christensen. Mary remained in Belfast, and Al returned to Chicago. My beloved Kathleen and I were married in London and sent telegraphs to Kathleen's parents in Belfast and to my parents in Pangman.

Marriage—A Beautiful Romance

Holland is sandwiched between England and Germany and is a trilingual country; Dutch, German and English are all spoken there. We felt very much at home in Holland. We were welcomed with open arms. Since I was deeply in love, I might have been anywhere and it would have felt the same to me, but Kathleen was homesick. She dearly missed her closely knit family. She was just twenty-two and had lived her entire life at home. The transition to marriage meant both laughter and tears for us. I was used to much traveling and the accompanying physical and emotional hardships. Kathleen was not.

We stayed in Holland for three or four days and were impressed by the cleanliness of the country. Everything was immaculate and in its proper place. For us, it was like walking into a Christmas postcard. Kathleen's mother's name, as stated earlier, was Wilhelmina. She was named after the queen of the Netherlands. All the men in the family were named William, after King William III, who conquered former King James II of England. This was typical of many Protestant families in Ulster. Kathleen's father and brother were called Bill. Her uncle and her cousin were "Big Bill," and "Wee Willie." We named our first son Bill, after Billy Graham and my Uncle Bill White. Our grandson is named William Sebastien White.

After leaving Holland we went on a romantic sea cruise. The ship was headed to Oslo, Norway. In Oslo, we met a Scottish evangelist who was known throughout Europe for his tremendous revivals of the 1930s. Jimmie Stuart was high strung and spoke to Kathleen and me for hours about these campaigns. He deliberated for a long time about the Hungarian and Eastern Block campaigns, for which his name became renowned throughout Europe. The numbers of attendees at one campaign reached 12,000. This was a vast crowd for those days. Jimmie was burned out at age forty-five from years of hard-hitting evangelism. He counseled me for hours on the practices of preaching.

Oslo rolled out the red carpet for us and offered us what was, really, some of the world's finest hospitality. Much to our surprise, King Olaf greeted us in the center of the street. He talked to Kathleen and me about the situation in the world since the reign of Adolf Hitler and the German occupation of Norway ten years earlier. This part of Europe was ravaged by the Nazis, and only now was King Olaf's country returning to a sense of normalcy.

Suddenly Silenced

I was a fervent evangelist, for even on our honeymoon I brought the Word of God. On the first Sunday of the eight days we were there, I preached before a few hundred people. Everything was delightful, and we left Norway with smiles on our faces and sped by train to Sweden.

Bluntly but fairly stated, Kathleen and I found the Swedes arrogant, and they were neutral on issues regarding World War II. The common man or woman did not want to speak about the hard times from which they were just now emerging. As far as the blight caused by the German occupation, Kathleen and I assessed it to be parallel to the situation in England and Ireland during the war. We found Sweden cold both in terms of the weather and the people. Of our voyages to various countries, our trip to Sweden was the least pleasant.

In contrast to Oslo, Norway, Copenhagen, Denmark, was a sinful city. The whole city was obsessed with sex. We spent three or four whirlwind days in a city ridden with women of the night and people given to all kinds of earthly pleasure, and nowhere could we see any evangelical influence. This city was burning with Epicureanism: hedonists everywhere!

Kathleen and I fled Copenhagen. We boarded a ship to Newcastle, England, and then we returned to Kathleen's native Belfast. We finally arrived back at the Calderwood home, to find a greeting that was, if you pardon the pun, fit for a king and queen. They listened carefully as we shared our tales of sojourn and the story of our honeymoon. Kathleen and I were definitely married now.

King George VI died, but London, England, was all atwitter, for it was the queen's coronation that June 1953. We were among the many thousands spreading out behind the ropes curbside. It was pageantry, pomp and ceremony.

Then out of Belfast we boarded a steamer, bound first for Liverpool. However, this time we were on an extended voyage from Belfast to Liverpool then Quebec to Winona Lake, Indiana. Much to our dismay, en route across the Atlantic we found ourselves detained for three days due to a severe storm. We were tossed to and fro on the high seas. Our ship was to us a mere cork bobbing up and down on the vast ocean. If this weren't bad enough, Kathleen was pregnant. Worrisome to me was the fact that Kathleen was seasick,

Marriage—A Beautiful Romance

morning sick, and homesick. This was a horrible voyage for her. Consequently, we were overjoyed when we reached land. Then rail to Quebec.

Kathleen was homesick again. Then came a respite at home via Winona Lake. My sister Betty and her husband, Elmer, drove back with us from Winona Lake to Pangman. Upon our arrival my family welcomed us warmly. My parents, Hugh and Aileen, Lewis and Clara and many warm neighbors greeted us openly with wide smiles. It felt good to see them again. These people were my roots. I must confess a hint of pride as I realized that the entire surrounding farm community was dazzled by my sky-blue azure-eyed beauty. Hugh played the old family piano while the whole family sang "I'll Take You Home Again, Kathleen." It was a party.

Kathleen and I purchased one of the original Buick Roadmasters in Chicago, a novelty in any era, and we drove it back to the farm. We offered it as a gift to my parents. You should have seen their faces. We were all delighted!

In September 1953, Kathleen and I ventured in a southwesterly direction to Montana and Wyoming. Youth for Christ rallies were held in thirty-four cities. These meetings, which ended in October, yielded scores of conversions to Christ.

Bill, Our first son, accompanied us as a baby. His second name is *Charlton*, after Charlton Heston of the film *The Ten Commandments*.

Kathleen, Homer James, Frank Nelsen, Bill and I crossed the continent to Charlotte, North Carolina, for the Leighton Ford and Jean Graham wedding in December. Billy Graham presided over the wedding at Calvary Presbyterian Church. It was an exquisite affair in the splendorous style of a Southern wedding.

I was late, so I was relegated to the position of head usher. In the wedding party at the front of the church Billy Graham made a mistake that nobody missed. Instead of saying "With this *ring* I do thee wed," he said, "With this *wing* I do thee wed." Billy's brother Mel burst out laughing, and I barely contained myself. Even Billy chuckled!

On Sunday morning I spoke. After the service Billy's father, William Franklin Graham I, who had a great wit, approached me. Catching myself up I remarked, "Your daughter's husband, Leighton, is brilliant and has the style of a master orator, like Billy."

Suddenly Silenced

But Billy's father turned smartly to me and said, "Ten years will tell the tale!"

In January 1954, our family, Homer James, Lester DeBoer and John Duff's Gospelaires team drove to Orlando, Florida. For the next eight months we campaigned throughout the Bible belt and up and down the Florida panhandle, all the way to Key West.

My friend Clarence Carter was a visionary. He organized a series of meetings for me to preach at and the Gospelaires to sing at, in the deep South, from Key West to Mobile. It was Clarence Carter who arranged for churches in these areas to run Billy Graham's film *Mr. Texas*, a World Wide Pictures production.

I was deeply humiliated when I was visited by Leighton and Jean Ford, who were on their honeymoon. As would be expected, they anticipated the usual thousands of people attending the service in Ocala, Florida. When the headcount was taken, there were twenty-seven people on the benches.

Our Christian singing group, the Gospelaires, traveled around the southeast. The Gospelaires began laying down plans for six months of meetings, beginning in September. Our first tent was constructed to fit one thousand people, but we attracted maybe thirty people.

Kathleen and I traded in our old Lincoln for an old house trailer. I was a proud husband and a new father, but we were really struggling. Times got so tough that Kathleen boarded a freighter from New Orleans back to Belfast. Then I experienced a kind of loneliness that was brand new for me.

If that weren't enough, a hurricane bore down on our tent, and the deluge tore it to shreds. I was in such a state of despair that I almost packed up and went home to the farm. I fasted and prayed day and night. The Gospelaires and I could claim few converts. For about six or seven months, I wandered around my wilderness.

An evangelist walks many pavements in his life, some of them very bleak and lonely. I was impelled to a solemn empathy for Winston Churchill's identification of his dark depression as his "black dog." There are times when all roads lead straight into the wilderness. And frequently it seemed that I was following in the footsteps of my namesake—into John Wesley's "wilderness" of the eighteenth century.

There have been many who have wandered into the wilderness.

Marriage—A Beautiful Romance

Moses was in the wilderness. Elijah was in the wilderness. John the Baptist was in the wilderness. Jesus Christ wandered in the wilderness for forty days and forty nights. I suspect that since the beginning of time, actors, athletes, politicians and evangelists have experienced the fiery kiln. It is the emotional crucible we have forged from our own conviction. In my low moments I suffered a depression so debilitating that it threatened my work. Subsequently, the unfortunate secondary affliction of this melancholy was a raging hypochondria.

The fall came fast, and I found myself in Belfast again. I picked up my lovely Kathleen. This time we held a three-week-long city-wide campaign at Wellington Hall in Belfast. Later that fall, we crossed to Scotland.

Then we held crusades in Glasgow, Edinburgh and Cupar. At a hotel in Glasgow we met Dr. Gordon Hendry and his family. In the 1940s we had been sponsored by the same committee of interdenominational professionals, which was comprised of wealthy businessmen.

Our team drove through the narrow roads of that country, forty miles due north of Edinburgh. We campaigned in a new and spacious Church of Scotland. It was packed. Many souls were saved here.

According to the front page of the *Toronto Star* (March 13, 2000), the region of Cupar, Scotland, is thought to be the ancestral home of the infamous Pontius Pilate. The growing belief is connected to a gnarled old yew tree that stands in the churchyard outside Cupar in a tiny hamlet named Fortingall, which boasts a population of thirty.

Archeologists have dated this widely acclaimed oldest tree in the country at an estimated 3,000 plus years. The historic medieval Holinshed's *Chronicles of England, Scotland and Ireland* cites Fortingall and this yew tree as the location of a Roman peace mission at the time of the reigning Caesar Augustus approximately 2,000 years ago. Pontius Pilate governed Judea from A.D. 26 to 36. This was the time when he presided over the trial of Jesus Christ and sent Him to His crucifixion. Tradition holds that Pilate and Herod both committed suicide in the Alps.

Our three-week campaign culminated in a meeting in Glasgow, in Scotland's largest theatre, where 153 souls were gloriously born again—in one night. The number was 153—as in the number of fish in the post-resurrection miracle of Jesus Christ (John 21:11).

Suddenly Silenced

Douglas McDougall, a nineteen-year-old astute and searching biological scientist, confronted me at Glasgow University. Out of nowhere, he began a classic creation versus evolution dialogue with me. During the progress of our discussions I invited him to attend our meeting to find out what I was talking about. His curiosity got the better of him. He showed up, listened intently, received the Spirit and gave his life to the Lord on the same night that 153 were born again. This too was the very hour that John Wesley White Jr. was born in Belfast. Ten years later Dr. Douglas McDougall, regarded as a leading nutritionist, appeared regularly on BBC television. He gave his testimony at our crusades whenever we came to Britain. Since his conversion Dr. McDougall has been a lay Methodist preacher.

Beginning in the new year of 1955, we journeyed across to Ulster and held back-to-back crusades that were sponsored by the interdenominational committee across Ulster for the Youth For Christ tour. These meetings were held consecutively to the middle of March in Belfast, Carrickfergus, St. Stewart, Coleraine, Omagh and Lurgan. This was a season of genuine revival that swept through swiftly, like the crowds of people who fled to the front to receive salvation.

The revival spread to Omagh at the west of the Loch. Of the many conversion stories of that time was a small eleven-year-old boy's decision for Christ. He went on to Trinity University, and then to Trinity Theological College. He was ordained as an Anglican curate and moved up the ranks to become the rector of the prestigious Drumcree Anglican Parish. He was a dedicated evangelical and a distinguished churchman. For years we corresponded in writing, and during our John Wesley White Associate Evangelist Tour in 1986, we visited the Rector John Pickering and his wife, Olive, in Ulster at Drumcree Parish. John sponsored and arranged scores of meetings throughout Ireland in the 1980s. The Reverend John Pickering's attempts at peace for the Orangemen have made the headlines of newspapers and television worldwide for over a quarter of a century.

In a Presbyterian church in Lurgan, I stood before swollen crowds that spilled into the aisles. They were Presbyterians, Methodists, Baptists, Anglicans, Pentecostals and Roman Catholics. Many teenage boys were converted. They later went on to theological college.

During the tour of 1986 I ministered to seventy clergy in Belfast.

Marriage—A Beautiful Romance

Among the ministers were the Reverend John Findlay from Coleraine and Pastor James S. Gray. The Reverend Doctor Harry Upritchard, an eminent Presbyterian theological minister, and I have also been in communication over the years.

I never forgot my roots, nor the precious love that I had for my mother and father. For ten years I had written to my parents faithfully each week. Then during one frantically busy week I was notified that at age sixty-nine my dear mother had died of a sudden cardiac arrest. Without hesitation that March 1955 I dropped everything and fled across the Atlantic for home. A new aeronautical invention called a jet winged me to the place of my youth, to Pangman, to bury my beloved mother. As the pall set in at the funeral home that my mother was no longer with me on this earth, I tuned in to the scriptural text that was based on the words of the 120-year-old Moses: *"The eternal God is your refuge, And underneath are the everlasting arms"* (Deuteronomy 33:27). My mother said repeatedly throughout the years that when little Roy died in 1919, Elisha A. Hoffman's classic hymn "Leaning on the Everlasting Arms" was sung. It was once more sung, by me, on this solemn occasion.

Leaning, leaning, safe and secure from all alarms;
Leaning, leaning, leaning on the everlasting arms.
(Elisha A. Hoffman, 1887)

Yes, and in the 1960s our young sons, Bill, Wesley, Paul and Randy, sang and trumpeted that same classic hymn on TV and on their own LP record album.

During that brutally cold winter we had to dig through four feet of snow and six feet of frozen ground to lay Mother to rest. The tombstone was set in place. Its inscription read "Martha Jean White—1887–1955, *'Until the day break, and the shadows flee away'* (Song of Solomon 2:17)."

I was grieving.

CHAPTER VII

The Left Side of the Road

In 1965 in New England, I was abruptly pulled over by a trooper who had, to his dismay, glanced across the street to see that I was driving on the left side of the road. When he approached me I was embarrassed. I did, however, realize my folly, and I said, "I really must apologize. I'm used to British roads."

The trooper, who had been writing up my ticket, suddenly had a change of heart when I pointed out the large billboard across the street that read "Dr. John Wesley White Crusade" and displayed a larger than life-sized picture of yours truly that was as clear as day. After a pause the trooper replied, "Okay this time, mister, but just remember you're in America now!" He ripped up my ticket.

Flash farther back to March 1955. The Gospelaires left for various locations in Canada and the United States. I had a wife and two boys. I journeyed to the Calderwood home to focus on the boys. This was a specific difficulty that I could correct. But again, I was tired to the bone. Moreover, my conscience began niggling me concerning my family responsibilities.

Kathleen and I left for a six-week Billy Graham Crusade, starting at Kelvin Hall in Glasgow, Scotland. Billy was now preaching before crowds of 15,000 nightly at the Tell Scotland crusade, which was chaired by Tom Allan, who was a highly respected member of the Church of Scotland. Billy concluded the series of meetings with 100,000 people at Hampton Park. The Billy Graham team featured scores of North American preachers. Tom, who had been involved in my crusade in 1954, did a terrific job.

Suddenly Silenced

The Tell Scotland crusade reached every level of Scottish society, even down to the John Brown Shipyard. The associate evangelists T.W. Wilson, Grady Wilson, Joe Blinco and Leighton Ford joined the Graham team. The team and I brought the Word to the rough shipbuilders and to the steelworkers at the steel mills in Hamilton, which sits between Edinburgh and Glasgow. In the sullied streets we preached to the unwashed masses. We took the message to many at soccer stadiums, theatres and open-air plazas throughout Scotland.

Meanwhile, Billy and his team were carrying the gospel to much of Scotland's high society and to royalty. Billy Graham's team leaders, including Cliff Barrows, George Beverly Shea and T.W. Wilson, stayed at the North Hotel in Glasgow, but the Queen's Park Hotel was the headquarters for the crusade, and this was where the majority of the team resided. In 1955, our family was ensconced in the hotel that Dr. Gordon Hendry and his family of physicians owned.

In March 1955, Billy Graham held hands with a frightened and anxious world as it broke into a cold sweat. These were the days of the hydrogen bomb. The H-bomb harnessed exponentially more explosive power than the atomic bombs that annihilated Hiroshima and Nagasaki only a single decade before, drawing a swift and frightening conclusion to World War II. From the atomic bomb there rose a noxious mushroom cloud that was witnessed by the world.

News of the escalating cold war between the United States and the USSR was everywhere. Newspaper boxes on the street corners of every city in the world displayed headlines that struck fear into the hearts of citizens going about daily tasks. People scurried home from work to place their ears to the radios and their eyes to the TV sets. They held their breaths as they learned that first the Russians, then the Americans, were conducting ominous tests with a bomb so powerful that it was said to have the capability to blow up the world. There now loomed the ever-present threat that should the incredible power of the H-bomb be released it could mean the end of the world.

On April 18, 1955, radio airwaves and television stations around the globe were flooded with the news that "Albert Einstein is dead." I rushed the message to Billy. He was shocked. The great evangelist sent me off to construct an illustration that might make sense of this tragic death. I hurried back to the hotel to get to work. The following is a quote from my illustration concerning Albert Einstein's passing, which Billy then delivered to an awe-inspired crowd:

> Albert Einstein is dead. About thermonuclear weaponry, Einstein reasoned, "The ghostlike character of this development lies in its apparently compulsory trend. Every step appears as the unavoidable consequence of the preceding one. In the end, there beckons more and more clearly general annihilation." Certainly nothing has happened in recent years to reverse this pessimism. The Canadian physicist Dr. Allan Munn says that the thermonuclear devices now with us "might cause the world and all in it to disintegrate in less than a minute."

Peter the apostle, who suffered an inglorious death at the hands of the Roman emperor Nero, foretold another shocking event to take place at an unknown time:

> *The day of the Lord will come as a thief in the night, in which the heavens will pass away with a great noise, and the elements will melt with fervent heat; both the earth and the works that are in it will be burned up. Therefore, since all these things will be dissolved, what manner of persons ought you to be in holy conduct and godliness, looking for and hastening the coming of the day of God, because of which the heavens will be dissolved, being on fire, and the elements will melt with fervent heat?* (2 Peter 3:10–12).

Just as dramatically, the century-old apostle of Jesus Christ, John, similarly warned the world when he revealed the second coming of Jesus Christ. "*'Behold, I am coming as a thief...' And they gathered them together to the place called in Hebrew, Armageddon*" (Revelation 16:15–16). And in post-modern times it was General Douglas MacArthur, the champion of the second world war, who boldly stated before his death, "We have had our last chance. The Battle of Armageddon comes next!" Indeed, we were gazing through the windows of heaven straight into Armageddon.

Thus I ascended to the position of which I had previously only dreamed, a researcher and illustrator for Billy Graham. Perhaps equally

Suddenly Silenced

moving to me was the now certain fact that as a writer I would follow in the footsteps of my childhood hero, the one I discovered in that caboose on the farm. I was thrilled that I was an R.A. Torrey. I thought distinctly about his tome *Anecdotes and Illustrations*. Even more than that, I would become Billy Graham's primary sermon illustrator. I would stand humbly alongside the twentieth century's greatest evangelist, supplying him with words to speak to untold numbers of Spirit-thirsty people.

I was thrilled about the success of the Tell Scotland effort. I suggested that we leave Scotland and trek across to Belfast. I enrolled at Queen's University in Belfast for one year and at Trinity College in Dublin for a second and third year.

While I was enrolled at Queen's University, I held city-wide campaigns. Now I was preaching in large and small Presbyterian and Church of Scotland churches in Ulster and Scotland and had a larger plan for my life in evangelism.

The time had come to consider the daunting task and great intellectual journey of my post-graduate work. I began by scanning a hundred newspapers that I found in libraries throughout these regions. My compass was set on *The Influence of North American Evangelism in Scotland and Ireland Between 1830 and 1914, Beginning with Charles Finney and Proceeding through D. L. Moody, R. A. Torrey, Wilbur Chapman and One Hundred Evangelists Who Had Crossed the Atlantic.*

I compiled over 10,000 pages of notes on my thesis topic, collected over a three-year period. I condensed these stacks into my graduate thesis. Ultimately, I arrived at a master's of literature degree at Trinity University in Dublin, the third oldest British university.

Kathleen and I were as proud as punch to buy our own home in Wellington Park near Queen's University in South Belfast. Paul, our third son, had been born in the Calderwood home in December 1955. Sadly, in March 1956, my father died, and I returned to Pangman. My father had been converted to Jesus Christ in 1913 during that tent revival, but my second parent was gone. This time all that I could hear ringing in my ears was Isaac Watts' classic hymn "At the Cross":

The Left Side of the Road

Alas, and did my Savior bleed,
And did my Sov'reign die?
Would He devote that sacred head
For such a worm as I?
At the cross, at the cross
Where I first saw the light,
And the burden of my heart rolled away
It was there by faith I received my sight,
And now I am happy all the day!
(Isaac Watts, 1707)

Upon my return to Belfast, I purchased a teeny-tiny little car, a Morris Minor. My family and I spent time taking drives down the left side of the road, having squeezed into our Minor. Our house was situated in a respectfully quiet upper-middle-class suburb of Belfast. I am still astounded when I think back on how Kathleen, our three boys and I cohabitated with no less than seven boarders at a time in this big old house. We were always very fortunate to rent rooms to rather dignified professionals, who held the greatest respect for our home.

We shared meals with them. I presided over our suppers, beginning with a drawn-out grace. I recall one boarder. He was a lawyer who sat statue-still while I asked for the Lord's blessing at our dinner. In contrite reverence the lawyer closed his eyes. He never even blinked as our middle son, Wesley, climbed up on the table and crawled over to this gentleman's plate. The lawyer never saw that his lamb chop was being grabbed from his plate and indelicately gobbled up by Wes. When grace ended and the lawyer opened his eyes, he could hardly bring himself to ask for another lamb chop. In realizing what had happened, our faces blushed with embarrassment. There was little we could say to console the famished man. We couldn't do much to assuage the lawyer's hot head or his empty stomach.

On another front, the American evangelist Jack Shuler had been the music director for Cliff Barrows in the 1940s. Jack had also been with the crusades in Belfast that had been sponsored by the Youth for Christ movement in the spring of 1956. I joined Jack Shuler's team as an associate evangelist for a six-week crusade. Jack was one of the three great evangelists of the era. Billy, Charles Templeton and Jack Shuler were known throughout the four corners of the globe for their dynamic evangelism. Jack possessed the striking good looks of a Hollywood actor, which, when combined with his dramatic and flamboyant style, captivated audiences everywhere he preached. He preached before crowds of 8,000 to 10,000 per night.

I was still preaching in the Presbyterian, Anglican, Baptist and Pentecostal churches and, as always, in the streets, at the stadiums, and in the shipyards. I read the Scriptures and the prayers on the platform at Jack's crusade meetings, and then I savored the brilliantly arranged words of a master orator.

Kathleen and I were in the process of redecorating our home. We had purchased royal blue carpet and found that we were left with a considerable amount of extra material. It occurred to me that the extra piece of carpeting would suit the two stairs to the platform at King's Hall where Jack Shuler held his crusade. So we laid the brand new carpet on the stairs. It looked regal—very attractive.

One evening after the crusade meeting, Kathleen, wee Wesley and I came to the stairs. We just marveled at the beauty of our new carpet. Kathleen stood atop the stairs while I gazed up from the bottom. Wes's tiny frame teetered up there. He was just far enough from his mother that she hadn't noticed her toddler son's curiosity over the imperial gallon of cream-colored paint that likewise balanced on the precipice of the stairs. Suddenly, there was a commotion and a roar came up. Wes had toppled and tipped the paint straight down the stairs, enveloping the bright new royal blue carpet in creamy paint.

The next sound that was heard was that of wee Wes feigning tears. I shouted up to him, "You're going to get a spanking this time, mister!"

In defiance Wes retaliated, "No, Daddy! Mommy already spanked me." Kathleen had merely tapped Wes' bottom with a feather. It was time for elbow grease and turpentine. The cleanup began!

In contrast to the evangelist Jack Shuler, who had been distant and, in all honesty, arrogant, the evangelist George Sweeting from Moody Bible Institute, though similarly dashing in appearance, possessed a modest, humorous and compassionate personality. George and his evangelistic team had flown from New Jersey to Belfast for a series of evangelistic meetings. This was very exciting for me. I had an insatiable thirst for North American evangelists. During George's visit I took

The Left Side of the Road

many opportunities to discuss a variety of topics with the North American evangelists who had come to town.

George Sweeting had his spiritual roots in the Scottish evangelist Jimmie Stuart. It was Jimmie Stuart who triggered my obsession with North American evangelism. It had been that way since my honeymoon in Norway. I was researching all the time. In fact, I was gathering information for my thesis when George arrived. George Sweeting was a specialist in the works of Moody and Sankey. He was therefore interested in and easily able to absorb himself in my work. He focused on my topic intensely and carefully. This meant a great deal to me. George and I developed a wonderful camaraderie in Belfast.

Kathleen and I invited George and the team to our home, where we shared precious fellowship and many more discussions. Indeed, George was full of illustrative stories that I found fascinating and edifying. One night he spoke of rock and roll legend Elvis Presley's life as being lonely and empty, though he found his way to any stage light available. His life had been a tragedy, even though he had acquired almost everything that the world seeks. Materialism had not brought the hip-gyrating icon what he most desperately needed: peace of mind. Only Jesus Christ delivers that.

Finances were scarce for Kathleen and me, and our house was filled with old furniture that we had purchased at auctions. On one particular afternoon, George Sweeting was comfortably seated at the head of our dining room table. He was a distinguished gentleman who gained the attention of everyone at the table. Then suddenly, during a serious discussion, George's chair crumbled beneath him. With a look of astonishment engraved on his face, he collapsed straight down and landed flat on his back! Kathleen and I were again embarrassed. We thanked God that George wasn't physically hurt, but he must have developed new questions about his amiable hosts.

From 1956 to 1976 Dr. George Sweeting was the president of Moody Bible Institute. He hosted Moody's annual founder's conference. Thousands of evangelicals attended this conference. I was one of the speakers there. In my introduction to the crowd I confessed the story of how twenty years earlier, President George Sweeting had been "let down!" Gales of laughter rose from the crowd. Dr. Sweeting is not a man who ought to be let down.

Suddenly Silenced

One night while I was preaching, I got to the main point late in my sermon. I was dealing with the topic of death and heaven. I found myself reminiscing about my son Wes. I recalled Wes' reaction when the boys' great-grandmother died. There was a Plymouth Brethren cemetery in Belfast. Wes and Bill insisted on coming to the funeral with me, even though they were two and three years of age respectively. When the pallbearers lowered the coffin, it was raining. Somehow Wes got loose from my hand and sauntered over to the grave. As he looked in, he slipped, and I grabbed him barely in time to keep him from falling in.

A few days later our canary died. Wes and Bill came out to the back garden to bury it. Wes had in mind the burial service of his great-grandmother and how his Grandpa Calderwood pronounced the final benediction at the committal: *"In the name of the Father, and of the Son, and of the Holy Ghost." So* when we buried the bird, as Bill dropped it into the hole, in a loud voice Wes exclaimed, "In the Name of the Father, and of the Son, and into the hole he goes!"

In the south of England I was preaching in a gospel tent. Wes was three by then, and he thought I had spoken long enough. A pooch wandered into the tent and headed straight for Wes. Neither Bill nor Paul ever admitted that they dared him to do it. Anyway, Wes gave the dog's tail one terrific twist. The ear-piercing barking that ensued certainly hastened the windup of that meeting!

In the spring of 1955 the Reverend David Alderdice, a Presbyterian minister and witty orator from Banbridge, Ulster, hosted my two-week crusade in the beautiful countryside of Ulster. Hundreds witnessed the eloquent and witty words of this master preacher. At the breakfast meetings David was nothing if not hilarious. We all sat overcome with David's funny anecdotes and strings of Irish jokes that flew from his mouth in rapid succession.

Joseph Scriven was born into David Alderdice's parish. He immigrated to Ontario, Canada, in the 1850s, where he wrote perhaps the world's greatest hymn, the consoling "What a Friend We Have in Jesus." This favorite gospel song is sung on the seven continents of the world and in 100 languages—it is loved by Christians everywhere! The tragic truth is that "What a Friend We Have in Jesus" began as a poem that he sent back to his mother in his native Banbridge. The poem was written after a year's grieving. Scriven's fiancée had been killed in a win-

The Left Side of the Road

ter accident. Scriven joined the Plymouth Brethren, helping the aged members of the community for the rest of his life.

Forty-three years later, in summer of 1998, Ulster's worst massacre of innocent civilians in thirty years occurred in the city of Omagh, which was populated by a mere 20,000. One afternoon, thousands of well-wishers turned out for an open-air service for the twenty-eight slain. Two hundred were injured in the bomber's blast. "This is a time for prayers, not speeches. A time to be quiet and to listen to a 'still small voice,'" exclaimed the mayor, son of the Reverend David Alderdice.

In Gosport, England, in 1956, I met Colonel Orde Dobbie. He was one of the British army's elite. He was born into good army stock. His father, Sir William Dobbie, had been appointed the governor general of Malta by Winston Churchill during World War II. The governor general lived alone as a widower in his son Orde's home. Colonel Dobbie's wife's name was Florence. She was a saint. She was one of the high-ranking British establishment. Her father had been a British army general in India. Orde was the strongest chairman of the John Wesley White Crusades in England. He was also one of my closest confidants. He organized my crusades, strategically modeling them after his World War II campaigns. He headed up the Church of England (Anglican) in the south of England, from Southampton to Portsmouth. He was one of the elite and a powerful leader of the Church of England. Orde organized campaigns in 100 churches. He also united Methodists, Baptists, Congregationals, Plymouth Brethren and Pentecostals into a month of crusade campaigns at one military venue.

Reverend Hugh Walker, a Presbyterian minister, was England's version of Cliff Barrows. He was a musical director and a beautiful singer with a charismatic personality. He emigrated from Ireland to Alberta and then moved to England with his family. He was my partner for three years. He became the musical director for the John Wesley White Crusades.

During the Gosport campaign, Hugh and I fasted and prayed. Orde and his campaign committee arranged "Operation Andrew" with the churches. During that campaign, 630 decisions were registered for Christ. In 1993 Mick Taylor, one of the 630, wrote to me about the Gosport area campaign. Mick had attended the crusade when he was seven years old, and he was converted there. He is now preaching in

Suddenly Silenced

England. In his letter to me he claimed that my book *Thinking the Unthinkable* was put into his hands by my close friend of many years Arthur Stephens. Arthur Stephens founded the All England–John Wesley White Crusades in the 1950s and early '60s.

In the late 1950s and early 1960s our strategy involved "Ringing Bournemouth" and surrounding areas, then "Ringing Exeter," and "Ringing Torquay." We then marched north, "Ringing Luton," and on to "Ringing Lincoln," "Ringing Worcester," and back to "Ringing Newport." We crisscrossed this part of Great Britain for eight years.

John Innis joined us as our pianist at our rally in the town hall at Bradford in Yorkshire, England. He went with Hugh Walker and me to Bournemouth. John was a doctor's son who had a great stage presence and a great talent for music. He was just seventeen years of age then. John and I spoke often of my recommending him to the Moody Bible Institute. Then John enrolled at Wheaton College in Chicago. Upon graduation from Wheaton, John enrolled in the Chicago Conservatory of Music. He was there for three years. He played the keyboards in the world-renowned Moody Church in Chicago. For the past third of a century he has been one of the two or three keyboardists with the Billy Graham Crusades. He is a success story and is well loved by those who know him.

During the period of 1955 to 1963, we followed a high-density itinerary and held hundreds of meetings. In Wales, we preached to large crowds—up to 1,800 at a time. Hundreds came forward. We held prayer meetings around the clock. Wales was on fire in revival. It was just like the Great Revival of 1905. We worked to save souls night and day.

Hubert Everson, a world famous gospel singer, and I met at a breakfast meeting at the Billy Graham Crusade in London in June 1989. Hubert recounted an event that had taken place over thirty years before in one enormous Congregational church in the city of Merthyr Tydfil.

Interestingly, Garnett Williams, the champion rock and roller, Howard Winstone, the world featherweight boxing champion, Jackie Collins, the international soccer hero of the Wales team, and the "Monkey Parade" of "beatnik" street fighters were all converted at the same time. We held five years of meetings, campaigns and crusades in England during my time at Oxford.

The Left Side of the Road

At the dawning of a new decade, the 1960s, we drove to Oxford in South Wales, where I evangelized door-to-door. I found myself in what might have been the poorest and most squalid coal-mining village in all of Britain. I would be preaching each night for a week in a tiny chapel there. Each day I would go house-to-house and ask the dwellers, "Does Jesus live here?" If He didn't, I'd try to explain how He'd like to move in and transform their lives.

One afternoon I was knocking on doors and came to one that was ajar. When I knocked, it swung open. An old man named Jones answered the door. Immediately I could see that he was worn out from a lifetime of grinding it out in the coal mines in the bowels of the earth. This man was alone. His wife had died, and his family had abandoned him and moved to London.

Old Man Jones' off-white whiskers matched his mane of grizzly gray hair that hung over his tired eyes, which were noticeably blinking above a sad and toothless smile. He knew me. He had hobbled around to the little chapel the night before. With lungs devoured by a lifetime of inhaling coal dust, he squeaked, "Come in." With a big, rough, shaky hand he shook mine and led me over to a creaky table, sitting me down on a wobbly bench beside it. Off to his right was a coal fire and hanging over it a black-coated chain suspending a soot-covered kettle. Removing it, he poured its contents into two rusty tin cups of tea leaves. A shake of sugar and a splash of milk later, tea was served. With a dull knife, worn nearly in half, he hacked off a couple of pieces of bread from a nearly spent loaf and squeezed chunks of cheese onto them. It was the miners' staff of life.

He wanted me to eat and drink with him, and I did. But when I asked him if Jesus lived here, he replied that He didn't. However, since the meeting the night before, he had thought of nothing else. How could he invite Jesus into his life and know that he was His?

I said, "Friend, just as when I knocked on your door you asked me to come in and sit down and eat with you, so Jesus knocks on your heart's door, and when you invite Him to do so, He comes into your life and sups with you and shares bread of life eternal with you."

There and then he asked Jesus to come into his heart. When I left, there was the freshness of new spiritual life on his face. The otherwise gruff old man had been well and truly born again!

Suddenly Silenced

Early the next morning, I felt the urge to go around and see Old Man Jones again, and when I turned into his street, there was a slow, soupy rain falling. When I reached his grubby door, it was tightly shut. After knocking and hearing no movement, I looked through the window. The drape was drawn, but not quite all the way. Through the opening, I saw a plain pine coffin, the kind the British government provides for those who cannot bury their own. The lid was up, and there was my friend, and on his face I thought I saw an expression of peace that read *"To live is Christ, and to die is gain"* (Philippians 1:21).

CHAPTER VIII

The Oxford Years

Kathleen was pregnant again. It was the night following St. Patrick's Day in March 1959, and our fourth son, Timothy Randolf Dean White, was born. Now we had four young boys and three miniature poodles.

I had been accepted at Oxford University. This was due, at least in part, from the letter of recommendation that Earle Cairns, my history professor from Wheaton College, had written. I was thrilled. Yes, we were excited, but money was tight, and we had to find a way to make an income to get us all through.

We were moving—moving to Oxford! The all-consuming question on our minds was how we were going to get to Oxford. We took it to the Lord and waited in faith. Then, like a brilliant light had been switched on, we could see the answer to our problem. We had a friend, Billy Paul, who had been converted three years earlier at the Jack Shuler Crusade at King's Hall in Belfast, where I had been an associate evangelist with Jack. Billy Paul owned a car dealership and took trade-ins. Not forgetting the great blessing of his salvation, Billy was forever grateful to us for carrying the good news of Jesus Christ to him. As a kindly Irish gesture he found it in his shamrock heart not to loan us a truck but instead to give us a truck, an "Old Rumbley." Kathleen and I smiled at Billy's generosity. But our smiles were drooping at the corners a bit, maybe because we sensed the enormity of the task that lay before us or because we had the rather disconcerting premonition that the Old Rumbley was a forerunner of the truck that we would purchase later and on another continent.

Suddenly Silenced

At three o'clock in the morning, Kathleen and I found ourselves still headlong into the move. We were cramming our belongings into boxes, bags and suitcases. What we could not pack into containers we managed to stack onto our Old Rumbley truck. We managed to sell most of the antique furniture that we had been using, and for the first time in our lives we were able to buy new pieces of furniture, which we stacked high in the truck.

When Kathleen and I rolled our Old Rumbley onto a ship out of the Port of Belfast, bound for Heysham, England, I was reminded of my experience on the "Rumbley" tractor. The sea, I remember, was itself thrashing about. We tossed and dipped and heaved. This time the trick was to avoid looking up. It was like being high atop the Leaning Tower of Pisa.

From Heysham we drove to Oxford. Upon arrival we dismantled the chaotic assemblage of everything we had brought with us. Gravity did most of the work, actually. With creaky knees we descended the cab and down onto the sideboards of our old, rickety truck, into our new life at Oxford, on Cumnor Road. Our house, although modest, was the answer to our prayers.

I was fortunate enough to be accepted into what many refer to as the greatest English speaking university in the world. In the fall of 1959, I enrolled at Oxford University. I reduced my evangelism involvement to a mere 200 meetings per year. Dr. John Walsh, who would later become my mentor and overseer of my thesis, bent the rule that an Oxford student could not travel abroad during his crucial years of study.

Eventually, as an evangelist, I covered every corner of Great Britain with God's good news. However, my studies now demanded that I spend a great deal of time in research in the London Museum Library and in Bodlean Library at Oxford. It was Mansfield College at Oxford for me, but John Walsh resided in Jesus College. Dr. Walsh appeared to me to be the most brilliant modern history scholar in the world.

My first encounter with John Walsh was rather auspicious. One anxious day I stood before this dignified, feisty, kindly and brilliant gentleman. Following a protracted silence I sat before him to be interviewed. He was an Oxford don. I trembled. After all, Dr. John Walsh was the first cousin of the world-renowned preacher and author Dr. Leslie Weatherhead and a personal friend of C.S. Lewis. I could barely sit still.

The Oxford Years

The interview was a blur, and when I returned to my room, Kathleen was wringing her hands, awaiting the result of my hour-long session. I threw up my hands. "It's hard to say," I mumbled.

"John, whatever do you mean?" she retorted.

I bellowed, "He stutters!" Dr. Walsh often responded to most situations by using his favorite phase: "T-tr-trans A-At-Atlan-Atlantic v-v-v-ver-verbos-verbosity, trans-Atlantic verbosity!" John Walsh was irreplaceable to me.

In 1963 I was preaching at the packed Bristol Temple on a Sunday evening. Our boys were singing and trumpeting for the Lord. The text for that evening was on David and Bathsheba and the prophet Nathan. I was particularly emphatic on that occasion as I announced Nathan's words *"You are the man." "You are the man." "You are the man"* (2 Samuel 12:7). Each time I spoke, I turned a little to face another section of the congregation. This had an impact on the crowd.

The following Tuesday I had to leave the seminar. I stood up and met Dr. Walsh at the front of the classroom and said, "Please excuse me, sir. I'm illegally parked. I'll be back in five minutes."

Dr. Walsh was taken aback, as a dozen students were snickering at me. Then it became clear to him what was going on. One of the dozen students stood up and announced, "John Wesley White is a Billy Graham evangelist. I saw him in The Temple; he is a Bible thumper."

Suddenly I walked back into the seminar, and this student began chanting, *"You are the man. You are the man. You are the man."* Everyone in the class broke up laughing.

Following his lecture John Walsh kept me back in private. He began stuttering, "Ya-ya-you a-a-a-are the m-m-m-m-ma-man. *You are the man*," and turning to his side, he exclaimed, *"You are the man."* Turning again he stuttered, *"You are the man."* He continued three times, until I was as red as a tomato.

Interestingly, in 2006, my facilitator, Stephen Trelford, happened to see a documentary featuring C.S. Lewis. John Walsh was interviewed with regard to his experience of Lewis. Amazingly, Dr. Walsh sped through his response, not stuttering once! Perhaps there has been a healing? King David prayed, *"O LORD my God, I cried out to You, And You healed me"* (Psalm 30:2).

Suddenly Silenced

As I began this phase of my life I kept remembering the strings of stuttering jokes that Ed Janecek sprung on me when we lived together on his parents' farm in Wisconsin in 1948. I began using his seemingly endless series of jokes. I kept people in my private and public life laughing for forty-eight years. I'm Irish!

On April 28, 1996, the strings of stuttering jokes stopped. I suffered my silencing stroke. When I began to speak again, I was stuttering. This led me to a profound empathy with John Walsh. It's difficult when people cannot understand what you say. For forty-eight years I had them rolling with laughter, around tables, in meetings, in halls and in arenas. Oh how it hurt when those strings of jokes stopped! That unforgettable first Monday morning after my stroke, through the tears I was still laughing, but I could not utter one word. Indeed, the only sound that came from me was the laughter I uttered as I recalled the years of hilarious humor. I was greatly blessed to so clearly recall the superb jokes that passed between Ed Janecek, Billy Graham, T.W. Wilson, Calvin Thielman, Perry Ellis, Harold Salem and me. It is difficult to overestimate the value of a good joke. They prayed unceasingly for a return of my speech. For the month I was in the Mayo Clinic, I reflected on those jokes: in my mind, it all paraded before me.

Kathleen, who had a decided flare for decoration, painted John Walsh's flat in Oxford in return for John Walsh's devotion to me. I assisted her. John was a dedicated academic, but in 1960 he married. In 1962 he and his wife had a daughter. As a baby shower gift and in a continued attempt to repay Dr. Walsh for his great kindness to me, Kathleen and I bought them a British style large-wheel carriage for their baby daughter. Oddly enough, when Dr. Walsh acquired a car, he selected me as his driving instructor. Can you imagine? I was still driving down the left side of the road.

Many scholars at Oxford had the privilege of sitting with John Walsh in the common room. I was one of those scholars. My research at the London Museum Library and the Bodlean Library at Oxford and through countless newspapers scattered throughout Britain resulted in 15,000 pages of notes. They grilled me all right, picking my brain for my understanding of my tome, still entitled *The Influence of North American Evangelism in Great Britain Between 1810 and 1914, on the Origin and Development of the Ecumenical Movement*.

The Oxford Years

Dr. Walsh organized and outlined the chapters of my thesis. He would spend days and nights in invaluable assistance to me, poring over my work, perusing my ideas and arranging my material. Dr. Walsh was painfully patient. Where this busy man found the time to spend with me this way I will never know. Yet he helped me to squeeze those 15,000 pages of notes into a scant 350 typewritten pages for my thesis.

Dr. Walsh would often leap into lengthy debates. The all-seeing John Walsh saw me through five years of study. He was strict and offered students "no free lunches." I was offered none. Preparing and writing my thesis took all the diligence and discipline that I could muster. There were times when I was so exhausted from study and revision that I literally dropped into bed. In excess of 50 percent of doctor of philosophy candidates were failing or were relegated to a grim destiny of continuous long hours in research.

In 1963, a tribunal of three examiners was appointed to oversee my arduous endeavor, the writing of my thesis. Upon entering the chambers I squinted ahead, glimpsing the tribunal perched on their bench high in the sky. I attempted to banish all thoughts from my mind. I stepped forward. I had to force myself to remember that I had prepared for this. My desire to join Billy Graham as an associate evangelist and researcher was a constant motivational factor for me.

From my point of view, these well-meaning academic gentlemen seemed to take my case personally. They may have believed that their decisions concerning my academic prowess would reflect either favorably or unfavorably on their standing as evaluators. I would stand wobbly-kneed before these academic drill sergeants in defense of my thesis. I kept fidgeting as drops of sweat beaded on my furrowed brow.

After half a decade of diligence and delight preparing my thesis, which was the summit of my scholastic effort, the day came that I was compelled to confront the academic tribunal for their crucial decision regarding my future. Would my work be accepted, or would it be vanquished as inferior? I was breathless.

This was the first time in my life that I donned a black suit with a clerical collar. Dr. Walsh apparently had taken pains to convince the panel of critical examiners that I was politically correct. He had made specific reference to my collar. He said, "A middle-sized collar is appropriate. A thin collar is Roman Catholic, and a wide collar is evangelical"!

Suddenly Silenced

For me, this was singularly the most crucial moment and my career determinant. I had fasted for a week before the inquisition. I had prayed day and night. I was powerless. I stood steadfast, immutably frozen. Alas, there was one singular option left for me. I was to wait in lonely desperation for the decree, the final judgment of the omnipotent panel.

A soundless eternity passed. Then Dr. Walsh did the unforgettable. He slowly and with a strained effort hoisted high the digested 1,500 pages of research, which were bound together in a giant black cover, and let it fall, plummeting, with its full weight crushing down upon me.

I slumped into a ball as the tumult of paper catapulted into my body. I fought to hang on. I crouched over, supporting the weight of the years at Oxford. My mind and spirit separated from my body, allowing me to sense the elation and the despair of the unknown. But this was the defining moment, the final examination at Oxford.

At once the trio of cloaked figures adjourned. They would be in recess for four hours—until about five o'clock.

The lapse of time between one and five felt like a cruel eternity. This was the longest four hours of my life thus far. Realizing that I would not learn of the decision until the next morning, I slept not at all.

At 10 a.m., I wandered wearily into the street and into an English telephone kiosk. I could wait no longer. One last thought paraded through my mind. Ironically, that crucial morning I had learned that the popular Pope John XXIII had died. The result of this news together with my academic anxieties meant that I was flooded with mixed emotions. I was as tense as "a cat on a hot tin roof." I felt like jumping off a cliff, or perhaps I was about to leap into ecstasy.

My stumbling fingers found themselves tripping over the holes in the telephone dial. I was dialing John Walsh's phone number. My mind seethed with the burning question.

Then, splitting the silence, Dr. Walsh answered the phone which was ringing. I broke out into a sweat. He began stuttering his remarks. For an entire minute I waited as he managed to thunder out the two most significant words in this era of my life: "Ya-ya-you-you're th-thhthhhrooo. You're through!"

I had my own two words: "Thank God!"

Believe it or not, Kathleen and I had a social life too. We made good friends while at Oxford. One of our friends springs immediately to mind. If *genius* is a valid term when describing someone, then my best friend, a native of South Africa, was a genius. He was Dr. Maxwell Cowan, a geneticist and biology professor. His wife, Margaret, was a pleasant woman, a nurse, and a native of Wales.

In the 1970s Maxwell's genius manifested itself in a highly controversial and unique event that took place in the human race: Louise Joy Brown was born. Louise was the world's first test-tube baby. Maxwell Cowan was a member of the team of scientists and engineers who made that possible. Maxwell and his team became known throughout the world. Now the world's first test-tube baby has a baby herself. Louise and her husband, security officer Wesley Mullinder, "conceived the baby the old-fashioned way" (*Toronto Star*, July 16, 2006).

On weekends and holidays during this period, Kathleen, the boys and I would climb into our station wagon and drive to the Youth for Christ rallies and to outlying churches. Our boys were developing their musical abilities. They performed a dozen Christian songs at the rallies and at the churches. They made their mother and father very proud as they marched on stage in their red coats and tartan knickers. Their bright red bow ties always received rave reviews. Our boys got their good looks from Kathleen. Their voices were simply the voices of angels, to their somewhat biased mom and dad.

Audiences always loudly applauded the boys. Two years later the boys acquired silver coronets, which they took pains to learn how to play. Eventually, this little trio sounded off for Christ across the Atlantic—from Edinburgh to California, from the U.K. to the USA. "The White Trio," as they came to be known, appeared on the BBC. The boys were heard in five countries: England, Scotland, Ireland, Canada and the United States. In every town, in every country, youngsters would swarm our station wagon, asking volumes of questions about the boys. I had to ask myself, was I playing second fiddle to the boys? I chuckle to myself when I think of this. I was the preacher and was hired as their spokesperson and personal trainer.

The endless strings of questions continued. I remember answering questions until my head ached. I remember acquiring a certain kind of empathy for Brian Epstein, the Beatles' manager, who suffered the same kind of inquisition and inundation.

I spent hours each day laughing, crying and praying. Other time

Suddenly Silenced

was spent bringing the boys' voices into perfect harmony. The boys' talents were accelerating. They were learning to "triple tongue" their silver coronets and trumpets.

Astoundingly, in 1963 two of the Beatles attended our Youth for Christ crusade in Liverpool, England. Liverpool was the bowel of working man's England. It was, as we say, "on the wrong side of the tracks." In years to come the situation would be reversed. Our boys would attend the Beatles' concerts.

Kathleen's unwavering faith was never so fully demonstrated as it was when concerned with our house in Oxford. She just knew that the Lord would tend his flock, and we were a part of his flock. We borrowed the money to buy one house in Oxford. This proved to be a boon for us. The house appreciated in value almost overnight. Our resources were slim when we started, and it took all our ingenuity combined with God's blessing to build our tiny empire into a comfortable living. It is expensive to attend Oxford and to support a family. Needless to say we were extremely busy, day and night.

I have never been a materialist ever since my days on the farm. When I did acquire material possessions, I usually left them scattered around. I have always had the tendency to be what some compulsive cleaners refer to as "messy." As a boy, my mind would always drift into flights of imagination whenever I was told to clean up my room. Kathleen is my opposite. She cherishes the sparkle of a well-dusted home. She revels in the grandeur of a tidy parlor. Tea must never be served in a messy sitting room. And the vestibule must remain uncluttered.

In view of our income requirements, Kathleen initiated a rather ingenious plan. It had to do with the purchase of a Shakespearean cottage on the Thames. It gives me goose bumps to recall the events that followed from the purchase of that home. As I have alluded to, Kathleen had developed an interest in the housing market. Specifically she enjoyed the preparation, reparation and decoration of old houses for tenancy. She had had success in this area in Belfast a couple of times, so it was natural that she repeat the pattern in Oxford.

The first of the cottages that Kathleen put her hand to was northwest of our house. It was in a small village where the Oxford Printing House operated. This splendid little Cotswold stone cottage with a thatched roof was built in the times of Sir William Shakespeare. And although it was fairly crude with its three-foot thick walls and mud basement, it radiated "old English charm," resplendent with alluring green grounds, colorful gardens and fully mature trees.

Upon entering the cottage one was immediately made aware that the people of 16th century England were short. Kathleen and I were forever conscious of the ceiling. It hung so low that it threatened to behead us with every step. To our astonishment, we found a creative way to retrench the floors. It occurred to Kathleen to send for Albert, our brother-in-law, in Belfast. He would help us with the retrenching. Albert was a burly Irishman. He was strong—so strong, in fact, that he could singlehandedly heft the old stone slabs that made up the flooring and waddle them from the house, through its narrow doors. In reconstructing the floor, Albert had to penetrate the rocklike earth ten inches down to replace the broken floor with a new base of concrete. A one-man construction crew, Albert was able to pour liquid concrete from a large bucket that was secured under one arm and smoothly distribute it so that it lay horizontal in the ground. It hardened virtually flat. This was an astounding feat. We use trucks for that same job today. The walls of the cottage were anything but square. From the supine perspective that one assumes when lying in bed, the walls reminded us of an ancient vertical winding English footpath. A square room is a modern luxury, we discovered.

It happened that the printer who prepared all the work for Oxford University lived next door to our little cottage. He was a culture vulture, and was he articulate! He was a connoisseur of good taste. After we had fixed up this cottage, this gentleman printer, anxious to keep the building in a semblance of its original form, offered to buy it from us. He could see that Kathleen had visions of placing the modern devices of the 20th century world into a 365-year-old structure.

At first, Kathleen was reluctant to sell it. She wanted to modernize it completely so that we could rent it for a profit. The idea of tearing down the centuries-old beams and gutting the living area appalled the printer, an aficionado of early craftsmanship. This printer who was a man of dignity had delicate sensitivities. In a fit of repulsion one day, he abruptly offered us twice the money we had paid for the cottage. Our move was hastily made!

Suddenly Silenced

Kathleen was inspired by our newly found fortune. She was absolutely decisive. Without hesitation she bought two connecting cottages in the village of Wootten, in the northeast of Oxford County. We modernized the first of the new cottages, and the White family moved in. Kathleen then modernized the second cottage. An honest description of these classic English cottages reveals that, although narrow, they were four stories tall, and they had served as a nunnery two hundred years earlier.

In the '80s our son Wesley was back at Oxford with his mother and me during a Billy Graham mission to England. He wouldn't stop needling us. He just had to see that cottage! So we acquiesced and drove up from London. When we arrived at the cottage, we knocked on the door. Much to our disappointment we found nobody home. Not wanting to discourage young Wes, we knocked on the door of the cottage across the street. To our surprise an English woman who was a loquacious talker answered the door. Almost without pausing to take a breath she informed us that the particular cottage in question had just been resold by a shrewd realtor to a rather gullible young couple whose objective it was to make a favorable impression on the social elite. The sale was on the basis that this very special cottage was one of historic significance because John Wesley had lived there. The price was half again as much as it would have been otherwise. The vendor exacted from them every pound he asked.

I knew, of course, that the great founder of Methodism had no more lived there than had Julius Caesar. But, as Wesley enjoyed telling the story, "The realtor had missed it by one. There had in fact been not one, but two John Wesleys who had lived there: John Wesley Sr. and John Wesley Jr.!"

The abundance the good Lord bestowed upon us was great, and we soon had enough money to purchase two more investment cottages. We also bought a house in downtown Oxford and two more in London. Kathleen was beginning to take on the characteristics of a "land baroness"! She managed our estates with the keen interest of a budding entrepreneur. Kathleen became deeply involved in the world of buying cottages and homes. She devoted much of her time to renovating them and selling them. God was really providing for us. It seemed that every time we finished a home, someone would appear with exactly the

The Oxford Years

money we asked for, and they would buy it. There were even several times that buyers would appear seemingly out of nowhere who were so hungry for our properties that we would be offered several hundred pounds more than we were asking.

I began developing an eye for property myself and would see a house that I thought was appropriate for the family. It usually needed work. On one occasion I attempted some renovation work. To be a part of this I had to get my hands dirty. Once done, I stood proudly back from one wall that I had finished. I pointed it out to Kathleen, anticipating her genuine approval. She stood there a minute and turned toward me and exclaimed, "John, this is all very well; you've displayed the utmost in creativity."

I replied, "Well, thanks." I said this in an appropriate recognition of my ingenuity. "But what do you mean by creativity?" I inquired.

With a quizzical look on her face, Kathleen crossed her arms, leaned back on my splendid wall and said, "Well, John, this is the first time that I've ever seen a room of this kind, or any kind for that matter, with the window put in upside down!"

From that moment on, I left the design and decoration of our homes to Kathleen.

Admittedly, Kathleen had developed a genuine flair for decoration. During one period she squeezed ten months of work into just four. In the months surrounding the summer solstice, two shifts of men a day worked on her prize home, Tralee House. From daybreak to well beyond darkness, crews were driven to toil on this magnificent English home. Kathleen would hire crews to build to specification, and then she would bring in interior decorators to fashion ornate and beautiful interiors. So gorgeous was this building, Tralee House, that world famous ministers and conference leaders stayed with us while venturing abroad.

A slight description of this unique edifice and its splendid features is required here, in order that the reader gather a mental picture of the degree to which Kathleen's creative flair for decoration was evident in our greatest home.

From the road looking toward Tralee House that had been owned by our next-door neighbor, Lord Harvey, our glamorous estate was guarded by a stone wall. It ran the perimeter of the property. It had been constructed by hand from the selective gleaning of stones from ancient Roman roads. The windows, ornate as they were, were framed in solid oak and offered a spectacular view whether inside or outside of the building.

Upon entering the front of Tralee House, one would be captivated by the visual elegance that the long, flat, evenly-cut stretches of parquet flooring provided. The floorboards were hewn from pure, refined mahogany. The color of the wood resembled the red skin of a fresh Georgian peanut. The living room displayed an entire wall of magnificently chiseled fieldstone, which gave the room the feel of timeless strength and of immensity. The builders had managed to blend the features of absolute and assured stability of structure with the epitome of English country charm. The wealth of Kathleen's passion for interior design and decoration were represented in the brilliant highlights that accented the excellence of the many rooms of Tralee House.

When one stood back and gazed out of our back windows, he or she beheld the splendor of our English apple orchard. Shiny red apples hung as ornaments gleaming from mature trees lined in ancient rows delighted the senses and beckoned the adventurous or the hungry. The fragrance of this orchard was indescribably wonderful. The olfactory sense ushered in a yearning for a bygone era. The rear property with its undulating character appeared to stand out above the surrounding region, much like I have seen in creative oil paintings brushed by English landscape artists. Such a painting might hang above a living room mantel in the castle of a king or queen. Our time residing in Tralee House offered us the gentle combination of joyous and cultured living.

Many people of notoriety came to witness Kathleen's handiwork. Both our cottages and our homes reflected the creative ingenuity that she had engineered. However delicate and demanding the work, during this period of our lives we seemed to get things done fast—and well. Money has never been our goal, but we both have a feeling that if Kathleen had stayed in the home redecoration business, we would be wealthy today.

In Tralee House we lived just two miles from Sir Winston Churchill's country home, Blenheim Palace. It must further be mentioned that Prince Faisal of Saudi Arabia, along with his personal harem of gorgeous Arabian women, resided for two years at the Tralee House in Begbroke, Oxfordshire. Prince Faisal had studied at Oxford, you see. In retrospect, it can be said with absolute certainty that any risks that the bank manager had originally taken on us paid dividends—royally!

CHAPTER IX

The Green Monster

In 1961 at the Grosvenor House in London, Billy Graham's voice fell prey to the evangelist's nightmare—laryngitis. It was on account of this that my close friend and Billy's brother-in-law, Leighton Ford, stood in for him at Manchester.

One of Billy Graham's assistants, Doug Judson, re-introduced me to Mr. Graham, who was lying in bed at the time. At the left of Mr. Graham's bed was an MP of the House of Commons, seated in a chair. At this time Billy spoke to me about the queen and her belief in Jesus Christ.

Billy also talked to me about illustrations. In light of my job writing illustrations and research material for Billy, I quote what Harvard-trained biographer Bill Martin published in his book on Billy Graham, *Prophet with Honor*: "Associate Evangelist John Wesley White has long been Graham's primary sermon illustrator." Who could have foreseen that I would come to be referred to as Billy Graham's "primary sermon illustrator"? God had indeed anointed me in my work as an evangelist.

In the January 2006 edition of *Decision*, my friend Cliff Barrows wrote the following: "Saskatchewan-born evangelist John Wesley White was instrumental in the growth of BGEA's ministry...John Wesley White was a great help in research and in finding illustrations that seemed to connect well with people."

Leighton Ford had been a close friend of mine for eleven years, since Wheaton College. Leighton's friend Calvin Thielman, a Texan, was Billy Graham's pastor. I was overjoyed when I crossed the Atlantic to stay in a Manchester hotel during the Manchester City Stadium Crusade. Thirty thousand people attended. At the hotel I was introduced to Calvin Thielman, and a great friendship was born. Calvin and I spent our time talking together about the BGEA.

Leighton, too, was exceedingly busy. He preached about "The Pearl of Great Price." Many decisions were made for Christ. Leighton's adopted father was a jeweler in Chatham, Ontario, and therefore Leighton was intimately familiar with the price of pearls.

After the two-week Manchester crusade that Billy preached at, Billy's team shifted to Cardiff, Wales, where Leighton Ford preached. Cliff Barrows, George Beverly Shea and Tedd Smith performed. Following this event Billy and his team crossed the Atlantic to crusade in Philadelphia. Jerry Beavan arranged my debut preaching assignment with the BGEA.

I was euphoric at the very thought of what was about to happen. A dream of a lifetime was about to come true. Fantastic moments of preaching flashed through my mind. There are only a handful of evangelists around the world who receive this kind of a calling. I remained steadfast and modest as I prepared for the work that stood before me.

In June 1963, Kathleen, Randy and I met Billy Graham and Dr. Robert Evans in Paris. We had taken the ferry from England to France. We drove from Paris to Lyon in our new golden Vauxhall. We talked for hours about evangelism and about researching sermons and illustrations. We also prayed. We shared the stories of our greatest experiences as evangelists. We talked and laughed. I could hardly believe that the dashing and charismatic Billy Graham, who had taken my breath away at the Washington Crusade and at Kelvin Hall in Glasgow years ago, was sitting in our car, confirming my appointment as an associate evangelist! This was an inexpressively exhilarating moment for me.

Billy and Leighton preached in Lyon. Then Kathleen, Randy, Leighton and I left Lyon and returned to our rooms in an old historic hotel situated in the picturesque wine country of central France. This historic hotel had been the castle where Napoleon and Josephine resided. During the eighteenth century, the French were known for their elaborate architecture—ornate in every detail. In modern times this very complex edifice carried with it the spirit of a bygone era. While effusing the charm of the Old World and the elegance of French royalty, it could not be denied that emanating from this structure was an air of impending doom, perhaps reminiscent of those days when France underwent siege and strife.

Over the years dark and mysterious rumors proliferated about the old castle. Alarmingly, there were rumors that our hotel was haunted! None of us really believed in ghosts, but hearing this rumor put us all slightly ill at ease. So went that dark night in that old hotel.

We were all making our personal transitions from the Old World to the New World. In the summer of 1963 our family immigrated to North America. We had been living in the grandeur of Tralee House; now we were to live more modestly. We stayed in an apartment in a northern suburb of Denver, Colorado. We were nestled in the cradle of the Rocky Mountains. Our personal transitions put a good deal of stress on us individually and as a family. Firstly, Kathleen had to give up her budding career as a house builder. This avocation had really become a passion for her, and she missed the house business badly. Secondly, the boys were required to accommodate brash new groups of friends.

In Oxford the boys had made friends with the sons of upper-middle-class professional people. Youth donned neatly pressed knickers and wore perfectly parted hair beneath tartan tams. The boys now befriended America's western mountain cowboys clad in tough blue denim, shin high leather boots and ten gallon cowboy hats!

British children had ridden old bicycles to school that featured book packs and carefully draped school jackets in their baskets. Now the boys witnessed the squeal of forty-four off-road vehicles delivering strapping young Americans to school. The English schoolboy found involvement in academic and social clubs to be an interesting pastime, and cricket, rugger and soccer were the sports of choice. The American youth liked to hunt, fish and play baseball, basketball, football and then hockey, when they weren't bird-dogging chicks. Yes, the boys knew change, and we all paid the price of the readjustment to the New World.

In the fall, Mark Bubeck, a Conservative Baptist and a close friend of mine from the days at Moody Bible Institute, arranged fourteen weeks of back-to-back campaigns at fourteen of Denver's churches.

In January 1964 I had a new job: a Billy Graham evangelist! Kathleen, the boys and I left Denver for Toronto for my first crusade with the BGEA. It was held in Charles Templeton's church on Avenue Road. Following this, Billy had an assignment for me that involved research and lecturing at Harvard University.

Reverend John Dillon was the director of the associate program in Minneapolis. From 1964 to 1984 he was the director for the BGEA associate evangelists. He was born in Williston, North Dakota. He has always been a humorous Irishman with good judgment. To this day John Dillon remains my friend. He started the program and organized my early crusades.

That summer I moved the family to Winnipeg, Manitoba, where we could be within shouting distance of my family. We just got settled in when I was assigned a crusade in Pocomoke City, Maryland.

Most of my early crusades were small. This concerned me. I wanted to put my best foot forward and show Billy Graham that I was an outstanding evangelist, but the crowds that gathered were small. I put it down to the fact that I was just getting underway in North America, and I was busy getting my feet wet in the evangelism of the BGEA.

At the Pocomoke City crusade the chairman was Perry Ellis, a Texan who stands a gargantuan six-feet nine-inches tall. He is brilliant and witty and has a larger than life personality, too. He was the chairman of the Southern Baptist Church. Perry has a beautiful wife, Robbie, who is a celebrity. When I visited Perry's house, I was exuberant about the possibilities that the future presented, but I was deflated about the small numbers that attended the crusade. Perry Ellis' pretty daughter Autumn was one of those who made a decision for Christ at one of my crusades. She married Larry Ross, who has been in advertising and promotions with the BGEA.

Billy Graham held a three-week crusade in Columbus, Ohio, at Jet Stadium. Thirty thousand attended nightly. I was mind-boggled and thrilled about the success of this crusade, the largest of its kind that I had been involved in to date. In addition to the crusading, I was preaching and lecturing at Ohio State University. And I was refreshing Billy's sermons by splicing current events and illustrations into his work.

In January 1964 we held a crusade in Steinbach, Manitoba, south of Winnipeg. This is where my aunt Maggie Pocock was living in a Mennonite community. Winnipeg was frozen out during the coldest

The Green Monster

winter that anyone could remember. Our spirits were decorated with icicles, and by the spring we'd had enough!

We made a family decision to pack up and head back east to "The Big Smoke"—Toronto. I considered buying an old International truck I'd seen. I'd always had a fascination with this kind of rugged old truck, ever since our "Rumbley" truck moved us from Ireland to England. Pondering the purchase of the $175 International relic provided me with a kind of warm nostalgic feeling. This metallic gem, I surmised, would carry the White family and our belongings to Canada's metropolis, Toronto.

The truck, although twenty years old, seemed solid enough to me. It was an open two and a half ton with a cab. Yes, this would do fine.

Kathleen took an immediate disliking to the idea and was adamant that I not even consider this "old wreck," as she not-too-affectionately referred to it. She was busy making plans to have our fine French Provincial furniture moved to the East via the reputable Allied Van Lines. She was secure in the knowledge that this trusted old company would ensure that our delicate furniture would arrive entirely intact.

Days passed, and I became more and more convinced that what I needed to do was to transport the White family together with our furniture in the old International. We could handle this move ourselves. We had moved from continent to continent and back again, hadn't we?

One day I rose up to my full height and, bursting with courage, I walked right up to Kathleen, who was standing at the kitchen sink doing the dishes. I declared, "Well, I did it."

Kathleen slowly twisted her body toward me and with an increasingly displeased expression inquired, "What, John? What did you do?"

I explained sheepishly, "I bought the truck."

"What truck?" Kathleen grimaced.

"You know, the green one," I reported.

Kathleen doesn't often scrunch up her face. Her face doesn't often turn as red as Rudolph's nose. She isn't very often loud enough to be heard halfway down the block, and I'm not often terrified when I look into her sky-blue azure eyes. But at this moment I could feel cold terror. It was the kind of terror that I felt when I was a small boy and had blatantly disobeyed my parents.

Suddenly Silenced

For the sake of saving Kathleen's reputation as a delicate and distinguished woman of exquisite taste and serene deportment, I'll waive any further description of the not-so-genteel monologue that followed. Suffice it to say, Kathleen was furious with my decision. Anyway, I was the head of the household, and I really believed that the old International was up to the job.

I implored Kathleen to "Please just trust me," and I began struggling to convince her, without further inflaming the situation, that the truck was roadworthy. With great and imaginative vision, I offered, "We'll throw a tarp over the furniture."

An uncomfortable pause came between us. Then I continued, "It will be carefully arranged and stacked in the truck by an expert furniture handler and mover." I was certain this would assuage my dear wife's anxieties.

Kathleen fell into a nasty silence. Her objections were no longer heard; they were felt!

When the twister had passed, I began preparing for the long, cold journey. Most of our belongings were strapped into place on the back of the International. The day we tied the tarps was a frigid day in April—there were whiteouts!

The next morning, the boys woke up early and jumped out of bed. Imagine a trip all the way to Toronto—by truck. Excited, I thrust myself onto the stiff bench seat in the cab of the truck. From my lofty perch I commanded Kathleen, the four boys and our two dogs to follow me in our tiny blue Vauxhall.

We started down the road and made it to the Trans-Canada Highway. *So far so good*, I remember thinking. Yet, burning into the back of my head, I could still feel the disapproval that shot from Kathleen's sky-blue azure eyes, which had been steel blue since she'd made up her mind to trust me.

Onto the highway I turned, and away I went. Blue clouds of smoke billowed from the exhaust pipe and rose like erupting volcanoes, further diminishing Kathleen's ability to see me. Alone in the cab, I had to admit to myself that this was a difficult undertaking, but I reasoned that Toronto wasn't too far away—just 1,300 miles!

I barely had time to relax before I had to slow down for a car that was crawling down the highway in front of me. I had to slow right

The Green Monster

down. To my horror I found that the brakes had all but completely given out. *I mustn't panic* raced through my mind. If I gingerly squeezed the brake pedal to the floor and back, it would gently rise. Up and down, up and down I pumped until I found myself stamping vehemently on the floorboards.

I finally rolled to an awkward stop on the shoulder of the highway. The old International sputtered and clanked and let fly with a bang. Blue smoke engulfed the wreck. I knew exactly what this meant—the engine had seized! As Kathleen and the boys pulled up behind the truck, I had a moment of dark despair.

Kathleen lurched out of the Vauxhall, and she screamed with anger, "Okay, John, what do you propose to do now?"

I fell silent. Not wanting to turn back, having already begun the journey, I simply and matter-of-factly stated, "Just trust me."

Kathleen bared her teeth and hissed at me, "We did trust you, John, and now look at the mess you've gotten us into!"

I couldn't deny that we were just east of Winnipeg and helplessly stuck.

I was suddenly struck with an idea. I knew that we were still on the outskirts of the city. In the still of the moment while others were in shock, I shifted Kathleen over in the Vauxhall, and I took the wheel and headed back to the city.

Kathleen finally broke the long anguishing silence and spoke. "John, whatever are you doing?"

I replied, "We'll rent a truck."

More silence!

We stopped at Hertz in an uncomfortable silence. We made arrangements to rent a yellow enclosed truck with dual rear wheels. The man who rented us the truck asked about our situation, and Kathleen piped up, "The Green Monster died."

"I beg your pardon, lady?"

"The Green Monster! Our truck! The one I told my husband not to buy just ground to a halt on the highway!"

The rental agent simply replied, "We at Hertz wish you and your family a safe and comfortable trip." I can still hear Kathleen's sardonic mutter to this day.

When we got back to the "Green Monster" I realized that something

Suddenly Silenced

had to be done with the Vauxhall. Kathleen and the boys stood in silence beside me as I got into the yellow truck and headed down the highway. In a brilliant, perhaps defiant, decision of leadership, I commanded Kathleen and the boys and our dogs to follow me in the Vauxhall.

When we stopped just down the road I maneuvered the rental truck into just the right position. From this point, I could angle the Vauxhall in just the right way so that I could drive our little blue car into the truck. Again, Kathleen flailed her arms and yelled her grievances in vigorous protest. The boys, now in a huddle, snickered. Straight away, I proceeded to drive the Vauxhall right into the back end of the truck. We couldn't believe that the truck now held a car!

I obtained an old tire and fastened it to the back of the rental truck. I acquired a logging chain somewhere and tied one end to the bumper of the yellow truck and the other end to the International. The idea was that in case of collision, the Green Monster would hit the yellow truck without damaging either vehicle. It was a stroke of genius. The kids cackled with glee at the adventure, the dogs barked, and Kathleen was about to explode!

With great and diplomatic skill, I persuaded Kathleen to haul herself up into the "Green Monster." I pled with her to simply "steer the truck."

Kathleen said, "I've never met a wife that would do this for a husband." She did this for me. Reluctantly, she hoisted herself up into the cab of the Green Monster. With the chain tensing and slacking with alternating jolts, jarring, then releasing, we bumped down the highway. The boys and the dogs rode with me. I kept glancing in the rearview mirror to see the strained look on Kathleen's face as she was determined to keep the tower of furniture atop the Green Monster from tumbling onto the highway.

Kathleen recalls how her arms ached from wrenching that huge steering wheel into position. There was neither heat nor power steering in the twenty-year-old International. Every time we hit the slightest curve in the road, Kathleen braced herself on the hard bench as she veered out into the oncoming traffic. From the Green Monster she couldn't see what was approaching in the oncoming lanes. Frequently instinct would take over, she later reported, and she would frantically press the horn—which no longer worked!

The Green Monster

I pressed on. The boys howled and rallied behind me. As I barreled down the highway I again glanced in the rearview mirror, to see Kathleen standing tiptoe on the running board, waving her arms wildly at the oncoming traffic. Clearly, she was overcome with fright.

I pulled over. Kathleen descended the International and came toward me. There was an exchange of words, and I agreed to change positions with her.

Now I piloted the Green Monster. Kathleen took time to adjust to the shifting of five gears and the jostling of four hysterical boys and two barking dogs. Back in the International I knew isolation, and I was steering the Green Monster with white knuckles.

It was growing increasingly colder outside and inside of the truck. Kathleen later told me that just before dusk, my face turned a deep purplish-blue. My radish-red eyes squinted to see oncoming vehicles, just as Kathleen said they would, and I prayed silently.

At dark we approached Fort William at the Lakehead in northern Ontario. In my solitude I took a moment to reflect. However ingenious my plan had been, I now determined to abandon my original idea; I'd had enough. Instead, I would load the family and our goods onto a freight train and take the easier route to Toronto.

When we stopped at a motel for the night, I approached Kathleen and the boys with a woeful expression on my face. I confessed that I had been stubborn headed about the whole thing and that we would pack it in and travel by rail.

To my great surprise, the boys began a collective protest. They begged me to go on. And, unbelievably, Kathleen confessed to having acquired a certain knack at handling the yellow truck. She had even become adept at silencing the troops, she declared. The dogs, well—they barked. She had nevertheless managed a slight grin; this time I was outvoted. So incredibly, the decision was made—the trip would continue.

Over the last year I had not spent much time at all with my family. Billy Graham had taken me far abroad often. But there developed a decided closeness among the White family members on this trip, particularly on those cold April nights in the motel rooms. I would sit with the boys and watch our beloved Toronto Maple Leafs, which featured Davey Keon and Frank Mahovolich, in captivating playoff games.

Suddenly Silenced

Kathleen would chat about the events of the day. To our great relief it appeared that she had simmered down.

Early on each of the four days on the trip back to Toronto, we ate a good breakfast and chuckled about what the day might bring. Kathleen, still slightly apprehensive, would gather herself and rise up courageously, signaling a return to the road. The boys scurried back into the yellow truck, the dogs leapt into position, and Kathleen—well, Kathleen climbed aboard the yellow truck, stationing herself behind the wheel. I ascended the Green Monster!

Throughout the highlands of northern Ontario our procession weaved and wobbled around the hilly bends of the mountainous region. Kathleen recalls one occasion when she had been following a slow moving logging truck for what seemed like hours. Feeling quite comfortable behind the wheel by now, she decided to pass the creeping truck ahead of her. We were perilously close to the sloped shoulder of the narrow two-lane highway that began a long and meandering curve. I could see Kathleen glance into the rearview mirror. I thought I caught her attention. I began shouting at the top of my voice, "Stop! Don't do it!"

My screams were in vain. I could feel her go! I gripped the Green Monster's wheel, and I cried out in fear. We sped up to pass, and I could feel the whirling sensation of free flight as the Green Monster, my old International, swerved to make a pass. I had no control over the truck. I felt my body being thrown to and fro as on the thrashing sea.

As quickly as it began we were through. We steered off the highway and up to a roadside restaurant to calm our nerves with some lunch.

We had just dug into lunch when a couple of country folks approached our table. Without invitation they shared how they had followed us when we passed that logging truck. The woman started, "I practically froze when I saw your huge green truck flip a good four feet in the air when it changed lanes to avoid a thick logging chain. It is a miracle that we're not all killed." Her husband was nonplussed. We said a quiet prayer and thanked the couple, assuring them that we would be careful and arrive alive.

The next day, the chain broke. I climbed under the Green Monster off the highway to fasten the chain to the front axle. We were conspicuous. An Ontario Provincial Police officer stopped to see what we were

The Green Monster

up to. By now, stubble had sprouted from my face, and my hair was matted with grease and dirt. I was a mess. The policeman leaned under the Green Monster, tipping his hat back, exposing his furrowed brow. He curiously inquired, "Who are you?"

Face to face with him now, with bloodshot eyes I indignantly quipped, "I am an associate evangelist with Billy Graham and an Oxford doctor of philosophy."

Silenced for a moment, he glared at me. He knew that what we were doing was illegal, but since there was no legal name for it, he wished us luck and bid us adieu. However, before we left, he pointed to a large mattress that he had picked up from the road. He simply said, "I believe that this is yours!"

Another pleasant night followed. We had dinner at six when darkness fell. In the dining room of the motel a man approached our table. I kind of turned away from him, realizing that I now sported a number of days' growth on my face and I appeared unquestionably disheveled. The man studied me for a moment and exclaimed, "Why, you're John Wesley White, aren't you?" Bashfully, I confessed that I was, and the man shook my hand, quite pleased at making my acquaintance. This really made my day.

The next day Kathleen, the four boys, the two dogs, the yellow truck carrying the blue Vauxhall, and the Green Monster and I rolled to a stop in Rexdale, a suburb of Toronto. Kathleen still remembers how her rich cousin Margaret, who was being entertained by her sister Jean, stood up suddenly, shocked at what she saw from the living room window, and cried out, "Look, the hillbillies! They've arrived at your house!" Just then a man, the neighbour, knocked on the door. Jean, with an apparent reluctance, answered it. The man, eyes straining, piped-up "I've never seen anything like it, and there's a woman driving it."

Jean blushed. She had to admit that it was only us, her sister and family, who had come from Winnipeg.

That weekend we had to break into our new home in Rexdale. When we arrived the doors were locked and we did not have a key. There was no way of getting in touch with our real estate agent, so we stuffed Randy through the milk box. He opened the front door, and we proudly marched in. We began unloading the Green Monster with the help of relatives who lived nearby.

Suddenly Silenced

The trip was truly over. Yet I had the dubious task of saying goodbye to the Green Monster. We thought about it for a while and decided to abandon the old International at the plaza. We said our fond farewells to our friend, the Green Monster. The boys recall the journey from Winnipeg to Toronto with great affection. They say that on that trip they experienced some of the happiest moments of their lives. The boys were tucked safely away in our new home Monday night as I preached that April 12, 1965, in Aliquippa, Pennsylvania.

At the team meeting in Miami in 1966, my good friend and colleague Irv Chambers, whom I first met in 1948, got me on the stage. Irv was with the Billy Graham crusades as early as that. My face was as red as a prime tomato this time. I was nervous and slightly embarrassed to tell the story of the Green Monster to 400 of my colleagues. Billy Graham, who was bedridden with a virus, had the meeting wired into his bedroom. He later recounted that when he heard me tell my story, he laughed so hard that he doubled over and fell right out of bed. Some things in life stay with you for an eternity.

CHAPTER X

The Right Side of the Road

On September 3, 1967, Canada's centennial year, Billy held a single afternoon rally before 40,000 at Toronto's Canadian National Exhibition. On this date in Sweden, an event grabbed the headlines of newspapers everywhere. All traffic changed direction in that country. They switched from the left side of the road to the right side of the road. I'd written an illustration about this event in the *Toronto Daily Star*. It seemed to me a perfect parallel to the lasting theme in the Bible that originated in the Garden of Eden, the elementary concept of right and wrong. Billy saw the fundamental truth in this illustration to persuade people to switch from the "left side" to the "right side" of the Lord.

Throughout the ages and the entire Bible, God has always drawn a definite line separating the wrong side of the Lord from the right side of the Lord. In the beginning man was instructed of God. In Genesis we learn that the Lord *"the Judge of all the earth do* ***right****"* (18:25, emphasis added). Of the hundreds of examples to be chosen from, I cite a few: *"Asa did what was* ***right*** *in the eyes of the LORD"* (1 Kings 15:11, emphasis added). Jehoshaphat did *"what was* ***right*** *in the eyes of the LORD"* (1 Kings 22:43, emphasis added).

In contrast, *"Ahaz...did not do what was* ***right*** *in the eyes of the Lord"* (2 Kings 16:2, emphasis added). Two examples *of* those who did not do *right* in the sight *of* the Lord are King Ahab and especially King Manasseh, who *"did that which was evil in the sight of the LORD"* (2 Kings 21:2 KJV). There continues in the Old Testament and through time a great list *of* kings and common folk alike who did not do *right* in the eyes *of* God.

Phillip received the singular gifting of an evangelist. He journeyed to Samaria. He spoke to a crowd, and many were converted to Jesus Christ. Then the apostle Peter, who received many *of* the fourteen gifts, proclaimed, *"They were ministering...the gospel to you by the Holy Spirit sent from heaven—things which angels desire to look into"* (1 Peter 1:12). Simon Peter warned Simon the Sorcerer, *"For thy heart is not **right** in the sight of God. Repent therefore of this thy wickedness, and pray God, if perhaps the thought of thine heart may be forgiven thee"* (Acts 8:21). It was time for the White family to move from the left side of the road to the *right* side of the road.

Of the fourteen gifts, I received that one gift, the gift of an evangelist. Paul announced that *"[Jesus] who descended is also the One who ascended far above all the heavens, that He might fill all things...He Himself gave some to be apostles, some prophets, some evangelists, and some pastors and teachers"* (Ephesians 4:10–11). Jesus commanded the twelve disciples and people everywhere. This, therefore, is the message that preachers and especially evangelists have carried to the world since the death of our Savior two millennia ago. Our Lord informed His disciples that those who hear the Word fall into four categories (Mark 4:3–9). First, those who hear, but the seed of the Word falls by the wayside. Second, those who hear, but the seed of the Word soon after falls away from the faith. Third, those who hear, but the seed of the Word is blown into thorns and thistles; they become Christians but live carnal lives. Fourth, those who hear the seed of the Word and become Christians and remain devout Christians.

According to the crusade statistics furnished by the Billy Graham Evangelistic Association, the findings are parallel to Jesus' statements. Approximately 5 percent of all listeners come forward to make a decision for Jesus Christ at the Billy Graham and associate crusades.

I am moved at this point to relay a rather ironic story that reveals the substance of the second category: those who hear the Word and come forward to make a decision, soon after to fall away from the faith. It was in the early 1960s. I ventured from Oxford to Wales for a crusade. On Sunday evening I was anointed, bringing a powerful message from the Word to the crowd via the Holy Spirit. At the invitation,

The Right Side of the Road

I was confronted by what I suspected was the sincerest of men. I personally counseled him, guiding him through the sinner's prayer: *"God be merciful to me, a sinner, and save me for Jesus' sake."* Abruptly, the man fell to his knees, himself in prayer. In my view this man had been properly moved in the Holy Spirit. For all outward appearances this dashing man, still in his twenties, I judged, was completely saved inside and out. He was full of tears in repentance for sins past and the certain renewal of his life now reaching into a definite eternity. I was touched. After a full half hour this young man rose to his feet and perceptibly to new spiritual heights. He had, I was sure, become a new creation in Christ. He had seen the light.

Following the crusade I journeyed for four hours back to our home in Oxford. During the night I was euphoric. The mental image of that young man kaleidoscoped in my mind, and it would not stop. I even found myself thinking that we had a new evangelist. If this were the case, something would have to be done.

Early the next morning Kathleen, the boys, the poodles and I packed up and prepared for a crusade in Scotland. I was tired but overjoyed at the apparent rebirth of that handsome young man whom I had counseled and led to the Lord. Finally, and with all the necessities of life brimming from our bags, we headed to Scotland.

We had no sooner landed than I was called to the phone. To my astonishment, it was my neighbor, who delivered an alarming message. Kathleen's sky-blue azure eyes steeled again as that neighbor informed us that that very same handsome and talented young man, the one who had tossed his life into the arms of Jesus, had been tossed into jail. "What?" I exclaimed over long distance telephone.

The neighbor gathered up all her courage and let fly with the news: "He robbed your house!"

My smile vanished. Then a verse crossed my mind. The apostle Paul informed his pupil Timothy, *"The solid foundation of God stands, having this seal: 'The Lord knows those who are His' and, 'Let everyone who names the name of Christ depart from iniquity'"* (2 Timothy 2:19). The apostle John as an old man wrote, *"They went out from us, but they were not of us; for if they had been of us, they would have continued with us; but they went out that they might be made manifest, that none of them were of us"* (1 John 2:19).

Suddenly Silenced

Another passage flooded my mind. *"From that time many of his disciples went back, and walked no more with him. Then said Jesus unto the twelve, Will ye also go away? Then Simon Peter answered him, Lord, to whom shall we go? thou hast the words of eternal life. And we believe and are sure that thou art that Christ, the Son of the living God"* (John 6:66–69). I was rightly appeased.

In the spring of 1965 we held fifteen days of glorious crusading in Morristown, Tennessee. The chairman of this crusade was John Wallace. John had been one of the most capable and dedicated crusade chairmen in his years with the John Wesley White Crusades. He had been a close friend and chairman of the American Join the Family television ministry. We held a two-week John Wesley White Crusade, which involved fifty churches. The final Sunday night 5,000 people were in attendance.

Of the many decisions made at this crusade was that of a brilliant medical student named Charles Lindsey, who later became an ophthalmologist. On January 24, 1993, Dr. Lindsey gave his testimony in a large First Baptist church in Morristown. He spoke of his conversion at the Morristown crusade in 1965, where he had given his life to Christ.

John and Paula Wallace built a spacious new home, the largest I'd ever stayed in. This sprawling home rolled out upon the hill on which it was built. This was a Southern mansion.

We held a two-week crusade in Richmond, California. The White family was present and participating. A moving testimony was delivered by a San Francisco Giant, Philippe Alou. For years Alou was the manager of the Montreal Expos. Many came forward that night. My boys performed at the beautiful Richmond Auditorium and were applauded. When it was over, the crusade committee passed a rather large hat around, and each member contributed silver to send the boys 400 miles south, to Disneyland. This moment was hilarious; it typified the feeling we were all sharing about the success of the crusade. Needless to say, the boys were excited. When we arrived at Disneyland the boys forgot all about performing and enjoyed countless trips around Disneyland, via rides that Kathleen and I could only describe as terrifying.

Upon tearing the boys away from Disneyland we toured to the Mennonite Bethel College Auditorium, in Newton, Kansas, which held

The Right Side of the Road

a crowd of 3,500. In August we packed the place by featuring the actress and blues singer Ethel Waters. The highlight of her testimony was her singing of the song "His Eye Is on the Sparrow."

Then the White family rushed to Rexdale in Toronto, where the boys went back to school full-time. I departed for three crusades in British Columbia, in western Canada, at the Kamloops arena, from September 10 to 19. The chairman of that crusade was a surgeon named Dr. Osborne.

On Saturday a Presbyterian minister felt an undeniable urge to get a man named George Girvan into the crusade meeting. That night he had him in for supper, and the man, not without reluctance, came along. I preached Jesus words *"This night your soul will be required of you"* (Luke 12:20). George heard an inner voice say, *"His is the way; walk you in it."* There was a fierce spiritual battle going on in his will. But eventually he broke loose from the devil's hold, and from high in the stands he made his way forward, where he prayed the prayer of decision for Christ, that he might be born again.

Sooner than for most, Jesus called, *"This night your soul will be required of you"* to George. That very night, in fact, he was alone in his home. The gas main broke, and his house blew up. He was rushed to the hospital with third degree burns. Dr. Osborne, the crusade chairman and Presbyterian minister, stood over him. George apparently regained consciousness only once before he took his flight home. The beloved physician heard him mutter almost inaudibly, "Doc, I'm glad I did it! I gave myself to Jesus." And born again as he was, he went to be with Christ.

I drove to the Trail area, where from September 22 to 29 I crusaded. In an auditorium in Nanaimo, I held another crusade from October 3 to 17. Then I lectured to the students and the faculty at the University of Victoria in British Columbia. I took the opportunity to visit my brother Hugh and his wife, Aileen, who lived in Victoria. They mentioned that their son Brian was in his first month at the University of Victoria. During the Nanaimo crusade he had come to the front of the platform while I preached. Brian dedicated his life to our Lord Jesus Christ.

When Brian received his final marks in June that year, to the delight of his parents it was discovered that he had achieved the highest marks of any male student in British Columbia that year. He was so bright that after his undergraduate work was completed, he was exempted from his first year of premed studies at the University of British Columbia. Today, Brian is a capable and well-liked Christian physician in Nanaimo, B.C.

The April 1966 issue of *Decision* recalled an important night for evangelism. That night was November 9, 1965, when a sudden power failure near Niagara Falls plunged the northeastern United States and parts of Canada into darkness. Pilots struggled blindly to find runways, and thousands of people were trapped in darkened elevators, frozen between floors. I was preaching and was in the middle of my message when the lights went out. It was pitch-black dark and white-knuckle cold. I boldly called to the crowd, "Come out of the darkness into the light." Scores scrambled to the platform, ascending into the everlasting arms of Jesus.

In May 1992 at a Franklin Graham–John Wesley White crusade I returned to the platform for the first time since my heart attack two months earlier. Wendy Wade, a woman of thirty-six, thanked me after the meeting and informed me that at nine years of age she had been at Worchester, Massachusetts, and had given her life to Jesus. She'd heard the radiant testimony of the reigning Miss America, Vonda Kay Van Dyke. In 1992 Wendy was rejoicing in Christ.

We purchased a new home in Willowdale, Ontario. Willowdale is a suburb of Toronto. We had lived in many houses in many places—now we had a home. (It has been our home for forty-four years!) We could settle in and dig in to a life.

We had just begun to acclimatize when our boys joined us for fifteen days of fruitful crusading in Gibson City, Illinois. Notably, the November 1966 issue of *Decision* illustrated the essence of the superb meetings that we held at this time. The small town of Gibson City yielded 700 decisions. George Beverly Shea, the great baritone, was accompanied by Don Hustad, who had been the keyboardist at Moody Bible Institute fifteen years earlier. George Beverly Shea composed a song that the boys sang and trumpeted in Gibson City. Their horns and voices announced "The Wonder of It All." This Sunday evening performance ended the crusade before a crowd of 5,000.

Dick Kemple was an insurance salesman and the wealthiest man in Gibson City. His name was plastered on every billboard along the six

The Right Side of the Road

highways that converge on the city. During the middle Sunday evening of the crusade he came to our meeting as a nominal Christian. There he was convicted in the Spirit of Christ. So intense was his conviction that he drove around his city until the wee hours of the morning, anxiously ransacking his life.

He stopped at his minister's manse in the middle of the night. In a fit of temper Kemple frantically pounded on the minister's door. The minister threw on his coat, and the two men made their way through the darkness to the church next door. The minister instructed Kemple to fall to his knees. The two men prayed the sinner's prayer: "*God, be merciful to me, a sinner*," for Christ's sake. Kemple accepted Christ there on his knees, but it was still necessary for him to make a public confession. This he would do the next Monday at our crusade.

Kemple came forward from the back of the crowd. He had been hiding there, experiencing the essence of Dale Carnegie's greatest and classic book *How to Make Friends and Influence People*. This gem has sold over 1,300,000 copies worldwide. "The fear of embarrassment is the curse of the mind," said Carnegie in his book, and Dick Kemple was under the spell of embarrassment. Kemple, a salesman like Carnegie, used the book's positive affirmations to rise to success in sales. Dick Kemple made his public confession.

That Thursday morning Kemple paid for the breakfasts of seventy-five local men. They met at a local restaurant. There these citizens heard a remarkable testimony and confession for Jesus Christ.

Following his courageous confession, Dick accepted a full-time position as a director with Youth For Christ. He threw fame and fortune aside, victorious in Jesus Christ, to serve his new Lord and Savior by crisscrossing the globe. For twenty-five years he shared his powerful testimony with citizens of the planet. Then, in October 1992, he talked to me at a Franklin Graham–John Wesley White Crusade, declaring his continuing love for Jesus Christ. His was a stunning conversion to Christ!

After Gibson City, we sped to Worthington, Minnesota, for a fifteen-day crusade. It was hot—sweltering hot! The Gibson City crusade had been held in a ballpark outside, whereas the Worthington crusade was held in an indoor auditorium. There were 4,800 people who congregated that Sunday night. Hundreds of decisions for Christ were rendered!

Suddenly Silenced

By this time the White boys were itching for some summer recreation, and we were fortunate enough to have the use of the cottage of a former graduate of Wheaton College, physician Dr. Peter Stam. Thus began the glorious days at the lake. Day after day the sun rose as a blazing orb, raising the temperature alarmingly. It was here that the boys learned to water ski. Our sons have always liked sports, and water skiing was no exception. They got so good on the skis that they even slalom-skied backwards!

From the shore, Kathleen yelled her caution to the boys, who were parading breakneck stunts before her. Her pleas were in vain as the boys, trailing the boat, were occasionally ejected from their skis. Each in their own turn would plunge headlong into the water, sending shivers of fear through their unfortunate and helpless mother stranded on the beach. The boys dared their mom to "be quiet and just try it, before you judge it."

Kathleen could take the chiding no longer and finally gathered up all of her courage and decided to see what all the fuss was about. She determined to try the skis, even though she was a non-swimmer. It seemed like a day had passed until she managed to jostle into place, squatting herself into what she thought was just the right position.

The roar of the motor came up, and she was off. Scant seconds later she slumped over into the fetal position. She flopped off the skis, slapping the waves. I could just glimpse into her sky-blue azure eyes long enough to see that she was terrified. She held onto the ski rope for dear life. Then I watched the boys' mother as she was dragged through the wake of the boat for what must have seemed to Kathleen an eternity.

She gasped for air as the torrent of water swelled around her. We horrified onlookers screamed, "Let go!" She continued to hang on until her strength gave way and her fingers could grasp the rope no longer. She was swallowed up in a whirlpool and went down—out of sight.

The water went deathly still. When Kathleen surfaced, limp, she was blue in the face. The boys were really frightened, but we were relieved when we returned Mom to the beach breathing and with color returning to her face. We were grateful that she survived this episode of the adventures of the White family. Now she could once again begin exercising her lungs from a safe distance on the burning sands of the lake. For thirty-

The Right Side of the Road

five years Kathleen has been plagued by occasional flashbacks of those summer days when she went under while water skiing.

Bill, Wesley, Paul and Randy sang and trumpeted for the Lord. They played songs from their recording arranged by Dr. Edward Thomas from Minneapolis. The album was entitled *Trumpets of the Lord*. It was pressed in the fall of 1966.

From Minnesota the White family piled into the car and headed for Toronto. Of the dozen crusades in 1966, there was only one remaining. It was held in Billings, Montana, in the fall. Throughout the event it was brutally cold and raining, terrifically contrasting with the oven conditions at Worthington. Now it was fall, and the wind and driving rain pelted us on the platform at the baseball stadium. On Sunday, the first evening, I was anointed and preaching. A full 8 percent of the drenched crowd made decisions on Sunday, though the rain stung their optimistic faces. This was a miracle!

Two teenagers, Vince Frank and Steve Ryan, came forward. For over a quarter of a century now these two men have pastored large churches in Idaho. On Monday, the conditions became so deplorable that we were forced to move the crusade indoors, to the Shriners' Auditorium.

One night we featured Paul Andersen, the man who had recently won the strongest man world championship in Moscow. The strongest man was casually clad in workout sweats as he bellowed down his love for Jesus Christ. Who was going to argue with this man's attire—or his message?

This modern-day Samson waved his brawny arms above the craning necks of the crowd. "I want twelve of the toughest cowboys to come up on the platform and seat themselves at the picnic table," he barked. The giant then lay down, face up, on the platform, beneath the huge table on which the goliaths were seated. Then with a mighty groan he hefted the table with his arms and legs, high into the air. The cowboys could only sigh in amazement as they found themselves airborne, well above the platform before an awestruck crowd. Goliath then proclaimed his love for Christ Jesus, and his demonstration of strength was complete.

That July Kathleen and the boys joined me. We drove the American South and into Mexico. Then, July 30 through August 2, the boys trumpeted and sang while I preached at the annual Campus Crusade conference, at Arrowhead Springs, California. Here I accepted the invitation to speak with Dr. Bill Bright, the founder and president of the Campus Crusade Ministries, about the previous year's congress in Berlin.

That summer the White family ventured to Twin Falls, Idaho. The first night was "Youth Night," and 157 young people came forward. One convert was twenty-year-old LaVonne Jostlin. In March LaVonne was married to Eric Jostlin, who was one of the original Rolling Stones. Eric had been saved in a Baptist church. He and LaVonne toured around the western United States evangelizing. Eric had turned from Satan to the Savior!

In stark contrast, a woman rushed me at one of the Twin Falls crusades to tell me about her husband. She cried, "He has been moved to tears by the Holy Spirit and he weeps in conviction but remains stubborn." He was a potential convert but refused to relinquish his will.

He threw a final party for his friends the very next night. At 11:30 a.m., he was killed—eaten by an auger, a grain-grinder. He suffocated. His mangled body was found prostrate in the grain hopper. John Corts, who would be the president of the BGEA in the '90s, discovered the man's picture on the front page of the local newspaper. The man's death tolled the alarm, and the town's folk flocked to our crusade!

Russell Wells and his wife, Lois, and Kathleen and I have been close friends for over the past third of a century. Russell was born an only child, in Moose Jaw, Saskatchewan. During his youth, his family moved to Prince Edward Island. Russell joined the Royal Canadian Air Force during World War II. After the war, Russell took up broadcast journalism in Toronto. He was fortunate enough to be the protégé of the senior and great Canadian voice of the CBC, Lorne Greene. Russell and Lorne became close friends. Under the tutelage of Lorne Green, Russell found his start on radio.

Russell has been kind, mentally stimulating and consistently supportive to me, particularly since my stroke. Every possible Saturday morning for thirty-three years, Russell has come to our house. He and I have discussed world affairs, current events, politics, economics, social issues, theological positions, biblical problems and most anything that comes to our minds. He is my intellectual brother. When I

The Right Side of the Road

had my silencing stroke, Russell was crushed. That never stopped him from visiting though—even when I could barely speak. Russell is a special friend.

On June 13, 1969, we took the family to a crusade in New York City. Accompanying us were our close friends the Wells family. Russell and Lois had three boys and two girls. That made four adults, nine kids and four poodles. What a zoo! We were off to Manhattan, all of us...as if they needed more people.

This crusade was held in a crowded Madison Square Gardens. Billy was brilliant. As I have said, Billy reached his peak energy in the 1960s. It was obvious to the world that he was greatly anointed—called and strong in the Lord.

The Whites and the Wells crusaded with Billy Graham in New York until June 22, 1969. After the long crusade and suffering the fast pace of New York, I found myself most anxious to get home. I needed to get my feet up. I guess I didn't look down at the speedometer often enough in the old Cadillac, and the rearview mirror was blocked by the boys, the dogs and the other things—we were crammed in.

My foot was leaden on the accelerator, the conversation was brisk and the New York State Thruway was as frustrating as always. It was bustling in the blazing heat, and its pavement was black and blistering. We were all overheated and on edge as we sped down the New York State thruway at 80 miles per hour. The speed limit was still 60 or 70 miles per hour (I can't remember).

Then it happened! I heard the screaming sirens. Leaning over in my seat, I caught a glimpse of the whirling red light in the side mirror. I was fit to be tied!

When I could finally find a spot to pull over, the policeman lifted the brim of his hat and leaned on my five-year-old Cadillac. He looked at me with deep, penetrating eyes and said something with Yankee earnestness like, "Well, mister, you wanna get somewhere in a hurry, don't ya? I've gotta mind to..." He glanced around the inside of the car, and seeing that it was hopeless, he scratched me out a ticket. This was only the third or fourth speeding ticket of my life.

I could feel my blood pressure blast off as I pulled away from him. The boys' chuckles stung my ears. Kathleen's Irish sky-blue azure eyes were fire and ice, and the dogs were yapping hysterically. This is when

Suddenly Silenced

I yelled my one-word sentence: "Silence!" Sweat was pouring down my brow, and my temper was flaring again.

As graciously as I could I acknowledged my temper and promised that I'd try to control it. However, it was still hundreds of miles to our home, and I was getting increasingly exhausted. I wanted to get home! A little flippant thought kept whisking its way through my mind. I kept thinking, *I couldn't be unlucky enough to have it happen two times on one trip, could I?* I stepped on the accelerator peddle again—I just refused to look at that speedometer!

I hunkered down in my seat, and I guess I buried that little red needle, because it wasn't long until I sensed a repeating incident on the burning thruway. I scrunched up my face, gritted my teeth and peeped into the rearview mirror once more. Another red light was spinning and honing in on me!

My blood flowed like ice in my veins. This time I had been caught in a speed trap. I can't imagine what this second policeman thought when the message came across the radio concerning my first speeding ticket of the day, but he didn't look at all amused to me. When he let me go, I merely slunk down in my seat, stuffed the speeding ticket into my pocket and crawled down the New York State Thruway. There was no way I could stop the gales of laughter pouring over me from the back seat. Have you ever felt lonely in a crowd? Then you know what I mean. Even the dogs howled at me. This is the true life of an evangelist!

At the Canada–US border I met Russell, and he had only one thing to say to me: "Two tickets, John?"

It had been twenty years since those glorious and inspiring days at Winona Lake. I was called there for a series of meetings from June 30 to July 3, 1969. The entire White family was there. The boys trumpeted for the Lord, and I preached nightly. Kathleen looked on with, I think, some pride. I couldn't help but acknowledge that I was feeling sentimental. I kept thinking about those great men who were connected with Youth For Christ back in the forties: Billy Graham and his team, Cliff Harrows and George Beverly Shea, T.W. Wilson, Torrey Johnson (president and founder of Youth for Christ), Bob Pierce, Chuck Templeton, Jack Shuler, and the many others who were involved in the early days. July 4 to 6, Billy Graham concluded the Winona Lake conference.

The Right Side of the Road

It was then that the Winona Lake meetings were closed for good. Half a century—then gone! A wrecking ball had been taken to the Billy Sunday tabernacle at Winona Lake. We grieved! Billy Graham was in tears. The Youth For Christ headquarters was moved to Wheaton, Illinois. This was truly the end of an epoch.

Ted Cornell accompanied my team as we headed for Sioux Falls, South Dakota. Ted was one of twelve musicians who made the trip that August. Ted Cornell was the youngest student ever to be admitted to the Julliard School of Music in New York City, the premier music school in the world. Over the past thirty years Ted has been involved in over 200 crusades with my team. In his native Saskatchewan during a Billy and Franklin Graham crusade to a crowd of over 20,000, Billy pronounced Ted Cornell the world's leading evangelistic musician. Ted stands a towering six foot six inches tall and commands the listeners' ears wherever he plays. He has been blessed with a charming wife, Zandra. In the '80s Ted's son, Ted Jr., made a decision for Jesus Christ at my crusade in Hawaii. Ted's daughter, Britney, made her decision for Christ at my crusade in New England. How greatly blessed we all have been!

The Sioux Falls meetings were held at Wood Stadium. This crusade set a record number of decisions for any associate Billy Graham crusade anywhere in North America—2,053 decisions. Nine thousand people attended on the last Sunday night alone!

Nels Stewart was a lady who came to Christ at Sioux Falls, South Dakota. She was an aristocratic and cultured woman. On the first night of the crusade, Nels' ten-year-old son came to Christ. The following Monday morning that same ten-year-old made the front page of the local newspaper. On Tuesday night, her fourteen-year-old daughter responded. Thursday night, Nels herself came forward and gave her life to Christ!

At a reception, Nels spotted me in a corner of the room. She approached me in reverence. Quietly, but with very deep emotion, she told me the following story:

> My late husband was the most prominent lawyer in this part of the country. He was brilliant and wealthy, but he always had to be number one—so we had the first color television in this state. The day it was installed we sat down together to watch an

Suddenly Silenced

evening of programming. Billy Graham came on, and Dr. Graham spoke about sin. My husband jumped to his feet, stomped across the room, snapped the television off, and angrily shouted, "I don't need to take that from Billy Graham, or God Almighty!" Immediately, he doubled up like a jackknife. I panicked. I ran next door and brought in a medical doctor, who pronounced him dead.

Today, Nels is a dedicated Christian!

We held eleven crusades in 1970, and we were introduced to Tom Bledsoe, who was song leader, soloist and head of the choir. He and his talented wife, Terry, provided stirring gospel songs that crowds came to appreciate everywhere the John Wesley White crusades held sway. Terry had crisscrossed North America as a featured soprano soloist with the internationally acclaimed Robert Shaw Corral. Tom was dashing and possessed a charismatic personality. Over one-third of a century he logged millions of air miles to various meetings as he carried evangelism to the world. He was a superb musical organizer with the Billy Graham crusade team. For over thirty years Tom, Terry, Kathleen and I have been very close friends.

During the 1980s and 1990s Tom functioned as the capable assistant to Cliff Barrows, as well as being the head musical organizer with the Billy Graham team. In addition, he also provided his services for the Franklin Graham–John Wesley White crusades and festivals. Tom Bledsoe has been indispensable.

Our most memorable crusade in 1970 was in Greeneville, Tennessee. A quarter of a century later, I fell to a stroke in Greeneville, Tennessee.

On Main Street that summer in 1970, the crusade committee hung a banner that announced the "Dr. John Wesley White Crusade." Elvis Presley just happened to be touring on his bus at the time. His bus stopped in downtown Greeneville. Amazingly, off the bus strode Elvis himself. He was accompanied by his entourage. The media swarmed and filmed his every move. The newsreel aired this event around the world. But appearing immediately behind the "Rock and Roll" legend and in plain view was my crusade banner. Jesus was with us. A decade later Kathleen and I were flipping through the channels one evening

The Right Side of the Road

when, lo and behold, we came upon the Elvis special again, and again our banner flew proudly over his shoulder.

Of the hundreds of conversions at the Greeneville crusade, one stands above all the others in my memory. Onto the track in front of the stands a seventy-one-year-old man rolled up in a wheelchair. He was blind, deaf and mute. His sister tapped my words out in Morse code on the back of his hand.

At the end of my message, I asked those who wished to respond to Christ's call to repeat the sinner's prayer after me. She asked for assistance in pushing her brother forward to be with the other inquirers. Her brother tapped out onto his sister's hand the prayer of commitment to Christ. He intimated that he had been born again. I was almost speechless. What a miracle!

On July 28, 1993, I was speaking at the Billy Graham School of Evangelism at the Cove in North Carolina when a Baptist preacher informed me that the blind, deaf and mute convert had moved on to heaven, where he could see, hear and speak the praises of his beloved Jesus Christ. In Greeneville, I was silenced in awe of God's work in this man's life. In Greeneville on April 28, 1996, I was silenced.

In September 1971 we pitched a tent for 2,800 in Spindale, North Carolina. With us on our crusade were Tom and Terry Bledsoe and Myrtle Hall, who sang. Bill Fasig played the piano. T.W. Wilson had come to Montreat to welcome Billy Graham and his secretary, Stephanie Wills. Johnny Lenning, from *The Hour of Decision*, coordinated this crusade. Johnny's boy Scott was among hundreds that had come forward to the Lord at Spindale. In November 1980, in Reno, Nevada, Scott Lenning's mother came forward at the invitation.

In the 1990s Scott joined the Billy Graham team as resident coordinator of the crusades. Scott's most memorable crusade was held in the TWA dome in St. Louis, October 14 to 17, 1999. Attendance averaged 45,000 per meeting, with an average of 2,500 individuals responding each evening to Billy Graham's invitation to commit their lives to Christ. In 2005 in New York City, Scott Lenning finished his five years of organizing Billy Graham crusades. Today he has moved on.

Another of the crusades that sticks in my mind was held in the arena in Collingwood, Ontario, Canada. A beautiful teenage girl named Rhonda Bell came to the front to give her life to Jesus. Shortly after, she married a TV manager. I met Rhonda again at People's Church in 1990. She was nostalgic about her conversion story of almost twenty years earlier. It was October 14, 1990. I was speaking at The People's Church in Toronto to celebrate the 50th anniversary of Paul Smith's call to the ministry.

The mayor of North York, the fourth largest city in Canada, was the Jewish Mel Lastman, a politician with a charismatic personality. He referred to his city as "the city with a heart." Mayor Mel stood by with me as arrangements were being made concerning the seating on the platform. Mel leaned over and muttered into my ear, "Who is the guy we're here to see? Who is the speaker, this Dr. John Wesley White?"

I responded, "It is me!" We chuckled. Later, Mel became the mayor of all of Toronto in 2003.

In 1972, we held ten crusades. Three were particularly interesting, I think. The first took place in April. I spoke for five days at Briercrest Bible College west of Moose Jaw, Saskatchewan. I was preaching a series on "The Signs of the Times: the Second Coming of Jesus Christ." Saskatchewan's premier was in the audience. Ross Thatcher was a nominal Christian who went to church Christmas and Easter. But he fell convicted in the Spirit and made a decision for Christ. Two months later he collapsed from a fatal heart attack, on a sidewalk in the streets of Regina.

Premier Thatcher's sudden death made the top story on the 11 o'clock CBC news and was delivered by Canada's most popular news anchor, Lloyd Robertson. Ross Thatcher died to this world, but he is alive in heaven.

The next memorable crusade of 1973 took place in Nampa, Idaho. Most of our crusades over the prior ten years were a standard fifteen-days long. Sterling Huston, our crusade director, made the tough decision to limit the length of our crusades, beginning with Nampa, to ten days. At this crusade on Sunday evening, 9,000 people attended. Of those 9,000 people, 1,700 made decisions for Christ.

Billy Graham's motto, for half a century, has been "*You will show me the path of life; In Your presence is fullness of joy; At Your right hand are pleasures forevermore*" (Psalm 16:11). We the evangelists preach Christ and the cross; that Christ, God incarnate on earth, died once for all; that He came not for the righteous but for the sinner, so that the sinner may be saved and not die but have everlasting life.

The Right Side of the Road

At the close of the Bible, Jesus' Way is revealed by that century-old apostle John, exiled on the Isle of Patmos, in the reflections of a life devoted to Christ Jesus. *"Blessed are they that wash their robes, that they may have the right [to come] to the tree of life, and my enter in by the gates into the city"* (Revelation 22:14). It was *right*.

CHAPTER XI

International Evangelism:
7 Continents, 100 Countries,
in 5 Years

Jesus proclaimed the gospel to Nicodemus and to all of the world: *"For God so loved the world that He gave His only begotten Son, that whoever believes in Him should not perish but have everlasting life"* (John 3:16). The apostle Matthew quoted Jesus regarding His instructions to His disciples: *"All authority has been given to Me in heaven and on earth. Go therefore and make disciples of all the nations, baptizing them in the name of the Father and of the Son and of the Holy Spirit"* (Matthew 28:18,19).

It happened in June 1961, in London, England, in the Grosvenor House Hotel downtown. I received my commission from Billy Graham to go into all the world and preach the gospel. I had fallen under the furnace force of the Holy Spirit, and I was altered forever. Henceforth, I was catapulted on an evangelistic journey that has led me to 7 continents and to 100 countries in the world. Evangelism, I have discovered, is not something that one leads oneself through. Instead it is an act of the Holy Spirit that tugs one through each day of one's life.

In London in 1966 my work as research and illustrator proliferated. I supplied hundreds of illustrations for Billy Graham during the twelve weeks of crusading in London as Billy's personal researcher.

At one of the fifty-two meetings Cliff Richard, the world-renowned Christian rock and roll star, teamed with me. He sang; I preached. And our meeting bore fruit. Among those who came to the front at the invitation that evening was Peter Tso, a scientist from China. In the '80s, I learned that Peter had become a supremely spiritual Christian, significant because he emigrated from London, England, to Ontario.

Suddenly Silenced

I made preparations for my trip aboard a large international jetliner headed for Berlin, Germany. In Berlin, in 1966 I attended the World Congress on Evangelism. An astounding 1,200 delegates were present from 100 countries. The theme of the congress was "One Race, One Gospel, One Task." It was none other than Billy Graham who presided over this congress. The next great congress was held in Lausanne, Switzerland, in 1974. In 1983 and 1986 the congresses were held in Amsterdam. These great evangelical events culminated again in Amsterdam at an international congress of 10,000 evangelists in July 2000. After the formal conference meetings in Berlin in 1966, Oral Roberts, Anglican bishop A.W. Goodwin Hudson, Calvin Thielman and I gathered around a table in a small cafe in Berlin for four hours of discussion. We embarked upon conversation that was so engaging that in retrospect I view that gathering as the theological and evangelical highlight of my life.

In November 1966 Billy Graham's singer Jimmie McDonald and I took a side tour to East Germany, Poland, and Moscow. Identifiably, there was only one Baptist church in Moscow. Christians were severely persecuted in the USSR. The situation pertaining to religion had remained unchanged since the Bolshevik Revolution of 1917. But I did preach in the singular Protestant church in Moscow. Upon entering this church I could see that it was packed like a can of sardines. I would give them what they were so thirsty for. I shared the pulpit for four hours with President Frank Peters of Sir Wilfred Laurier University in Kitchener, Ontario.

Jimmie McDonald was black and charismatic. His singing was effusive. It contained the passion of the great gospel singers of the American South. Some consider Russians subordinate people. Their tyrannical upbringing in an oppressive political environment is legendary, but Jimmie had the congregation in tears when he sang "How Great Thou Art" in the Russian language. Immediately following his singing, Jimmie pronounced to the applauding crowd, "I have sung your song for you." It was clear; Jimmie had been greatly anointed that evening.

Our 1967 tour took us on a trip to Bogota, Colombia, nestled in the enormous surrounding Andes mountains. Of necessity, we stretched our lungs in the thin air of the towering heights. Suspended atop the

International Evangelism

summit of this great stone was a statue of Jesus. In contrast to the cross of Bogota, this Jesus extended His arms wide open, beckoning God, that God commission Him to go into all the world (including South America) and preach the gospel.

It could be seen for vast distances. A capital city knelt at the feet of the giant Jesus. Beneath this monumental statue was illuminated the Spanish word for Christ, *Christo*. From our preaching precipice, we descended down the mountain to Rio de Janeiro, the "Marvelous City." Rio is one of the five most scenic cities in the world. It compares with Vancouver, British Columbia; San Francisco, California; Auckland, New Zealand; and Vladivostok, Russia. It was here that I beheld Rio—the real Rio, the one on the postcards. This thriving megametropolis stands on a shimmering bay at the mouth of the great Atlantic Ocean. Surrounding the city, a singular mountain jutted straight up out of the water above our heads—into heaven.

On our ten-day itinerary was a conference near Rio that June in 1978. Four hundred sacrificing missionaries stood by awaiting our message. These great men and women hailed from north Los Angeles. John MacArthur, a relative of the famous General Douglas MacArthur and a great radio personality from Southern California, and I twinned on the crusade trail in Brazil. John would preach the mornings, and I would preach the evenings.

Upon departing Rio De Janeiro we trekked through the wilds of the South American coast to evangelize in Buenos Aires, Argentina, a city that boasts the longest and widest street in the world; to Santiago, Chile; to Lima, Peru, the home of the Incas; to Bolivia, and on to Panama, where the two vast oceans, the Atlantic and the Pacific, converge at the notorious Panama Canal. Then on to Guatemala we went. We finally stopped in Mexico. Upon returning to Toronto, I reflected on the Lord's palette, His handiwork—this beautiful semi-hemisphere.

Then we flew to the glimmering Caribbean, where during the last week of April and the first week of May 1967 we held meetings in Nassau, Bahamas. Sterling Huston was the coordinator of this crusade. He was brilliant and a superb organizer. He has personally counseled me for a third of a generation and coordinated my crusades for seven years—with the kind of attention to detail that allows a crusade that is a large and complex event to run smoothly. I was able to repay Sterling

Suddenly Silenced

for his devotion to my ministry by recommending him to Billy himself, at his home, "Little Piney Cove," in Montreat, North Carolina. Billy then promoted Sterling to director of Billy Graham's North American crusades. As stated, Sterling was singularly talented and a hard working individual: a "five star general." In 1973, he received his well-deserved appointment with the Billy Graham Evangelistic Association. I was further able to recognize Sterling's immense contribution when as the chancellor of Richmond College in Toronto I conferred on him an honorary doctor of letters degree. Sterling and Esther and Kathleen and I remain close friends to this day.

The July 1967 issue of *Decision* stated, "The evangelist Dr. John Wesley White declared that he had never experienced such a movement of the Holy Spirit" to date. The weeks of April 9 to 23, a total of 52,000 people came to the Nassau meetings. This crusade had the unfailing support of the governor, the premier, the Anglican bishop and nearly all of the clergy. What made this event remarkable was that the final night, 9,000 people attended, half of them being unable to jam into the airplane hangar we used. An outstanding 1,700 decisions had been made for Christ!

During our trip to the glamorous islands in the Caribbean Sea in December 1978, the John Wesley White team crusaded in Montego Bay, Jamaica. This region of the country featured a wide variety of peoples.

Then in December 1985 we returned to Jamaica. This time we went to the eastern part of the island for a crusade that was coordinated by Dan Southern. For the second half of the '80s, Ted Cornell and Steve Musto accompanied us on our crusades, from Alaska to Jamaica. Steve spent much of that time with Grady Wilson. Steve possessed highly developed oratory skills. He was most assuredly articulate. I was grateful when Steve accepted my invitation to read the "talking book" version of my publication *Re-entry*.

Next, we held a circle of meetings from Port Antonio, Jamaica, around to Kingston and through the Blue Mountains, which stood a gargantuan 7,000 feet tall. As I call to memory the events of this period of my life, one meeting stands out above all the others. It was held in a small Spanish town. Nine thousand Spirit-thirsty people attended the crusade. The platform was pressed up against the wall of the local penitentiary. No doubt the high wall and its barbed wire restrained the

International Evangelism

prisoners from their long-sought treasure, the freedom to flee from their concrete captivity to the neighboring pastures of tropical splendor.

Flashing forward to 1999, three years after my stroke, Franklin Graham held a festival again in Jamaica, from March 11 to 14. Kathleen and I attended. The festival, as Franklin had come to refer to them, was named "Celebrate Jesus '99 With Franklin Graham." Ruth Graham had begun a relief program for the suffering children in Third World countries. The program was called "Operation Christmas Child." The genius of this program was that each child would receive a shoebox stuffed with toys and useful articles. Upon getting their Christmas shoebox, these poor and pathetic children broke into wide smiles. Our hearts were touched, and we praised God that we'd been given the chance to shed a little light into the loving eyes of the children. Over a year of diligent planning and much prayer by over 2,000 churches and over 1,000 pastors had provided the means by which over 250,000 people could attend this festival. And more than 16,000 of them made decisions for Jesus.

I packed for an extensive world voyage, including that region. I left for Europe and points east. I toured London, Rome, Greece, Israel, Jordan, Iran, Afghanistan, Pakistan, India, Burma, Thailand and Vietnam. In October 1967, the Vietnam War was raging in Asia. The infamous Tet Offensive loomed. This was the most devastating battle of the senseless war. Americans were taking it on the chin. It is said that it took five American soldiers to defeat one North Vietnamese. There just weren't enough American soldiers to do the job. A tired and homesick military floundered in the tall grasses, waste deep in the mosquito-infested canals that bred disease and mortal discontent. The morale of the common soldier was at an all-time low during the Vietnam scuffle. My journey also included Hong Kong, Taipei, Tokyo—about forty countries in all.

My experience in Japan sticks with me. Japan was particularly secular. They were proud of their technological developments. There seemed to be an unspoken belief among the Japanese at the time that the solution to the world's problems was in the development and distribution of the emerging technologies. Japan stood in stark contrast to the rest of the Orient, the island was so underpopulated with Christians.

Arrangements had been made for the Billy Graham crusade in the Budokan, an arena in Japan. One morning I was speaking before the

Suddenly Silenced

congregated 3,000 ministers, missionaries and Christian workers. I recall that Billy Graham called and informed me that I was to be sent on an errand—I was to speak in the town hall in Sapporo, in Northern Japan. The evening crusade meetings in the Budokan were relayed nightly to Sapporo, Hokkaido. The weather gets cold up there. It's like parts of Canada. Little known in the Western world, this region enjoyed some notoriety as the world turned its eyes to Sapporo, Hakkaido, for the 1997 winter Olympics.

I often reflect on one particularly outstanding account of Christian dedication that was relayed to me by an American missionary named Richard Goodall. Goodall recounted, "When I got out at the airport in Sappora, I was met by Mr. and Mrs. Mitsuhashi." Mr. Mitsuhashi, spastic in his limbs, was riding on his wife's back and looking happily over her shoulder. As they greeted me, I tried not to stare, but I was astonished at this arrangement. Astonished, not just at the piggybacking, but by the beaming and infectious smiles which lit up the faces of Mr. and Mrs. Mitsuhashi, like the flashes of the nearby airport beacon.

When I had a moment to be alone with Richard Goodall, I was curious to know the story behind this amazing couple. He told me that Mrs. Mitsuhashi came from a well-to-do Buddhist home. She was a professional nurse. She had worked in a hospital where a dying Christian missionary led the young nurse to Christ. When she told her parents, they disinherited her. But she was so full of the love of Christ that she resolved to spend all day, every day, going from house to house telling people about Jesus Christ. This woman was famished from lack of food, but she was full of Jesus Christ. Some days she subsisted on as little as three apples yet witnessed all day long about her love of her Lord Jesus.

She met her husband one day when she went to a Christian gathering in a home. There was a testimony meeting. Then came a time for prayer requests. A small invalid man of great grace and zeal asked for prayer, "not for healing, but for a wife." During the prayer, the nurse sat down beside him. Not long after that they were married!

Taking me to their dilapidated car, they drove me to the meeting. A chain of miracles had made it possible for the town hall relays to be held. They left no stone unturned. Mr. and Mrs. Mitsuhashi went from house to house all day, him on her back, and they'd witness door to

International Evangelism

door. As you may know, the Japanese people do not readily invite into their homes strangers who simply arrive on their doorsteps and knock. But who could say no to a wife carrying her invalid husband on her back, both with faces lit up like Tokyo neons? One thing that Mr. and Mrs. Mitsuhashi found out again and again was that as they went from house to house, they seldom had a door closed to them. This is how these magnificent people led scores of people to Christ.

A new year, 1968, was ushered in. On March 31, we flew to Brisbane, Australia, to hold a crusade until April 6. I preached five days to Billy's three days. We preached in a cricket field. As it turned out, this was my link to my long awaited opportunity to preach with Billy Graham.

On the first Sunday afternoon I preached to a crowd of 15,000. On the Friday night Billy preached to 48,000. Then, on the second Sunday and last day of our crusade, Billy preached before 60,000 spirited Australians. We had successfully reached Australia with the gospel!

One of the decisions made in Australia was rendered by Bob Davies, from Brisbane. This is of personal significance to me, as Bob later immigrated to Toronto to join Richmond College as its controller. Half a world away, and a new job for Bob! I was hired as the college's chancellor.

Then I journeyed to Brisbane and on to Sydney, Australia, to be with Billy Graham and his team. While I was with the eminent archbishop at his cathedral in Sydney, Australia, Kathleen was shoe shopping in Toronto. Kathleen likes to buy my shoes. She's chic—very stylish. She buys me French shoes, the ones with the high heels. I agreed to wear a pair of these shoes while I was preaching at a high Anglican cathedral in Sydney. This beautiful and historic cathedral displayed ornate stained glass windows that depicted the saints winging their way through heaven. And the cathedral was exquisite. It was elaborate to the minutest detail.

Twenty of the world's nations were represented in the pews as I preached. I was delivering a particularly articulate sermon. I was clad in the finest of robes, and I was in the finest of forms. I was elevated, high in the pulpit. I felt that I could almost reach out and touch the hand of God. There *are* such moments as a preacher, you know.

I finished preaching and left the pulpit, pacing each step of my descent. The exhilaration of pomposity had come upon me. As the audience applauded, every eye was trained on me. It was my grandiose moment.

All at once, I stumbled down the finely carpeted stairs. My finely polished French high-heeled shoe was caught in the carpet. For one desperate second I wrestled with it, my ankle twisting and pulling. Then I tripped and flopped on my face, tumbling down the stairs.

At the bottom of steps, I struggled to haul myself up on my feet. My face flushed, I was disgraced. In a trance-like state I thought that I could look through another kind of hole—a hole in the earth that led straight home to Toronto. I could still hear the gasps of the great congregation. Then in a moment of silence a little dark-haired altar boy walked over to me. His tiny hands gently reached down to help me up from the marble floor. I was almost dizzy.

I began hobbling down the aisle. As I squinted through straining eyes, the aisle looked so long that it seemed like the world's longest street that ran past the entire population of the world and on into eternity. The enormous cathedral was in a hush. Red faced, I began shaking hands. I thought, *If could just lose myself in the shaking of hands.*

Seemingly out of nowhere, a spunky Irish canon accosted me, proclaiming, "Dr. White, this great cathedral is in the business of saving souls." I glanced down as he held out his hand to me. He spouted, "This is your heel!"

In 1979, I spent twenty-two days of glorious crusading with the team. I was becoming prolific at writing illustrations for Billy. The Australian newspapers would publish the topics of Billy's sermon, and I would regularly spend nights with the light on, researching and creating suitable illustrations for Billy's message the next night. Early in the morning I would creep quietly to Billy's room and slip the illustration under his door. I would then go back to bed and sleep until the late afternoon, when I would go to the crusade site to join the team.

The next time that I saw Australia was in March and April 1996, just prior to my stroke. I had been with the father, Billy Graham; now I accompanied the son, Franklin Graham, on his first international festival in four cities: Sydney, Cairns, Townsville and Brisbane.

Flashback to March 1968: I made my way to South Africa to spend three weeks visiting the missionary fields. I averaged an exhausting one country per day. I moved from Prestoria to Bloomforteim to Capetown,

International Evangelism

then from Lesotino to Durban to Swaziland. Then I crisscrossed the country to Mozambique to Tanzania to Zimbabwe. In Zimbabwe I saw the world's tallest waterfalls—what a magnificent sight they were! Then on to Angola to Zaire to Cameroon to Gabon I went. And into the country of Nigeria's capital, Lagos, I ventured. Then I went to Benin to Toga to Ghana and on to the Ivory Coast. Then pushing on to Liberia I met with missionaries from Moody Bible Institute. I was in beautiful Sierra Leone before departing to Guinea to Senegal to Mauritania, then to Algeria to Morocco, then to the Canary Islands, and finally back to New York.

In 1969, we left one of the coldest days and most severe blizzards in Toronto that I could remember. When we landed in Melbourne, Australia, it was a scorching 110 degrees Fahrenheit. It was blazing hot! We held a month long Billy Graham crusade in the large Music Bowl amphitheater. I was thrilled to be writing Billy Graham's illustrations. Then, I held a crusade in Canberra, Australia's capital.

After I finished preaching on the last Sunday morning, I flew to Sydney, then on to Mauritius in the South Pacific. Then I flew to Madagascar, the poorest country in the world, and finally I made my way to Johannesburg. Here I preached a Sunday evening service. How could I do all this in one day? Well, the time zones allowed me to do it. We crossed enough time zones to save us eight hours in one day. This was a personal record.

In Pinetown, South Africa, I held a Billy Graham crusade (March 24 to 31). For the crusade Pinetown's churches united under the supervision of the Church of England, which was headed up by Bishop John Stephens. This crusade was so well attended that we had to use a neighboring facility for the overflow. The Holy Spirit was really at work!

Apartheid was at its worst thirty years ago when I was in Durban, South Africa. Deep into the South African countryside Bishop Stephens and I drove in a jeep along the bumpy surface of the sun-cracked and parched roads. The Zulus lived here, in their mud huts.

Apartheid was dismal. The Zulus were living in squalor in the stinking heat. They worked in crowded gangs teetering on steep hills and often in gold and diamond mines fourteen hours a day. Men, women and children slaved out the miserable days of their lives.

Suddenly Silenced

I recall Bishop John Stephens and I visiting one of the large families. There were a dozen clinging children in their one-room mud hut. The sight of their fractured little existence brought immediate tears to my eyes. These hardworking black people had cavernous lines etched in their faces. Their hands were gnarled and scraped. The men sometimes had one arm that was longer than the other from pulling in the mines. The faces of the men, in fact their entire bodies, were covered in blisters and sometimes open sores. Many of them hobbled around in pain, battered and bruised.

The mines in which they toiled day after endless day were little more than cylindrical shafts burrowed thousands of feet into the earth. Men crawled through the dank and dark underground world virtually blind. Archaic equipment meant that artificial light was undependable at best, and these men had to find ways to make the most out of the few devices they had. Their hours were spent clawing at black walls, attempting to expose the coveted metal of materialism, the lust of fat cats—gold—and for the dearest friend of affluent girls—diamonds.

Bishop Stephens and I presented a little homily before the family with twelve children. We offered the most powerful Bible verse we knew—John 3:16. Then heaven itself sprung open in a symphony of sound; it was the downtrodden black Zulu family breaking into a five-verse version of "Jesus Loves Me, This I Know."

For minutes the bishop and I stood riveted as the sound of these simple and loving souls singing ushered musical rivulets of love into their foul little hut . The love of Jesus flooded the place, and we were all drowning in the Spirit. *Humbled* is an entirely inadequate word, but it's the best I've got to describe how we felt. I was almost envious, embarrassed even, at the great passion these Zulus displayed for their Savior.

When the simple child's Sunday school song ended, the bishop and I were both exhausted and elated. Jesus' Spirit of love filled the teeny-tiny little mud hut!

Following this campaign we ventured across land to Johannesburg, then on to Kenya, Nairobi, to Ethiopia and through the Sudan to Cairo, Egypt. Then we jetted to London and civilization.

I was tired after my sojourn around half the world. It felt like years since I'd seen my family. Through bleary eyes, I squinted out of the jet's

International Evangelism

window as I headed for home. I returned to my home in Toronto, where I had the opportunity to spend time with my family, who'd had to spend most of the winter without me. It was precious to reunite with Kathleen and the boys. Soon we would share a dip in the pool!

An evangelist's itinerary is often demanding and disruptive to his or her personal life. Off I went again, this time to South Korea. Five a.m. came early each morning when in 1973 the believers in Christ gathered in the churches of South Korea to pray. From May 18 to 24 we held a remarkable crusade in Taegu, Korea. An astonishing and enthusiastic 40,000 attended these meetings. This spirited crusade culminated on the Saturday afternoon when 35,000 gathered to hear the Word of God, according to the August 1973 issue of *Decision*. Then on Sunday afternoon we traveled to Suwon, Korea, where another 35,000 people were in attendance. Wednesday to Sunday the Billy Graham team drew historic numbers of people. One Sunday afternoon at the Billy Graham team meeting after the crusade, a head count was taken. The count revealed that 1,100,000 people had come to our crusade. On *The Tonight Show*, Johnnie Carson had Billy Graham as a guest. Johnnie announced that this Korean crusade had made history.

In 1974 I preached at twelve of my own crusades. That spring at Baguio on the northern Philippine island of Luzon, hundreds of decisions were made for Jesus Christ. This is where we met Olga Brady. Olga came from an elitist family—well-to-do and well known. Her husband, the owner of a German gold mine, suddenly died, and she fell into a melancholic trance. Olga and her husband had been swingers, enchanted by the glittering allure of the nightlife, and now she felt completely empty. She withdrew, and as it is suggested in the Frank Sinatra song, she wanted to just "curl up and die."

One day she was invited to attend a gospel meeting at the Baguio high school gymnasium. She saw it as a means of escaping her deep depression, where suicide loomed. That evening Tom Bledsoe's singing was brilliantly inspirational. High in the gym's balcony, Olga heard a knock on her heart's door. It was Jesus. She was profoundly moved, and her heart responded. The light was switched back on. Her depression lifted, and her soul flew. She returned to the gospel meetings with her doctor, who was likewise saved, and Olga began lighting up the whole spiritual sky with her testimony, revealing the power of the Risen Christ.

Suddenly Silenced

Moving on from Baguio we took our crusade to a soccer stadium in the then capital city of the Philippines, Quezon City. The stadium had been erected very near the world's largest prison. I think that the closest I've ever been to heaven and, ironically enough, hell was during this visit.

Another Olga, Olga Robertson, was an Arab woman who had been disenfranchised by her wealthy upper-class parents when she married an American by the name of Robertson at Clark Air Force Base, during World War II. Olga had been in a full pregnancy with twins when Robertson suddenly departed for home, the United States. Olga never set her embittered eyes on him again. It was a cold, forsaken feeling that she packed with her when she descended to the Pacific to cast herself and her babies into the unforgiving tide of the Pacific. En route to the endless waves, she heard music and went into a mission. There in a moment of thunderous transformation, she gave her life to Jesus.

While praying, she felt a call to take Christ into that most ominous prison. Now, thirty years later, she was that prison's beloved chaplain. After our meeting, Olga took me to the electric chair room and to death row. This was an experience that I will never forget. I was shocked to realize that I stood before the scene of execution. A peculiarly dark feeling exudes from a place where men are put to death.

Olga reported that a young man named Billy, who had recently been executed for murdering two people, had prior to his execution been led by Olga to Christ during a last-minute meeting on death row. Before Billy died, he donated both of his eyes to an eye bank. Then he was shaved and hooded, and with the electrodes screwed down tight into his head he sang, *"Yea, though I walk through the valley of the shadow of death, I will fear no evil: for thou art with me"* (Psalm 23:4).

For Billy, death had lost its terror. It was now merely a faint shadow. His final earthly utterances were exultations: "Dear Jesus, I thank You that I am in Your care and that You have prepared a place for me in heaven and I am going to see You face to—"

Before Billy could finish the sentence, he was in heaven. The death switch had been thrown, and several thousand volts of electricity had thrown his body into convulsions. A final death rattle was heard, then—silence.

After the electric chair room, Olga marched me to death row, a

International Evangelism

place where the condemned wait in quiet isolation, reflecting on their misbegotten lives and awaiting the deadly jolt that would shock the breath of life out of the mortal shell. Each condemned man awaited the same fate, some soon, some later on. But each one knew the terror of a certain kind of death at the hands of man.

The numbers of such men were staggering. President Marcos was catching up on a backlog of executions. Olga was parading me through what seemed like a disparaging and demeaning human zoo. There in the misty twilight, sounds of crying and groaning pierced the otherwise eerie silence. Bitterness and hate festered like the open sores that multiplied on the carcasses of the condemned. A low ceiling added a perceptible claustrophobia to those within the tomb that caged the captives. A stench and a ferocious heat—100 degree Fahrenheit—helped to putrefy the atmosphere, and a tremendous humidity made it feel like it was raining when it was not.

The miserable inmates drifted in and out of alpha waves. Every now and again they rose to consciousness at the painful beckoning of stomachs that barked audibly for food. What crumbs were thrown to the men, they pinched from the slimy bacteria-ridden floor and pressed to the inner cheeks of desert-dry mouths. Sometimes skinny fingers would return with a tooth that had escaped bleeding gums. The arid stench of the mingled vomit, urine, perspiration and human excrement was indescribable. Hell is much too kind a description for the conditions in which these outcasts subsisted.

Olga called for the notorious death row "Jesus trio" to step forward. Until Billy's death this talented musical group had been a quartet. She told me afterwards that between them they had murdered perhaps 100 people. Out of that squalid, terrified company stepped Romeo, Gaugenzio and Boyzeo. One had a beaten-up guitar. They opened their dog-eared songbook and sang in such angelic harmony, it was as if they were already in heaven. And they transported me from what felt like upstairs from hell to the ground floor of heaven:

> Come, ye sinners, lost and hopeless,
> Jesus' blood can make you free;
> For He saved the worst among you,
> When He saved a wretch like me.

Suddenly Silenced

And I know, yes, I know
Jesus' blood can make the vilest sinner clean,
And I know, yes, I know
Jesus' blood can make the vilest sinner clean.
(Anna W. Waterman, 1920)

CHAPTER XII

George W. Bush

November 1963 swept in like a hurricane. After what seemed like an eternity I received my doctor of philosophy degree from Oxford University. By graduation day at Oxford the White family had emigrated from Britain to North America. Our son Bill celebrated his tenth birthday in the brave new world on November 22 in Denver. The American president was John Fitzgerald Kennedy.

> John Fitzgerald Kennedy is dead—by assassination.
> Robert Kennedy is dead—by assassination.
> Martin Luther King is dead—by assassination.
> Ernest Hemingway is dead—by suicide.
> Marilyn Monroe is dead—by suicide.
> Jimi Hendrix is dead—by suicide.
> Jim Morrison is dead—by suicide.
> Janis Joplin is dead—by suicide.

A generation is wasted. Then the September 11, 2001, era crashed its way in. One generation passes, leaving the world to carry on. But it was November 22, 1963. It was the day that death stalked the world.

On this chilly November morning in 1963 in Denver I had been delivering the final of a series of lectures to ordination candidates. I was already deeply ensconced at the headquarters of the seminary of the Conservative Baptist denomination in Denver. The particular lecture of the day was entitled "Death, Judgment and Eternity." When it was finished, I left.

Suddenly Silenced

I climbed into our gray car. I leaned forward in my seat, still a little frigid. As I reached for the radio dial, frost nipped my fingertips. When I turned on the radio, a country and western song was playing. I had been listening intently to distract me from the icy onslaught of winter's certain arrival. It was scant seconds before the song was interrupted. The words "The president has been wounded in Dallas" shot from the speakers into my car and into my brain. As fate would have it, I had left a lecture on funerals and death and was about to prepare another.

In a surreal mental fog, I sped blindly through the streets of Denver. I just couldn't seem to accept what I'd heard. If my time calculations were correct, the drive from the lecture hall to our apartment took exactly twenty-seven minutes.

"The president is dead. John Fitzgerald Kennedy is dead" were the next penetrating words that struck me.

My heart nearly stopped. I felt sick. I felt as if I had been punched in the stomach. It was November 22, 1963. Bill's tenth birthday party was over!

Ominously, my close friend and tutor Dr. John Walsh also lost his world-acclaimed colleague. John Walsh had often referred to Clive Staples Lewis as the most brilliant intellectual in the English-speaking world. Lewis' specialization was in literature. The genius Christian scholar C.S. Lewis was dead. It was November 22, 1963. Heaven had taken this saint. This luminous British author, born in Belfast, wrote more than thirty books, including his Christian classic *The Screwtape Letters*. *The Screwtape Letters* is a mantle of literary genius that has been acclaimed throughout the world for its witty account of how men can lose their souls to the devil.

A secular, socially sophisticated and politically arrogant anarchist author also perished that day. Aldous Huxley, the world-renowned atheist, was dead. It was November 22, 1963. Huxley lives on in the minds of the literary world for his classic *Brave New World*. This dark and prophetic work depicts a totalitarian society that disregards individual dignity and worships science and the advancement and age of mechanical takeover.

Kathleen and I ventured to my first Billy Graham team meeting in Miami. Then we boarded a connecting flight to Dallas. In Dallas we witnessed the solemn crowds assembling. Kathleen stood on the very spot where President John F. Kennedy had been shot. We bowed our heads in reverence for the dark catastrophe that had befallen all of us.

In the mid to late 1960s and in the early 1970s, there was Haight Ashbury in San Francisco, Greenwich Village in New York, Yorkville in Toronto and Soho in London. They were supposed to be paradisiacal suburbs, home to the turned-on generation. As *Time* put it in 1968, "The times were out of joint and the young were into joints."

It was the '60s all right; the South American physician Che Guevara was dead. Guevara was the Karl Marx of the twentieth century. He was an icon to the student left. Left-wing baby boomers had his picture pasted on dormitory walls everywhere. The revolutionary 1960s were red hot, and they were upon us. The world was erupting in war. The escalation of the Vietnam confrontation was spearheaded by Lyndon B. Johnson, who believed that this "policing action" could actually be won. He sent 500,000 American youths to battle in the steamy fields of the stinking jungle and often to lose their lives in a conflict for which it seemed there was no easy justification. Young men, usually in their late teens or early twenties, returned to their native soil either in a pine box or quite defective and suffering the long-term effects of Agent Orange.

Americans at home during the Vietnam War rose in protest. The revolutionaries, the Black Panthers, the Freedom Fighters, the "Love In" people and Timothy Leary clenched their fists in anger. Yes, the icon of a million young people, Che Guevara, the bearded, beret-wearing revolutionary, was slain! He championed the left and, like others before him, faced his own special brand of crucifixion. He perished in the sweaty jungle trenches of Latin-speaking South America. The left wing would have to do without him. His life had been all that he had to give.

Emerging from the 1968 Democratic national convention in Chicago were the dynamic and demigod duo of an era, Jerry Rubin and Abbie Hoffman. They fought their ways into that rather vocal, rather defiant subculture of radicals referred to as the "Yippies." These two spokesmen of a remarkably short epoch scratched their names onto the pages of the age by attaching themselves to a group labeled "The Chicago Seven." In the light of hindsight, it needs be mentioned that if Hoffman and Rubin engineered any kind of program for the reconstruction of society after they smashed and grabbed it, they appear to have failed.

Another crowned rebel who rose to a dubious prominence during this period was the LSD prophet and ex Catholic priest named Timothy Leary. Leary claimed unabashedly to be a "christ." But what "christ" is it who condemns so many of his followers to lives of torment and disillusionment? Who exiles his beleaguered pawns to psychiatric hospitals and casts upon the masses the blight of a deepening angst—a continual gut-wrenching hunger for meaning—and living moment to moment, anguishing over whether personal survival would appear anywhere on the radar screen of human possibility?

In the 1960s body-painted and ponytailed youth seemed to get their kicks from, in the words of the Chambers brothers, "pychedelicizing their minds," beating their drums at social protests, and generally knocking the establishment. To be in, you had to be spaced out on drugs, make obscene gestures at the establishment and hate your parents. The road to paradise was to drop out; to hide behind a human hedge of hair down to your waist, front and back if possible; burn your draft card and wardrobe; push into a pair of tight jeans and wear them in perpetuity. Then you'd flop into a commune, spurn marriage, and hitchhike with Timothy Leary!

You were into Beatlemania with the Beatles. You'd roll with the Rolling Stones and applaud Jerry Rubin, who instructed the young to just "Do It." You'd be a groupie with Charlie Manson and groove on Rod McKuen. You'd get caught in a coffin before you'd salute a flag and cast a vote for free enterprise over Che Guevara, Mai Tse Tung, Fidel Castro or Ho Chi Mingh. It was all part of the scene.

At the end of April 1968 I flew to Ashland, Oregon, for one of my own crusades. Jerry Fabiano was an instigator of the nefarious and notorious San Francisco State College campus riots. That contagion spread around the world. I ran into some of the activists of this movement as far away as Australia. In Ashland, Oregon, there was a hippie colony lurking in the mountains nearby. Jerry Fabiano came up from California expressly to get them to join the Herbert Marcuse revolution. But our crusade was in the wind. As a propagandist, he thought he'd invest a night off in seeing how "the Billy Graham people do it."

So Sunday evening there he was, a way up in the farthest bleacher of the big gym. The last thing he expected that night as he crouched with his cronies behind beads and beards was that Jesus Christ would single him out and call him, so distinctly and unmistakably that only an act of human defiance could cause him to say no to the voice of the Savior. Jerry Fabiano testified to me that "halfway through your talk, I knew Jesus was calling me. For years I had been looking for a genuine Messiah to follow and a really exciting crusade into which I could fling myself. This was Christ the Messiah. This was the Kingdom in which I could work." At the invitation, Jerry gave his life to Jesus. The "street vibes" were for Jerry's troops, who had occupied that city.

In 1969, Jerry had been one of the leaders of the "Jesus People" movement and had been crusading throughout the West. I was also crusading in the West, and in August we were in Rapid City, South Dakota. Seven hundred made decisions in Rapid City. Charles Spurgeon's prodigal great-grandson from the West was one of them. This youth was brilliant but in the 1960s had lapsed into a sinful lifestyle. Hippiedom had led him away from Christ. But Christ made it right, and this fallen son was returned to the fold in Rapid City!

The 1960s bore the stamp of another genius artist, poet, and musician. Bob Dylan, the Jewish folk hero and street caller of a generation, lyrically annihilated society by placing a magnifying glass over its materialistic hypocrisy, as showcased in his famous song "Like a Rolling Stone." Flash ahead now to September and October 1975 in Hibbing, Minnesota, where our John Wesley White team held a crusade in an inner city auditorium. Flash ahead again. It's another twenty years later, in July 1995, and I hold a Promise Keeper's rally in the Minneapolis Metrodome before 61,000 men. Then in August of that same year, we held a Promise Keeper's rally in Hibbing, where 12 percent of the men in attendance made decisions for Christ.

Hibbing was a grimy blue-collar mining town just about seventy-five miles due west of Duluth. The area was populated with muscle-bound ironworkers. This was the town where the world famous Bob Dylan was raised. Bob's uncle Jack Zimmerman owned a radio station in Hibbing. It was Jack who bought Bob his first guitar. I was invited to be interviewed by Jack for three minutes on his morning program. To my surprise the interview continued for an hour. The subjects of our on-air and very public conversation were his nephew Bob Dylan and Jesus Christ.

Suddenly Silenced

Jack Zimmerman was intently interested in Jesus the Christ. He talked to me about our crusade. I informed him without hesitation that our crusade was interdenominational. To this Jack declared that he was devoutly Jewish. However true his statement was, it was also undeniably true that the spotlight found him perched nightly at the back of our crusade. Jack was not converted, yet he certainly began thinking about the Messiah, Jesus Christ.

Flash back now to our Concord, California, crusade in August 1976. We had encountered the "Jesus People." The Vineyard movement was charismatic, and to our delight it seemed much of the movement attended our crusade. It felt like a full-scale revival! We gazed across the sea of bodies and witnessed the waving of a sea of hands and heard the thunderous drone of voices, uniformly testifying their love of Jesus. We smiled.

In 1976 Bob Dylan was engulfed by the Jesus People. From a spiritual perspective it can be said that the most relevant Dylan is the Dylan of the late '70s. This greatest minstrel and balladeer of a generation experienced an protracted period of steadily increasing interest in Jesus as the Messiah and Savior. Then, strikingly, the heavenly angels sang, and Bob Dylan was born again.

The September 17, 2001, issue of *Time* was quoted as saying about the 1970s and Dylan, "He devoted the decade to touring and becoming a born-again Christian." His most notable Christian songs are "It's Alright," "Knocking on Heaven's Door," "You've Got to Serve Somebody," "Slow Train Coming," "Pressing On," and "Saved." *Saved* was his all-out Christian album. "There is his painting, his apparent continuing devotion to Christianity and his farm in Minnesota, where he loves to spend time with his family when not performing some 100 shows a year" (*Toronto Sun*, July 2, 2001).

In the 1970s there was a religious tidal wave referred to as the "Jesus People." It spread the Word first across the southwestern United States. Then the "Jesus Freaks" took the name of Jesus elsewhere in the United States and Canada. However, it was really the entire "Jesus Movement" that was transforming the lives of the drug-burned-out hippies in record numbers. The barbershops were back in business.

I preached many times in southern California. There were three hippy pastors whom I remember well. Mike McIntosh hailed from San

George W. Bush

Diego. In 1979, I spoke in Edmonton at the Billy Graham School of Evangelism. Mike decided to travel there to the crusade. This handsome man approached me smiling. He announced that he found my book *Re-entry* truly revolutionary. Later, Mike founded the megachurch Horizon Christian Fellowship. In 1983 I held a five-day crusade in San Diego, where Mike was the chairman. Six hundred people made decisions for Jesus Christ. We thank Mike, who donated $4,000 to our Join the Family Christian television ministry.

Then there was pastor Skip Heitzig of Southern California. He rebelled against the establishment and wore long hair down his back. Skip entered the drug world. He was empty. One day he turned on the TV, tuned in to the Billy Graham crusade and dropped out of hippiedom. In Albuquerque, New Mexico, Skip founded Harvest Christian Fellowship, which today has a member roll of 15,000. We are grateful to Skip for donating $5,000 to our Join the Family television ministry. Today, Skip has been with Franklin's Samaritan's Purse for over three decades.

Pastor Greg Laurie, now also a friend of Franklin's and with Samaritan's Purse for the same period, was a hippy. But he was converted to Jesus Christ while Chuck Smith preached at Calvary Harvest Fellowship Church. Greg founded his Harvest Christian Fellowship in Riverside, California. Recently, *Time* identified Greg's church as the twelfth largest church in the United States. Additionally, Greg has a radio program that airs Christian crusades across the United States.

There were three long-haired hippies who hailed from Willowdale, Ontario. Each in his own time, within a six-month period and a three-mile radius of each other, was born again. They were our son Paul, my facilitator Stephen Trelford and Benny Hinn. Three boys became men of God.

In 1969 one Sunday night 9,000 people attended our crusade in Sioux Falls, South Dakota. A record breaking 2,053 decisions were made. Then in rushed the 1970s like an evil tsunami. Our boys had fallen under the spell of the flower power era.

In the terrible wake of the hippie tide, Kathleen and I made the decision to lease out our house for a year and take the boys to St. Petersburg, Florida. We moved into a house across the street from a bishop. On Halloween, just two months after we had arrived, the bishop's wife told Kathleen that our house was haunted. We tried to settle there anyway. However, every time the floor boards creaked, the rafters shifted or the wind blew, we were sure that a certain Casper was lurking somewhere just out of sight, but never out of mind.

Kathleen became depressed. She sank into a funk. The boys continued to rabble-rouse, and I was fit to be tied. We were in the pit. After only half a year we returned to Toronto. For the remaining six months that our home was leased we rented a house in Don Mills, a few miles from our home. From the heights of spiritual ecstasy in South Dakota to the decent into the maelstrom we rode the roller-coaster peaks and valleys. My crusades, once large, had shrunk to small meetings. Bill and Stephen Trelford fled, thumbing across country in the summertime. They didn't stop until they saw the majestic Atlantic Ocean swelling before them.

In August 1971 Wesley, Paul and I traveled in our old worn-out Cadillac to Canon City, Colorado, where I would preach in a stadium. Of the three hippies from Willowdale, our third son, Paul, was the first to undergo conversion to Jesus Christ. On a Wednesday at my invitation Paul came forward to receive the Savior. Wesley, however, remained in his seat-unconverted. This caused me mixed emotions. My concerns over Wesley would be relieved, however. He came to be converted in the spring of 1974 when he read Charles Colson's *Born Again* about his conversion to Jesus Christ. Wesley got down on his knees beside me and asked the merciful Lord to save him.

In Canon City, my antiquated Cadillac had broken down. So, I replaced it with an antiquated Chevrolet Corvair. It was a compact car with the engine in the trunk.

One thousand miles due north of Canon City, Briercrest High School in Saskatchewan enrolled Paul. Interestingly, Paul's hockey coach, a former player for the Boston Bruins, had been born again. So Paul had been schooled in hockey and in the Lord. He had been the top scorer in the All-England hockey league. Prior to meeting Jesus, Paul had been an average student and hockey player, but once converted he excelled in hockey and his studies.

In June 1972, Paul traveled with me to the Dallas Expo, where Billy Graham addressed 80,000 youths. This was a "second blessing" for Paul. Paul fasted and prayed. Kathleen, who always saw the benefits of eating a good meal, was worried sick. That September, Paul entered Richmond College. Then in the summertime he made up his grade 12. Two years later at the age of eighteen Paul received his BA from Richmond College. From there he went on to the University of Toronto, where he received his honors BA.

Paul drifted into "the Catacombs." Pastor Merv and Merla Watson were the shepherds who presided over the Christian celebrants at the Catacombs. This was not a typical church but an exuberant throng of Christians that joined together every Thursday night in St. Paul's Cathedral, an Anglican church in downtown Toronto. During these very days Stephen Trelford and Benny Hinn spent time at the Catacombs. Merla was an accomplished guitarist who wrote captivating Christian songs. One such song was "My Provider, His Grace Is Sufficient for Me." They sang this song repeatedly.

Paul spent two years at the Catacombs, absorbing the spiritual atmosphere of Jesus Christ. Then he formed a trio to perform on *100 Huntley Street*. On that very Huntley Street program the former heavyweight-boxing champion of the world George Foreman gave his testimony.

Paul wished to complete his education, so he enrolled at the University of Waterloo, where he attained his master's degree in history. Then he traveled to Bristol University in England, where he was the leading goal scorer on the team. Soon after receiving his PhD in Calvinism and Shakespearean literature, Paul began his teaching career at Wheaton College. After only one semester he moved to Waco, Texas. At Baylor University he was a professor of English. Then he made his move to Purdue University in West Lafayette, Indiana, where he and his wife are both professors.

My facilitator, Stephen Trelford, and our son Bill began their friendship in the '60s and for forty years have maintained a close association. Stephen Trelford, too, is born again. Stephen, who was raised in North York (Willowdale), was born of two upper-class parents. His mother, Margaret Findley, was raised in Rosedale, across the street from her first cousin Timothy Findley, who died in France on June 21, 2002, of complications arising from hip surgery. Timothy Findley is recognized as one of Canada's foremost secular authors.

Interestingly, the main character of his Governor-General's-Award-winning book *The Wars* was based on Stephen's grandfather, Thomas

Suddenly Silenced

Irving Fredrick Findley, who was a decorated pilot, a war hero shot down during a European mission. Young Timothy, also a TIFF, would hide beside and under Thomas' bed in Toronto while his favorite uncle shared personal letters that he had written to Stephen's grandmother from the fighting front in Europe. The content of these letters served as the basis for *The Wars* and other best-selling novels. She was also related by marriage to Oswald J. Smith. Stephen's mother would talk to him about the early days at Peoples Church on Bloor Street. Sadly, Stephen's mother died when he was young.

Stephen's father, Edward Lee Trelford, was raised in the distinguished Forest Hill area of Toronto and attended the prestigious Upper Canada College preparatory school. In the 1960s Edward Trelford formed a company with Bill Templeton, the brother of Charles Templeton, Billy Graham's partner during the 1940s. Edward in 1971 was commissioned by the government of Ontario to build the prototype for the worldwide Imax movie system for their groundbreaking entertainment complex, Ontario Place. Edward Trelford engineered and constructed what was at the time the world's largest movie screen.

Stephen's father was strict and ruled the house with an authoritarian fervor. The freedom-seeking Stephen called Bill. The two long-haired boys met in Stephen's upstairs room and made a pact to hitchhike east across the country. Although they had just fifteen dollars between them, they would not stop traveling until they set foot on the Atlantic shores. They made it! When they returned from the East Coast they described cold, wet nights cramped up in ditches, under highway overpasses and in sopping fields. Yes, Stephen and Bill remain friends to this day.

In Toronto again and having seen just enough to be disillusioned with the ways of world, in September 1971 Stephen went with a close friend to a small Christian meeting at The House of Emmaus in downtown Toronto. He had been torn apart due to split between his father and him. But Stephen's wrestling went deeper than that. He was obsessed with perplexing questions surrounding the existence of God and the possible relevance of Jesus Christ. He describes his life as living in a continual state of existential angst.

But when Stephen opened the door to a small internal room in The House of Emmaus he saw something very unusual. About a dozen people sat around an enormous bowl of warm water on the floor. A "Jesus Freak" woman with partially braided hair to her waist invited Stephen and his friend to join them by taking off their shoes and socks to take part in the foot-washing ceremony. As a ruminating Stephen removed his socks and sat down he heard the woman explain, "If washing feet is good enough for Jesus Christ, then it's good enough for me." As Stephen's feet and the feet of those around the bowl were being washed, a few men stood behind the ceremony. They were speaking in something that sounded like a language. For the most part their arms were lifted up, and they appeared to be gazing straight into heaven. Stephen's mind raced. He was confused, but he was keenly aware of something else in that room, something so beautiful that he felt that he wanted to draw near to it.

Then the historic moment for my facilitator came. Stephen put on his socks and shoes and stood up and raised his head a little. He looked up. An urge came over him, and in a moment of complete surrender he asked his crucial question: "Jesus, if You are real, please let me know it." Within a moment too short to describe, the Holy Spirit of Jesus Christ entered him and swept him clean. Stephen describes this experience as a brilliant beam of light that scanned through him. He was cleansed of all his former doubts, fears and questions. Stephen knew that God the Father and His Son Jesus Christ were real.

All things had become new for Stephen. *"There appeared unto them cloven tongues like as of fire, and it sat upon each of them. And they were all filled with the Holy Ghost, and began to speak with other tongues, as the Spirit gave them utterance"* (Acts 2:3–4). This is the moment when Stephen Trelford began his spiritual life. He walked out through the front door of The House of Emmaus, and he remembers thinking, *Everything is different now. I am a believer. Jesus is Lord. But, what do I do now?* Stephen was born again. He was joyous beyond measure, for he knew that he was saved.

As the immediate days passed, Stephen sought the Lord's guidance concerning what to do about being a Christian and about what had really happened to him. He needed a context with which to think about his new life. Stephen knew that he had to study the works of the great Christian writers.

So, upon returning to school, the light of Christ and the lamp of learning was all the motivation Stephen needed. He accomplished straight A's in his first semester at Seneca College. He was at the top of his class. The next semester Stephen achieved straight A's again, except for in mathematics. So Stephen submitted his transcript to prospective universities.

The first university to respond to him was Bishop's University. This was an elite private Anglican school headed by professors from Oxford University who wished to preserve English style scholasticism in Quebec. The prestigious Bishop's University was located on the outskirts of Montreal. Stephen was delighted, not only to be accepted to the same university that his Anglican clergyman cousin John Whittall had attended a decade earlier, but also that he was awarded two monetary scholarships. One was to cover the costs of tuition and books; the other was to cover the cost of living in residence.

With the Spirit of Christ living in his heart and in his mind, Stephen excelled in his first year. He was elected the student representative for the Department of Religion. He earned monetary prizes for high academic standing. Additionally, Stephen received special academic consideration and was offered the opportunity to undertake research projects within the Department of Religion as substitutes for course credits. After two years Stephen emerged with his thesis, "The Atoning Significance of the Death of Jesus Christ." He attended the Graduate School of Education following his honors BA.

Following Bishop's, Stephen was hired to teach English at Seneca College. Since then Stephen has taught a variety of English and communication courses at Seneca.

For the past ten years Stephen and I have enjoyed a rich friendship. We have worked in close association on television and radio scripts, on speeches, on our monthly "Letter to Franklin Graham" and countless other letters and "White Papers." Of course we have collaborated on our ten-year project, my autobiography. Stephen has been invaluable to me as my right-hand man.

Yes, the third of the three hippies was Benny Hinn. In his autobiography *Good Morning, Holy Spirit*, Benny explained, "My father was the [associate] mayor of Jaffa during my childhood. He was a strong man, about 6'2, 250 pounds, and a natural leader. He was strong in every way—physically, mentally, and in will." Costandi Hinn, Benny's father, was Greek, like Plato, Luke and Timothy. He was trusted by the

Israelis; hence he could become the associate mayor of Jaffa. Benny's mother, Clemence Hinn, was Armenian.

Benny is only five foot seven inches and approximately 155 pounds. He was born on December 3, 1952, in Israel. That same year Franklin Graham had been born in July. Later, Franklin would be born again in Israel. Benny was one of a family of six boys and two girls. Of the six boys, Benny is the eldest. In Jerusalem, Benny and his family attended the Greek Orthodox Church before emigrating to Toronto in July 1968.

From Benny's book *Good Morning, Holy Spirit* we read, "Life changed rapidly for me...I went to a public high school—Georges Vanier Secondary School." Our sons Bill and Wesley and their cousins Linda, Beverley, and Doug McVety and my niece Sheryl White attended the same school.

As a senior in high school in February 1972 Benny Hinn underwent the Baptism of the Holy Spirit.

> As I sat there... a small group of students walked over to my table. I recognized them immediately. They were the ones who had been pestering me with all of this "Jesus" talk.
> They asked me to join in their morning-prayer meeting. The room was just off the library. I thought, "Well, I'll get them off my back. One little prayer meeting isn't going to hurt me." I said, "All right," and they walked with me into the room. It was a small group, just twelve or fifteen kids. And my chair was right in the middle.
> All of a sudden the entire group lifted their hands and began to pray in some funny foreign language. I didn't even close my eyes. I could hardly blink. Here were students, seventeen, eighteen, nineteen years old—kids I had known in class—praising God with unintelligible sounds.
> I had never heard of speaking in tongues, and I was dumbfounded. To think that here was Benny, in a public school, on public property, sitting in the middle of a bunch of babbling fanatics. It was almost more than I could comprehend. I didn't pray. I just watched.
> What happened next was more than I could ever have imag-

ined. I was startled by a sudden urge to pray. But I really didn't know what to say... I had never been taught the "sinner's prayer"—not in all of my religion classes. All I could remember of my encounters with the "Jesus people" was the phrase, "You've got to meet Jesus." Those words seemed out of place to me because I thought I knew Him.

It was an awkward moment. No one was praying with me or even for me. Yet I was surrounded by the most intense spiritual atmosphere I had ever felt. Was I a sinner? I didn't think so. I was just a good little [Greek Orthodox] Catholic boy, who prayed every night and confessed sin whether I needed to or not. But at that moment I closed my eyes and said four words that changed my life forever. Right out loud I said, "Lord, Jesus, come back."...Did I think He had left my house or departed from my life? I really did not know...a feeling came over me...It went right through me. What I really felt, though, was that this surge of power was cleansing me—instantly, from the inside out. I felt absolutely clean, immaculate, and pure.

Suddenly I saw Jesus with my own eyes. It happened in a moment of time. There He was. Jesus.

Benny could never forget the day that he brought Jesus home. He reflected:

I walked into my bedroom, and, as if magnetized, I was drawn to that big black Bible. It was the only Bible in our home. Mom and Dad didn't even have one. I had no idea where it came from, but it had been mine as long as I could remember.

The pages had hardly been turned since our arrival in Canada, but now I prayed, "Lord, You've got to show me what has happened to me today." I opened the Scripture and began to devour it like a starving man who has just been given a loaf of bread. The Holy Spirit became my teacher. I didn't know it at the time...the kids at the prayer meeting didn't say, "Now here's what the Bible says." They didn't tell me anything. In fact, they had no idea what had transpired during the past twenty-four hours.

Benny couldn't keep something of this importance from his mother. When he told her that he had been saved, she glared at him with a deep and questioning look and quipped, "Saved from what?"

His father slapped him in the face. Benny felt the pain. He had hurt the family. His father hated his eldest son's new faith and threatened to kick him out of the house.

His father had Benny see a psychiatrist. The psychiatrist reported that he was just going through something and that he'd return to normal.

Perhaps Benny's father had always envisioned an ambitious future for his son, which included enrolment in Osgoode Hall at the University of Toronto and a hope that Benny would one day enter the prestigious world of politics. His father became angry when Benny made his decision to preach. His father remained angry for a long time.

Benny's brothers persecuted him relentlessly, until he cried, "Lord, will it ever end? Will they ever come to know You?" For two entire years Benny's five brothers hated him for his conversion to Jesus Christ. Likewise, *"[Joseph's ten] brothers...hated him and could not speak peaceably to him"* (Genesis 37:4). It was hell for Benny Hinn.

However, there is explanation in the words of Jesus to His disciples. *"If anyone comes to Me and does not hate his father and mother, wife and children, brothers and sisters, yes, and his own life also, he cannot be My disciple. And whoever does not bear his cross and come after Me cannot be My disciple"* (Luke 14:26–27). Ten of Jesus' disciples were martyred.

After a while there was nobody in his family that Benny could talk to. He was alone with Jesus. The family situation was so inflammatory that Benny's elderly grandmother made a special trip from Israel. She told Benny that he was crazy and an embarrassment to the family name. Benny Hinn was truly ostracized from his family.

Benny Hinn admits to having felt quite the intruder when he agreed to join the prayer meeting at George S. Vanier Secondary School, but at the Catacombs he felt that he belonged. So had Paul and Stephen. The Catacombs was a community of teaching and worshipping. This house of worship was perhaps the pre-eminent place in Toronto for believers to come to join the flock in fellowship.

Benny had emigrated from Israel to Canada in July 1968. And it was thirty-four months and three days before Christmas 1973 when

Suddenly Silenced

Benny Hinn underwent the second blessing at a Kathryn Kuhlman meeting in Pittsburgh.

It was abundantly clear that Christ was channeling through Kathryn Kuhlman to perform His miracles. Many would come to the platform with broken appendages, suffering the loss of one sense or another, or with the affliction of myriad maladies, and they would depart the platform—healed!

Luke recorded,

> *Through the hands of the apostles many signs and wonders were done among the people. And they were all with one accord in Solomon's Porch. Yet none of the rest dared join them, but the people esteemed them highly. And, believers were increasingly added to the Lord, multitudes of both men and women, so that they brought the sick out into the streets and laid them on beds and couches, that at least the shadow of Peter passing by might fall on some of them* (Acts 5:12–15).

As I preached one Sunday morning at a little mission in Mason City, Iowa, in the '70s, my son Wes was with us. This little mission was where Kathryn Kuhlman spent much of her time in her twenties. She was alone, lost in an existential search for meaning in her life. Then Jesus Christ told her what to do. Throughout her life she had lived in Pittsburgh and had received the anointing of the Holy Spirit and the gift of healing. Over her distinguished career Kathryn Kuhlman spoke before many thousands of people. Her fame traveled swiftly through the Christian underground and into households throughout North America. Kathryn Kuhlman left a legacy of saved souls and healed bodies. She was a miracle—and a mystery!

Yes, in the early '70s following his experiences in the Catacombs, Benny Hinn caught the spiritual fire at a Kathryn Kuhlman meeting at First Presbyterian Church, which featured Jimmy McDonald, the world-renowned black tenor. In the 1960s he toured with Billy Graham, bringing countless souls to Christ with his voice.

Benny bussed with a delegation of believers from Toronto to see Kathryn Kuhlman and Jimmy McDonald. Benny had always spoken with a stutter, but following the Kathryn Kuhlman meeting, astoundingly, he began speaking without an affected tongue from the platform.

George W. Bush

In Toronto he preached under the anointing of the Holy Spirit, and he was as clear as a bell.

In *Good Morning, Holy Spirit* Benny wrote,

> In the *Toronto Star* in April 1975, a newspaper ad with my picture in it appeared. I was preaching at a little pentecostal church on the west side of town, and the pastor wanted to attract some visitors. It worked, Costandi and Clemence [Hinn] saw the ad. I was sitting on the platform that Sunday night. During the song service I looked up and could hardly believe my eyes. There were my mother and my father being ushered to a seat just a few rows in front of the platform. I thought, "This is it. I'm going to die." My good friend [Reverend] Jim Poynter [a Free Methodist] was seated on the platform next to me. I turned to him and said, "Pray, Jim! Pray!" He was shocked when I told him Mother and Dad were there...As I began to preach, the power of God's presence began to flow through me, but I couldn't bring myself to look in the direction of my parents not even for a fleeting glance. All I knew was that my concern about stuttering was needless. When God healed me, the healing was permanent.
>
> Toward the end of the service I began praying for those who needed a healing. Oh, the power of God filled that place. As the meeting was ending, my parents got up and walked out the back door.

Benny was a burgeoning preacher on the brink of a spiritual explosion. He was aflame in the Spirit. A generation earlier a dashing spectacle was Dr. Robert Lee of the First Baptist Church in Memphis. He wore an eye-catching white suit. After witnessing Dr. Lee at work I became a member of that esteemed church and have remained so for the past fifty-five years. A generation later the flamboyant Benny Hinn, dressed in a white linen suit, presented a similarly striking spectacle on the stage of the Lord. *"While they looked steadfastly toward heaven as He went up, behold, two men stood by them in white apparel"* (Acts 1:10).

Prior to becoming world famous, Benny would hold huge "preaching and healing" rallies in "Hogs Hollow" on Yonge Street in Toronto.

Suddenly Silenced

It was here that he began making a name for himself as the word of his ministry spread like a spiritual tornado.

Kathleen's family visited our home to watch *Agape*, at that time the second most widely watched religious television program on Canadian television. Benny Hinn counseled my preaching. Then came that historic meeting in 1977 when Benny and I walked and talked and prayed together at the Jesus People meeting in Brantford, Ontario, that saw 10,000 young people sprawling on lawns and on the hill. Brian Kempster coordinated this rally. A lawyer, Brian incorporated our Join the Family Christian Ministries. In 2007, Dr. Rondo Thomas became the chairman.

On the Canadian scene, John George Diefenbaker, a staunch Conservative, held the prime minister's office from 1957 to 1963. In 1963 John Diefenbaker's prime ministerial duties were dead. It was the end of an era. John F. Kennedy was dead.

John George Diefenbaker's father hailed from Neustadt, Ontario. This hamlet was close to my father's birthplace. When John Diefenbaker was young, his family moved to the Saskatchewan prairies, like my father's family did. Diefenbaker was influenced by the Bible-preaching churches of the Prairies. His parents sent him to Saskatoon to acquire a solid university education from the University of Saskatchewan. John became a defense lawyer who gained renown for his spellbinding oratory skill. He championed individual rights.

John Diefenbaker eventually became the vice president of the Canadian Bar Association. He was Canadian through and through and struggled to maintain the Canadian right to retain sovereignty. Canada, he believed, should have the right to make its own decisions. Diefenbaker's counterpart in the United States was Dwight D. Eisenhower. Diefenbaker believed that the Liberals had gained far too much power federally and attempted to provide a political balance to the Liberal party, which had control of Canada for too long.

In contrast, later in the decade of the '60s emerged the bilingual socially-swinging champion of abortion and women's and gay rights, Pierre Elliott Trudeau. John Diefenbaker had rejected what he called a "hyphenated citizenship," with its emphasis on being Canadian first. Prime Minister Trudeau took a more "one world" view of citizenry. He loosened the immigration laws, enticing millions to flood into Canada.

George W. Bush

The rights of the individual immigrant to maintain a "country of origin" citizenship was upheld. Thus, Canada has become a cultural mosaic, versus the Diefenbaker vision of a Canadian melting pot.

Pierre Elliott Trudeau was heralded as the flamboyant and intellectually brilliant prime minister. He was a charismatic leader. He was on the elite left. He was a "freedom fighter" for human rights, yet Fidel Castro of Communist Cuba he held as one of his close political comrades. However suspect this uncomfortable truth was for the political right, Canada's young people adored Trudeau. The youth movement that swept a nation during the volatile 1960s proclaimed "Trudeaumania." Canadian youth fled through the streets and gathered in the parks. They crammed into spaces outside the Parliament buildings of Ottawa and the Liberal headquarters in Montreal and Toronto. They waved posters featuring headshots of Trudeau. These enthusiastic young people lined up, sometimes for days, when word leaked out that their icon of the political left was to make a press appearance or merely pass by behind the tinted glass of his limousine. In the 1960s, the world's young were searching for heroes, and the man with the red rose in his lapel fit the bill.

In February 1968 Trudeau was an unknown entity. But both the country and the man were positioned for the kind of liberalism that emerged. In the spring of 1968, Trudeau swept the vote. He declared a Liberal majority. With the exception of one nine-month period in the late '70s when Conservative leader Joe Clark was elected by the slimmest of margins, Trudeau held sway over Canada.

In 1968, Richard Milhous Nixon was elected as president of the United States. Before he entered his teens he had heard that personal call of Christ in his heart at the Amy McPherson Temple in Los Angeles, California, as the dynamic Paul Rader preached. When Paul Rader extended the invitation to confess Christ as Lord and Savior, among those who came forward was that destiny's child, the lad from Whittier, California.

Later, Nixon's rock solid conservative attitude was set in stone. North American youth, maybe even the youth of the world, responded to this symbol of over-control and eventually protested what appeared to them to be an angry, aggressively arrogant adversary.

A unique opportunity came to me one day in Portland, Oregon. It was May 1968. I accompanied Billy Graham, George Beverly Shea,

Suddenly Silenced

T.W. Wilson, Ralph Bell and Russ Busby to a fifteen-minute meeting that was extended to seventy minutes in Richard Nixon's office in a hotel. What made this meeting particularly enlightening was its scope, which included the comparison of organizing political and evangelistic crusades. There are many similarities between the two.

At some point during our meeting Pat Nixon, Richard's wife, kindly reminded us that we were running late. We had to get a move on, as we were about the business of assembling the large Portland crusade for 26,000 people.

Bobby Kennedy had scheduled a meeting with Billy Graham. Realizing he was running late, Billy asked me to take his place! The Bobby Kennedy that I met was on the campaign trail. He was pursuing the presidency of the United States. In the 1940s, Bobby's father, Joseph Kennedy, had been the American ambassador to the Court of St. James (the United Kingdom). The Kennedy boys lived in London for some time. There, Joseph Jr., who was later killed in WWII, John, Robert, and Teddy met London's young female debutantes—high society girls.

Bobby's girlfriend at the time was a luminous young thespian from London, Joan Winmill. At the famous Harringay Crusade in 1954, Joan Winmill came forward to give her life to Christ. That evening after the crusade she met with Billy's wife, Ruth, who led Joan to the Lord.

Joan Winmill was the star in a Billy Graham film produced by Worldwide Pictures, *Souls in Conflict*. It was Joan's life story. Once the movie was completed it was distributed to churches around the world. Joan promoted the film herself by taking it on tour.

At one of the first church appearances she made, she was met by the dashing film agent Bill Brown. It was a story made for Hollywood. Boy meets girl! Love at first sight! Bill was later heard to comment, "I always wanted to meet a Christian Broadway doll." Bill Brown became the president of Worldwide Pictures.

Joan gave testimony at my crusade in Belfast, in Wellington Hall, in the 1950s. In the 1960s, Joan and Bill became close friends with Kathleen and I. Joan was a star actress with Billy Graham's Worldwide Pictures.

In May 1968, in Billy Graham's room at the hotel in Portland, Oregon, I met with Bobby Kennedy. We held an in-depth discussion on

George W. Bush

the spiritual crisis in America. In need of some air, we went for a walk outside. As we walked, we talked. Accompanying Bobby Kennedy and me was the all-star NFL football player Rosie Grier. This friendly giant was Kennedy's personal bodyguard.

All at once, Bobby, Rosie and I found ourselves in a media storm in the streets of downtown Portland. The streets were dotted with cameras. Bobby responded by continually repeating the same phrase to the gaping onlookers. The phrase was taken from George Bernard Shaw: "You see things and you say, 'Why?' But I dream things that never were and I say, 'Why not?'" We were also swarmed by crowds of people. It was clear that our conversation was over!

In the 1970s on *Larry King Live* Rosie Grier told the world that, although in the 1960s he was a black icon, he felt empty. He was a rebel. But he was truly born again, and in the 1970s, Rosie was a revolutionary for Christ.

One of my treasures was a Scofield Bible that Bobby Kennedy signed with one of those twenty-five-cent pens. During September 1968, I drove to Hardin-Simmons University in Abilene, Texas, for a crusade. The historic Bible that Bobby Kennedy personally autographed remained in the abandoned and beaten old Chrysler that I had been driving, which died on the way to St. Louis. I simply forgot it. Somebody got a prize souvenir.

Tragically, that June Bobby Kennedy was assassinated in the Ambassador Hotel in downtown Los Angeles. In April, when we were in Australia, Martin Luther King Jr. had likewise been assassinated. An attempt had also been made on the life of Governor George Wallace at the Democratic National Convention, in Chicago. In 1999, George Wallace died in his mansion in Birmingham, Alabama. Franklin Graham spoke at the funeral for the dead governor.

In the 1960s the Federal Bureau of Investigation was concerned about the safety of Billy Graham. They offered protection, which Billy gratefully accepted. The FBI formed a human chain for miles in a radius around Billy and Ruth's mountain home in Montreat, North Carolina. German shepherd guard dogs surrounded the Graham home with teeth bared. They stood sentry against vigilantes and hit men. The FBI themselves stood sentry day and night, awaiting anything suspicious. What was America becoming?

Suddenly Silenced

From August 30 to September 8, 1968, we held a Billy Graham crusade in Pittsburgh, Pennsylvania. Anita Smith, the wife of our pastor Paul Smith of Peoples Church in Toronto, accompanied us. Billy arranged for the team to meet Richard Nixon in the afternoon. Kathleen, Anita and I joined the meeting. Billy reintroduced me as "a scholar from Oxford, his researcher, and his associate evangelist." As Nixon greeted me, his gaze was into Kathleen's Irish blue azure eyes. Who could blame him? He insisted that he had met Kathleen before—maybe in another life! She assured him that if they had met she would have remembered. Nixon replied that Kathleen must have a twin out there somewhere.

It was on the road again for the White family. We found ourselves in Aberdeen, South Dakota, for a crusade from July 6 to 20, 1969. Reverend Harold Salem was the chairman of this associate evangelist crusade. We employed Leighton Ford's team: Irv Chambers, the choirmaster, song leader and soloist, and John Innis, the organist and pianist.

JFK made good on his promise. On July 20, 1969, Neil Armstrong set foot on the moon! The time for the televised moon landing was originally set for 10 p.m. central time. But in the early days of NASA's space program, there were understandable delays. After our crusade meeting that night the air was still suffocatingly hot. It was the kind of night that a swing on a front porch glider, a tall glass of cold lemonade and a snooze might be very appealing. But a quiet little-town evening at dusk wasn't for us that night. This was a night for running. We, all of us, jumped into our cars and sped to our hotel room at the Holiday Inn.

We arrived at the hotel and dashed into the room reserved for the White family. Kathleen, the four boys, the four poodles, Irv, John, Harold and his wife, Beulah, their kids and I packed the room. Whose fingers would be the ones to turn on the TV? We perched ourselves on the two beds and sat cross-legged on the floor, anxiously awaiting the second most important moment of the twentieth century.

Then Harold started with his string of jokes. He had us buckled over with laughter as he clowned around. Harold pitched his jokes right through the great moment when the foot hit the moon—America's moment—a footprint and a flag for America!

Ironically, all was not well in America. Another well-known figure

George W. Bush

was in desperate straits that week. This was the week of Chappaquiddick. The eyes of the world were fixed on the man poised to run for the presidency of the United States of America in 1972. He was the head of the pack. But Teddy Kennedy, the lone Kennedy, had during a dark night on the Cape been driving drunk. He'd partied and picked up a woman in private. In secrecy, the two stole through the blackness. They raced across an old single-lane bridge on the windy Cape. Before either of them could come to, all control was lost. They crashed through the wall of the bridge, sending their vehicle airborne and sinking deep into the river, delivering Mary Jo Kopechne to her watery grave. Teddy's indiscretion virtually eliminated him from the presidential race.

The story stunned America. The morning's headlines bled the tragic ink of a rogue who had fallen from the favor of his country. This sad Kennedy saga stood in stark contrast to John Kennedy's dream come true, the great and lofty walk 263,000 miles from the third satellite from the sun. A footprint and a flag for the moon!

In 1972, there were three major bones of contention: the oil crisis building in the Middle East, the continuing Vietnam War, and the rising religious conflicts in Ireland. Nixon had attended the Moscow Baptist Church and then telephoned Billy Graham. He wanted to let Billy know that the president was behind him in his attempts to bring a solution to the chaos in Belfast. The call made Billy uneasy. The evangelist's coming to Ireland might be misunderstood. The sensitive Irish might believe that God's representative was acting as a political agent with an exclusively American agenda.

Kathleen, Billy Graham, T.W. Wilson and I connected with evangelist Arthur Blessit when he jetted from the star-studded Sunset Strip in Los Angeles to troubled Ulster to meet us. Arthur Blessit had gained the confidence of the "Jesus People" on Sunset Strip. He was renowned for dragging a fifteen-foot replica of Jesus' cross around the world, from Moscow to Mexico.

When we arrived in Belfast, Billy Graham and Arthur Blessit made their way on foot through both the Protestant and Catholic sectors. They handed out biblical tracts in hopes of bringing peace to the region. They were inundated by mobs of Irishmen, yet they managed to talk with countless individuals along the way. Hesitation posed many perils. They were in the danger zone. It was prudent to just keep moving, but for two and a half hours they stayed and talked.

The first Sunday in Belfast, T.W Wilson and I caught Ian Paisley preaching in his Free Presbyterian Church against Billy Graham's attempt at uniting Ireland. Ian Paisley's sermon lit a fire under the Protestants. The blaze and its smoke were directed at the Roman Catholics. It signaled that the time had come for a fight.

We held a dozen meetings in the interiors of back rooms and behind church doors throughout Ireland and Ulster. We urgently prayed for a message from God. We sought direction and a way to bring peace to the area that was grabbing the headlines of the world as a "hotbed" of religious feuding. It has been this way for the past quarter of a century.

We escaped Ireland relatively unscathed. Kathleen and I were invited to the Nixon inauguration on January 20, 1973. I teamed with Billy Graham, who offered the inaugural prayer. The Lord had blessed me with the great honor of contributing to the writing of this prayer. Kathleen and I chatted with Vice President Nelson Aldrich Rockefeller. Rockefeller was the governor of New York and had been appointed the coordinator of inter-American affairs by President Franklin D. Roosevelt. Kathleen and I found Nelson Rockefeller charming and interesting. And he seemed to have some interest in the Youth For Christ movement. It can be said that it was a "presidential" three days for us.

It was the leftists' key moment in history. Factions were taking aim at President Richard Nixon, and they had him in the crosshairs. They had him in the sites of a most powerful weapon, the smoking gun known as political insurrection.

In June 1972, the Committee to Re-elect the President (CRP) broke into offices of the Democratic National Committee in the Watergate apartment complex. The liberals held their collective breath, closed an eye and pulled the trigger. They hit the bull right in the eye. Repercussions of the Watergate break-in reverberated globally. The media stormed the event and told the world the tale of possible ethical and illegal cover-ups in the White House. The blast from the leftist arms had indeed ripped a gash in the highest office in America, and America began to hemorrhage profusely.

The shot would eventually prove fatal. A Goliath would again fall.

George W. Bush

Initially, during the frenzy, the comment to the press from the political "right" was that this was little more than an attack on George McGovern. He could not hope to defeat Nixon on the more important issues of the campaign, could he?

The Watergate affair was heating up to the boiling point, and, astoundingly, Richard Nixon kept a cool head. Eventually the Watergate plumbers and Richard Nixon himself were implicated in the break-in. The rest is history. It was resignation or impeachment for the 31st president of the United States. Richard Nixon acquiesced. The bell of resignation rang out, the reverberations of which sent a country and world shuddering into shock!

The oil magnates had permeated the Permian Basin (North America), the shallow shale where the black crude swales. They figured they had discovered enough oil to gush ceaselessly for thirty years around the clock. There would be hot geysers of oil endlessly shooting into cloudless sky. But these were the days of the Arabian oil embargo. The oil and gas prices trebled for 240 million disillusioned Americans, who despaired that the natural resources were insufficient to produce enough of the stuff for everybody.

On the surface it seemed ironic that, with the discovery of so much oil in Texas, the American people could get hit so hard at the gas pumps, for home heating and for all public consumption. But one has to understand the politics of global economics to see the cause and effect of the Saudi Arabian–American oil connection. Oil, like other natural resources and commodities, is internationally regulated, and its monetary value fluctuates with the rise and fall of the world markets.

When the Saudi government, a gigantic player in global economics, suddenly places sanctions on its oil reserves, America and other nations that trade with Saudi Arabia for their oil find that consumer costs correspondingly escalate. The costs incurred alert the sanctioned nations to the necessity of providing the technology, the manpower and enough oil to keep themselves in energy. It is like being faced with the challenge of birthing an enormous new business on the spur of the moment. Thus the citizens dig deep into their pockets, making up the substantial shortfall. Wars are fought over such matters.

On Sunday morning, August 4, 1974, our team held a John Wesley White crusade. Midland, Texas with a population of 58,000, is the oil

Suddenly Silenced

center of the country. Thus in the 1970s, it was the wealthiest city per capita in America. At the invitation of about seventy-five local churches, I preached a six-day associate evangelist crusade. On Sunday our team took the platform at First Presbyterian Church, where the Bush family regularly attended.

On Thursday the national television networks announced the news that President Richard Milhous Nixon would make a public resignation on Friday, August 9. When the infamous moment came, the great crowd became anxious. There was jostling in the seats at Midland's ballpark as I preached. Baseball caps and hats were tipped backwards as all eyes were transfixed on the screen. Jaws slackened as the fateful moment arrived in technicolor: the live spectacle of the 31st president of the United States offering his resignation and an apology to the American people.

Spectators froze in their seats. As hot as it was, I thought that I could feel a chill in the air. History was broadcast on a parching summer day in that ballpark. The spectacular announcement and resignation speech was made by Richard Nixon. The experience at that high voltage ballpark reminded me of this scene in Acts: *"Some among the multitude cried one thing and some another...[There was a] tumult"* (Acts 21:34). I thought that I could hear their voices rising above the din. Some Republicans cried, "Hail the Chief; let him reign," while the Democrats shouted, "Ah, kick the bum out!" My preaching was abruptly stopped. Richard Nixon was the first American no more!

A nation and the world now had just one word: "Why?" According to accounts in the August 27, 2000, issue of *The New York Times*, Dr. Hutschnecker, a New York psychotherapist Nixon consulted, described Nixon as having "a good portion of neurotic symptoms." Allegedly, the former president took the drug Dilantin, normally indicated for relief of "fear, worry, guilt, panic, anger and related emotions, irritability, rage, mood, depression, violent behavior, hyperglycemia, alcohol, anorexia, bulimia and binge eating, cardiac arrhythmia, muscular disorders." Dilantin has "potentially very serious side effect risks, like change of mental status, person becoming confused, loss of memory, irritability, definitely could have an effect on cognitive function."

As a former president of the United States, Richard Millions Nixon did much to recover his status as a respectable world leader. His public

George W. Bush

relations trips to China prior to that country's separation from the Soviet Union were notable, and among other things he succeeded in restoring relations between the "New China" and the "Western World." It has been reported that Nixon will be remembered more for the diplomatic efforts of his end years than for the debacle of his presidency. Only time will tell.

Nixon slipped away into relative obscurity and died at his home in Whittier, California, at the age of eighty-one. Billy Graham preached at Nixon's funeral. Presidents Gerald Ford, Jimmy Carter, Ronald Reagan, George Herbert Walker Bush and the sitting president, William Jefferson Clinton, all paid homage to a president of world renown. Richard Milhous Nixon is one of the most frequently written about presidents in U.S. history.

Interestingly, in 2004 Brian Mulroney, a former prime minister of Canada, gave a warm personal eulogy at the funeral for his close friend Ronald Reagan. They were two Irish peas in a pod. In the '80s, member of Parliament Len Gustafson, a close friend of the prime minister, was from the riding that the White family farm was in. He invited me to Ottawa to meet with Prime Minister Mulroney for half an hour. Our son Wesley and I flew from Toronto to Ottawa. Within the regal chambers of the prime minister's office in the parliament buildings, we compared the blueprints of Billy Graham's strategy for evangelistic campaigning with the strategies for political campaigning. It was a most enlightening and enjoyable visit.

I still chuckle when I recall our return flight. Wes exclaimed, "Dad, you hail from Saskatchewan. You know, Brian Mulroney looks like he does too."

I asked, "What do you mean?"

Wes quipped, "He has a 'Moose Jaw'!"

Puritanism began in the 1500s, and with it emerged some of history's most magnetic leaders. In 1608 the Protestants formed the "Evangelical Union" in Prague, Germany, just prior to the Bohemian Period. The Evangelical Alliance, formed in the UK in 1846, and the World Evangelical Alliance followed in 1951. The purpose of this alliance was to unify the Protestant churches.

These words of Jesus are written in the beatitudes: "*Blessed are ye, when men shall revile you, and persecute you, and shall say all manner of evil against you falsely, for my sake"* (Matthew 5:11). Jesus elaborated in the book of John, *"If the world hates you, you know that it hated Me before it hated you. If you were of the world, the world would love its own. Yet because you are not of the world, but I chose you out of the world, therefore the world hates you"* (John 15:18,19).

At the age of 100, the apostle John was tortured and then was exiled on the Isle of Patmos. There he wrote the book of Revelation. Denyse O'Leary wrote in "A Velvet Oppression" in *Christianity Today* on April 2, 2001:

> Michael Horowitz, a leader in the campaign against religious persecution worldwide, that for Christians has many parallels with Jewish experience. Evangelicals are the "new Jews of the 21st century," Horowitz says. "Every statement used to distance oneself from Jews is now being said about Christians. It's utterly striking how verbatim the same language is used in newsrooms, at fancy dinner parties, in faculty clubs."

Our men of influence must operate in the theatre of public persecution.

President George W. Bush's grandmother "Dotty" had an influence on young George's life. She read the Bible to George daily. She prepared him for a life of Christian spirituality. The strict Barbara Bush, George's mother, insisted that her brood adhere to a regular regimen of church attendance at a Presbyterian church in Midland. The minister of this church was Dr. Lynn. He was a prayerful and theological saint. When young Robin Bush tragically died of cancer, Barbara's hair turned from dark brown to gray.

George was born and grew up in the family mansion at 2703 Sentinel Avenue. His home borders on the ballpark in which we held our John Wesley White crusade during the Nixon resignation of August 9, 1974. As a boy, George was a Little League catcher. He loved the game. George saw hundreds of games in that ballpark behind his house, and he played hundreds of games there.

George W. Bush was educated at Yale and Harvard in New England but returned to Midland during the summers. Following his formal education, in the 1980s he made a major business decision. He bought the Texas Rangers baseball club. It was the right decision for George. Although he had attended two liberal schools in New England, George

George W. Bush

was on the political right and felt more at home when he returned to his native Texas. He has proclaimed that he wants to live and die and be buried in Midland.

It is of primary significance that for forty years George Bush Jr.'s closest friend has been Don Evans, a fixture at his evangelical church. Don's wife, Susan, introduced George to his wife-to-be, Laura. According to the August 7, 2000, issue of *Time,*

> 1986 is the mystical year when everything came together. The story is all about faith and redemption; it's the year he turned 40 and quit drinking and found his faith reawakened after a walk on the beach with Billy Graham. The process of finally growing up and calming down, of course, had really begun when he married Laura, "the best thing he's ever done,"... It was Laura who had issued W. the ultimatum about booze. "It's me or the bottle," she reportedly told her husband.

The way had been paved for George to take his famous and life-changing walk with Billy Graham. It was during this walk that George W. Bush found Jesus Christ. The *New York Herald Tribune* during his presidential race on August 29, 2000, made reference to George W. Bush's statement concerning Jesus Christ our Lord. The president declared, "He [Jesus] changed my heart."

With his familial influence, his education, his puritan evangelical influence, his spiritual walk with Billy Graham, his political experience and his disciplined and dedicated wife, the making of a president was complete. George W. Bush became the most powerful man in the world at the emergence of the third millennium. Since September 11, 2001, he continuously exerted his spiritually directed power throughout the world.

A dozen years earlier, in March 1986, as Billy Graham's primary researcher, I sat behind Billy, who was seated beside Vice President George H. W. Bush at the Washington, DC, crusade. As we chatted, George Bush Sr. informed us that George W. had taken a walk on the beach with Billy Graham, and there the junior Bush had been led to Jesus Christ.

In 1999 Kathleen and I traveled to San Antonio, Texas, to join the Billy Graham team for a crusade. The then governor of Texas, George W. Bush, gave his personal testimony there.

Suddenly Silenced

In October 2000, Kathleen and I attended the Billy Graham crusade in Jacksonville, Florida. At the hotel following the crusade, Billy discussed how he had announced his support for George W. Bush, who narrowly squeaked out a victory by a margin of 7,211 votes in Florida. It is surmised that Billy's support was enough to put George W. Bush over the top to become the next president of the United States. A walk on the beach, then the presidency. On the Sunday morning, Kathleen and I spoke with the pastor in Jacksonville about George W. Bush, the same morning the campaigning potential next president had been at the service.

History now records that in November 2004, President Bush defeated John F. Kerry following a hard-fought campaign that had the world in its clutches. John Kerry came out swinging, blindsiding the sitting president, but George W. threw crushing blows at the Democratic position, particularly on the war in Iraq. The president emerged the clear winner. Redoubling his efforts, Kerry, with the combined assistance of his wife, the liberal news media, and the support of elitist New England, fought back. However, as the world sat perched on the edge of many millions of seats, Bush held his position with the strength predicted by his father, the former president. George W. not only took the electoral college, but he also won the popular vote by a history-making three million plus votes, to begin his second term as president of the United States. In the March 8, 2007, *Toronto Star* it was written,

> Does it encourage you to know that [Vladimir Putin] had a born-again experience similar to [George W. Bush]'s? Remarkable enough that a man who would head the KGB's successor had a mother who was (for years secretly) a devout Christian. In 1996 (Bush saw the light in 1986), after nearly dying in a fire (Bush's demon was booze), Putin became a practicing member of the Russian Orthodox Church.

In the October 7, 2002 *Toronto Star*, it is written "the (White) House (resides) arguable the most fervent Christian president in U.S. history."

In 2003, I believed that Paul Martin was the best prime minister since John Diefenbaker. Martin appeared to be a champion and a statesmen and a nominal Roman Catholic. I hoped that he would bat-

George W. Bush

tle for the maintaining of the traditional definition of marriage. Unfortunately, he did not. Of some immediate consequence at the time, a definitive scientific study emerged that supported the idea that just 3 percent of the world's population was biologically gay.

Four predominant evangelical leaders attracted Canadian headlines: David Mainse, the founder of *100 Huntley Street* and Crossroads Television Network and champion of maintaining the traditional definition of marriage in Canada; Charles McVety, the head of the Family Action Coalition and president of Canada Christian College; Bruce Clemenger, the president of the Evangelical Fellowship of Canada; and Michael Coren, radio and television talk show host.

In Canada in 2006 there was perhaps no topic as red hot as the debate over the issue of same-sex marriage. There was a 50–50 split vote on this issue in the House of Commons, and the country took a ride on a dizzying and emotional roller coaster. There was uncertainty over whether gays would be granted equal legal rights with traditional married couples. Up rose a hew and cry for the incoming prime minister to firmly state his position concerning this hot-button issue, which could have determined Stephen Harper's destiny as concerned his leadership of Canada. King David declared, *"Exaltation comes neither from the east Nor from the west nor from the south. But God is the Judge: He puts down one, And exalts another"* (Psalm 75:6,7). So Paul Martin was defeated, and the once very much underdog candidate Stephen Harper was exalted to the esteemed office of prime minister of Canada.

In 2006, another evangelical took high office. Stephen Harper became the prime minister. He worships regularly in an evangelical Christian and Missionary Alliance church. At my brother Hugh's funeral in Ottawa, David Mainse gave his testimony and announced that Stephen Harper had been converted to Jesus Christ thirteen years earlier. He had been led to the Lord by Preston Manning. Apparently, Mr. Harper was keen on bringing himself as an evangelical to that high office.

Prime Minister Harper has, in terms of finance, health and moral integrity, really set the pace. He anticipates a majority government. Interestingly, Canada has become the world's lending market. Stephen Harper's economics appear to be right on the money.

On June 22, 1992, I spoke to 800 ministers and their wives at the

Suddenly Silenced

Billy Graham School of Evangelism at the Hilton Hotel near the Cove in Asheville, North Carolina. The title I had selected that day for my speech was the conspicuous two-word edict "Go Forward!"

I had prayed fervently prior to that meeting, and the Lord filled me with unction. My subject was "*I am not ashamed of the gospel of Christ*" (Romans 1:16). In synchronization with the alphabet, with my evangelistic finger extended, I repeated "Go forward" twenty-six times. The substance of each letter of the alphabet took approximately two minutes to deliver.

A: Jesus proclaimed, "*He has **anointed** Me To preach the gospel*" (Luke 4:18, emphasis added). "Go forward."

B: Jesus declared, "*The **beginning** of the gospel*" (Mark 1:1, emphasis added). "Go forward."

C: The apostle Paul rejoiced, "*I preach the gospel...**without charge***" (1 Corinthians 9:18, emphasis added). "Go forward."

D: Paul also commanded, "*Now this I **do** for the gospel's sake*" (1 Corinthians 9:23, emphasis added). "Go forward."

E: The century-old apostle John reflected, "*The **everlasting** gospel*" (Revelation 14:6, emphasis added). "Go forward."

F: To the church of Philippi Paul said, "***Fellowship** in the gospel*" (Philippians 1:5, emphasis added). "Go forward."

G: Then in elation he rejoiced, "*The light of the **glorious gospel** of Christ*" (2 Corinthians 4:4, emphasis added). "Go forward."

H: Then he revealed, "*If our **gospel** be **hid**, it is hid to them that are lost*" (2 Corinthians 4:3, emphasis added). "Go forward."

I: Then he courageously testified, "*I am not ashamed of the gospel of Christ*" (Romans 1:16, emphasis added). "Go forward."

J: Now he instructed, "*God will **judge** the secrets of men by Jesus Christ, according to my gospel*" (Romans 2:16, emphasis added). "Go forward."

George W. Bush

K: The taxman Matthew referred to *"preaching the **gospel** of the **kingdom**"* (Matthew 4:23, emphasis added). "Go forward."

L: Jesus taught His disciples, *"Whoever **loses** his life for My sake and the **gospel's** will save it"* (Mark 8:35, emphasis added). "Go forward."

M: Paul shared with his close friends that Onesimus *"might have **ministered** unto me in the bonds of the **gospel**"* (Philemon 1:13, emphasis added). "Go forward."

N: The prophetic Jesus announced, *"This **gospel** of the kingdom will be preached...to all the **nations**"* (Matthew 24:14, emphasis added). "Go forward."

O: Paul said that the Jews *"have not all **obeyed** the **gospel**"* (Romans 10:16, emphasis added). "Go forward."

P: Jesus commissioned us to, *"Go into all the world and **preach** the **gospel**"* (Mark 16:15, emphasis added). "Go forward."

Q: To the church of Ephesus Paul counseled, *"Having shod your feet with...the **gospel** of peace...taking the shield of faith...**quench** all the fiery darts of the wicked one"* (Ephesians 6:15,16, emphasis added). "Go forward."

R: Jesus exhorted, **"Repent,** *and believe in the **gospel**"* (Mark 1:15, emphasis added). "Go forward."

S: Paul clarified for the Romans, *"[I am] an apostle, **separated** unto the **gospel**"* (Romans 1:1 KJV, emphasis added). "Go forward."

T: In the first epistle to the Thessalonians Paul advised, *"We were...put in **trust** with the **gospel**"* (1 Thessalonians 2:4, emphasis added). "Go forward."

U: To the Galatians Paul revealed that *"the **gospel** for the **uncircumcised** had been committed to me"* (Galatians 2:7, emphasis added). "Go forward."

V: Paul reflectively revealed, **"Verily** *that, when I preach the gospel"* (1 Corinthians 9:18, emphasis added). "Go forward."

W: Paul admonished the Corinthians, saying, *"**Woe** is me if I do not preach the **gospel!**"* (1 Corinthians 9:16, emphasis added). "Go forward."

X: Then Paul said, "*How shall they preach, except they be sent?...that preach the gospel*" (Romans 10:15 KJV, emphasis added). "Go forward."

Y: Paul then instructed the Thessalonians, "*We preached unto you the gospel of God*" (1 Thessalonians 2:9 KJV, emphasis added). "Go forward."

Z: Finally, Paul said about the Jews, "*They have a zeal for God...But they have not all obeyed the gospel*" (Romans 10:2–16, emphasis added). "Go forward."

Most remarkable was the reaction of long-time friends Calvin Thielman and Harold Salem, who were seated in the front row of the auditorium. Calvin and Harold spontaneously stood up, ramrod straight. As I got to the letter *H*, filled with the Holy Spirit they shouted to the audience, "Go forward."

First a dozen or so people in the front row stood up in the exhilaration of the Spirit and then sat down again.

Then three minutes later fifty people stood up and in unison chimed, "Go forward."

Then they sat down. I would then quote by letter the next Scripture. All at once, many rows of the auditorium stood up spontaneously and declared, "Go forward."

Then they sat down. Then I wielded a few more Scriptures, and a full quarter of the auditorium stood up, shouting, "Go forward." Soon the entire auditorium was in tremors, with everyone on their feet, harmoniously chanting, "Go forward." "Go forward." "Go forward." They clapped and shouted and stomped the floor. To my ears all this sounded like the ringing of glorious tubular bells. It was Shekinah! And the light of Christ was everywhere.

Suddenly a bridge appeared between evangelistic campaigning and political campaigning. Only a scant three weeks following my "Go forward" message, on July 16, 1992, during the Democratic National convention, held in Madison Square Garden in New York City, the yet relatively unknown next vice president of the United States, Al Gore, took the platform.

Gore's pastor from Carthage, Tennessee, had been in attendance at that historic "Go forward" meeting in Asheville the previous month.

George W. Bush

The minister enthusiastically relayed to the potential next vice president the use of the term "Go forward" with its power to captivate and generate an excited response from a crowd. It seemed that Al Gore went with the decision to use the modified term "Got to go," referring to the Bush-Quayle team, to ignite the crowd at the convention.

As the sparkplug phrase powered its magic, Gore repeated, "Got to go." "Got to go." "Got to go." He repeated this little phrase many times. That evening the convention center was electrified. There was a charge in the air, and the crowd exploded into support for the Clinton-Gore administration. They spontaneously stood up, ramrod straight, clapping, shouting and stomping the floor until the auditorium was in tremors with "Got to go." Again, this time for Al Gore, it was tubular bells.

CHAPTER XIII

Agape

In 1972, I was facing fatigue. The strain of continual crusading and speaking and traveling was becoming too much for me. That November I was burdened in prayer. One day the weight of it all was so heavy that on the shoulder of a road in Peterborough, Ontario, I broke down and cried. Astonishingly, with my tears clearing, I saw a vision of Jesus on the hood of my car. Without hesitation I got out, and kneeling in the ditch I earnestly prayed, "Lord, which way shall I go? I am lost. I am just a child from the farm." This was a crisis! Jesus admonished, *"What, could ye not watch with me one hour? Watch and pray"* (Matthew 26:40,41). I was elated that Jesus had spoken to me. I rose to my feet feeling a renewed strength in the Lord, and I made a covenant with Him to spend one hour a day in prayer. I would talk with Jesus one hour a day on my knees, come hell or high water. This was my crisis in Christ!

I had been preaching that night in the Salvation Army citadel. The next morning that was it; I resolved to go to the hardware store to buy a chain and tether myself to the bed by the ankle. This time I was adamant. I would not be interrupted during my hour of prayer. I would spend one hour in fervent prayer each day, *"the hour of prayer"* (Acts 3:1).

Ironically, the telephone interrupted my all-out plight to pray early on. This particular day Kathleen walked in on me while I was praying. In astonishment, with those sky-blue azure eyes glaring, she admonished, "Well, John, here you are, my husband, tethered to a bed. Well, that's the devotion of an all-out evangelist for you. Anyway, John, the phone is for you. It's either Billy Graham, an angel or—the devil!"

Suddenly Silenced

Whoever it was, I continued praying, tethered to the bed. I recall the door closing behind me. The cold steel chain fastened around my ankle assured me that Jesus would be my priority and that no one could keep me from my promise. This practice continued for years. As extreme as this sounds, I believe that God honored this decision.

In December 1972 in Florida, I spoke to Billy's team of 400 people. Billy heard my forty-minute plea, my urgent burden for Canada. My topic was "The Signs of the Times: the Second Coming of Jesus Christ." The substance of my message was that the time for Christ's coming was drawing nigh. Many members of our team reported actually feeling the passion in my words. I was heavily anointed with the Holy Spirit that day. Billy appreciated my calling to Canada, and George Beverly Shea, the other Canadian on the team, was especially moved. This was a historic meeting and had a profound impact on my ministry in the 1970s.

In January 1973, I got the call from Billy Graham that President Lyndon B. Johnson had died. I was flown by Learjet from Toronto to Asheville, North Carolina. I drove to Montreat, where Billy and I had a private meeting at his country home, "Little Piney Cove," concerning the president's death. Three long days were spent in preparation for President Johnson's funeral. Calvin Thielman and I teamed in this effort. We researched the material for the funeral address, and Calvin carefully crafted it.

In a private meeting with Billy Graham, Johnson had disclosed that he was disillusioned, disheveled and burned out. He alluded to the fact that he was exhausted from traveling and lecturing; he was entirely disgusted with the Vietnam War. He just wanted to go home to his ranch. The weight of it all proved to be too much for President Johnson. When he swept the election in 1964, he was a youthful fifty-four-year-old. In 1973, he was an aged sixty-two-year-old. He died at age sixty-four.

During the funeral, Billy declared that while Lyndon Johnson was dying, he stated that he wanted him to preach his funeral. He explained, "Billy Graham, you will preach the gospel of Jesus Christ for half the sermon; the other half will be about me." Billy's speech was a resounding success. It made headlines around the world.

Billy Graham's television program and the thought of bringing Jesus Christ to my native Canada was never far from my mind. Billy informed me that he was enthusiastic about this idea and supported the plan that I appear on Canadian network television. At the time, Toronto offered only three Canadian television stations, and only two of those networks telecast nationwide.

At the turn of the twenty-first century in Canada, television experienced a media explosion. Household television viewers are offered 300 stations, in addition to Web TV and satellite dish television, which brings in hundreds of stations from countries around the world. I was greatly burdened to spread the Word of God across Canada, and the television program was born.

Billy's son-in-law Ted Dienert was a television producer and agreed to create a pilot program for this series. After much deliberation about what we should name the program we selected the Greek word that represents the special form of unconditional and spiritual love that Jesus offers mankind: *Agape*.

Billy was so positive that he appointed his own long-time friend George Beverly Shea, a Billy Graham Evangelistic Association founding member and baritone singer, to perform weekly on *Agape*. What a blessed addition he was. Rounding out the musical segment of *Agape* was the undeniably angelic Evie Tornquist. The teenager sang many contemporary gospel songs. She was not well known at the time. Kathleen had seen Evie's performance on television from the White House during President Gerald Ford's term in office. When we heard her sing we were immediately impressed, and we contacted her, asking her to appear regularly on *Agape*. Evie gleefully agreed.

The rich bass voice belonged to the photogenic Lowell Jackson, also a recruit from the BGEA. He was the point man. As an additional exercise in expertise Lowell coordinated our crusades from 1972 through 1979. Further connecting *Agape* with the BGEA, Billy Graham's son-in-law Dr. Stephan Tchividjian appeared on the program in three- or four-minute segments during each of the airings. The web was woven with even more intricate thread when Ted Dienert's mother, Millie, known around the world as an articulate Christian speaker, appeared in her own three- or four-minute spots each week.

From 1973 to 1978, *Agape* was picked up coast-to-coast in Canada and could be seen in New York City. *Agape* established an even higher profile after *Decision* ran favorable reports on it. In the 1970s, *Decision* had a circulation of five million copies around the world. By the mid-1970s, *Agape* became the second most-watched religious program in Canada. Billy Graham assured us that we were producing a quality program.

We taped in thirteen-week quarters, and we went into CTV studios in Toronto for one week each season. We would tape in remarkably large segments, ten hours of programming at a time. Ted Dienert then edited the material until we had our thirteen half-hour programs. I was researching illustrations for *Agape* all season long. Judiciously, I found that I could make the most of my research illustrations by using each of them a remarkable six times: for Billy, for my crusades, for *Agape*, for books, for articles, and for when I appeared annually on the *Hour of Decision* radio program.

My preparation for a fresh sermon was rather extensive. I would kneel beside my bed and pray while I arranged little notes and about thirty Bible verses. Then I would synthesize them into one Christocentric sermon. I would then meditate on the relevant Bible passages and the substance of my messages. It usually took me about four hours to get mentally and spiritually prepared to give my messages.

From *Just As I Am*: "With a D.Phil. from Oxford, John could have had a brilliant career in the academic world, but I have seldom met a man who had a deeper burden for evangelism. His unique brand of eloquent preaching is unforgettable." Reverend Lewis Blanchard was the coordinator for 132 of my crusades with the Billy Graham Evangelistic Association, which continued over twenty-five years. Lewis marveled at how I could come up with a new crusade sermon every time I spoke. "*Ye have an unction from the Holy One*" (1 John 2:20).

Another major advancement in my preaching technique was about to eclipse anything that I had previously used. Its genesis occurred one day at a crusade in Burlington, Iowa. In the adjacent room to mine, Bill Fasig, a keyboardist and sound specialist, heard me reading the scriptural passages for my message that night. He interrupted me with a unique idea—an idea that I consistently used for my speaking engagements over the years. Bill demonstrated how I could play a recorded message into my earphone from a tape player in my pocket.

I discovered that this technique could enhance the delivery of my message. I could deliver even more articulate and more detailed messages than ever before, because I could relay information verbatim that

Agape

I had previously compiled. Spontaneous facts and myriad details for illustrations could now stream into my ear at will. In theory, at least, this process would allow me to deliver messages according to exact time specifications.

The one caveat in using Bill's technique was that there was an approximate two-second delay between the time I heard the message and the time it took for my brain to coordinate the message with my eye movements. It became increasingly apparent to all who witnessed my efforts that I had to spend the time to retrain my brain to process the information I was hearing and synchronize it with my eye movements. This sensitive balancing of the senses is most assuredly an acquired skill. In fact, it took me a full two years of continuous practice to get it right. Yet, once I managed to coordinate my timing properly, my appearances on TV became exponentially more efficient.

Of the many thousands of letters that I have received, this is one of the most significant. In this age of pilots, airplanes and airline accountability, an airline captain from Prince George, British Columbia, wrote to *Decision*:

> Sunday, while I was alone in my apartment, depressed, hung over from the previous night's activities, fed up with life, trying to find a way out of it, I turned on the television set for want of something better to do. John Wesley White was just beginning his message about the vast emptiness that exists in the lives of those persons without God. This was my problem, so I began to listen. When the invitation was given for me to pray, I did, and praise the Lord. He saved me instantly. He made a new person out of me. I have been so happy that I cannot contain myself.
>
> I am an airline captain and have told most of the people I work with about my experience with God. I am praying that I may be able to lead many of them to Christ. In all the years that I have been flying, I can truly say that I have never been any higher than I am now with Jesus in my heart. The program *Agape* was the vehicle God used to bring me to Him.

It was during this period that Sam Hamilton, a rich baritone from Ulster, joined *Agape*. He was converted to Christ after he watched

Suddenly Silenced

Agape in the 1970s. His mentor was George Beverly Shea. Some say that Sam's singing resembles Bev's. Many people would say that Sam looked like Larry Hagman, J.R. of *Dallas*, an audience-grabbing television series of the 1980s. Sam was with us for twenty years. He also sang for The Peoples Church of Toronto in the 1980s when our program ratings hit an all-time high and our mailing list expanded to 17,000 dedicated members. It was also Sam's responsibility to respond to our most generous North American donors. Sam was always spiritually encouraging. He was a close and loyal friend of mine. He always had our ministry's interests at heart.

In 1962, David Mainse was a relatively unknown evangelist. For fifteen years David's evangelism ministry grew in Ontario. On September 3, 1967, I was introduced to him. In the third millennium David has been Canada's premiere evangelist for over a generation.

When I was in a library in Sydney, Australia, I spotted the cover of *Time*. It sported a full-page frontal picture of the "Golden Jet," Bobby Hull, in full flight. I flipped to the article inside the magazine. It declared Bobby Hull a supreme sportsman, every ounce muscle! I had introduced Bobby Hull to Billy Graham. Interestingly, Bobby Hull was a dead-ringer for David Mainse.

David spent his very young years in the eastern townships of Quebec. His father had been a missionary in Egypt. He returned to Canada for the first two years of David's life but accepted his calling to return to Egypt for the next seven years, leaving David to be raised by his mother, for whom it would have been too dangerous to accompany him. When David was just twelve his mother died of cancer while living in their new home in Renfrew, Ontario. David had always considered his mother very loving and his father strict.

At an early age David had to begin fending for himself and worked at odd jobs to make money. Later, David left a job at a gas station to work at a Chrysler dealership. The rebellious teenaged David became involved with a motorcycle club called the "Throttle Twisters." Every moment that he was not in school he would cruise around on his bike. Of his riding David writes in his autobiography,

> In spite of all the riding, there was a hollowness in me that no long-distance cruising seemed to fill. At least, when I was rid-

ing, there was always the possibility that things might be better at my destination, wherever that happened to be. Of course, they weren't but as long as I was en route, I could at least maintain the illusion that they might be.

Around this time David's boss was a zealous Baptist named Sid Healey. Jack was a close friend to Billy Graham. One of David's favorite cars on the lot was a big, new, blue Chrysler. By sixteen, David had earned his chauffeur's license and could transport vehicles from one city to another. One day Sid asked David if he would drive some of the young people from his church to a Jack Wyrtzen Word of Life camp in Schroon Lake, New York, for an evangelistic meeting.

As most young men would have been, David was thrilled with the opportunity to drive that great Chrysler. Sid had obviously thought this one through. Letting David drive the Chrysler would ensure David's arrival at Jack's meeting. However, David was determined not to be hustled by any evangelist into making a commitment to Christ.

As he beheld the meeting he was greatly impressed with the testimony of Gil Dodds, who would become the world's fastest indoor-mile sprinter and my coach and friend at Wheaton College. At Jack Wyrtzen's meeting, David was given a lot to think about. He was still unsaved!

Homer James had been on the Billy Graham team for a generation and was seen on CBC-TV across Canada. He had won the amateur hour contest with his program *The Caravan Hour*. Homer, who was the first cousin of George Beverly Shea's first wife, Irma, in the 1950s had been with the Leighton Ford team and the John Wesley White gospel singing group the "Gospelaires," who had crossed two continents in the service of the Lord. And Homer James performed at David's crucial meeting.

That night Jack Wyrtzen was powerful and anointed. He offered the cross of Christ as a plan of salvation to the crowd. At the invitation, it was Homer who came before the platform. Then it was Homer who compassionately put his arm around David, asking him gently, "Don't you plan sometime to give your heart to God?"

"Yes, I do intend to, Homer," David replied, "but not now." David realized that this was the first time he had ever said "yes" to Jesus.

Suddenly Silenced

"Doesn't it make sense that you should do it tonight?" responded Homer.

It was at this moment that the world changed for David Mainse. He went forward, and he heard a man declare Jesus' words *"the one who comes to Me I will by no means cast out"* (John 6:37). David Mainse had been born again!

David has taken his ministry across Canada, namely his television program *100 Huntley Street,* which began airing in 1977. This sparkling Christian program has enjoyed consistently high ratings nationally for thirty years. Since then, David's Christian brainchild has blossomed. It now reaches viewers all over the world, in sixty-five nations, with timely and inspiring programming. Again, it is the Savior beating Satan. Kathleen and I have been close friends with David and his wife, Norma Jean, for over a generation.

Television appearances became an increasingly important feature of my ministry. In addition to the *John Wesley White Program,* I have been on my friend David Mainse's *100 Huntley Street Program* many times over the past thirty years. Additionally, over a two-year period during the early 1980s, I was featured on the news each week.

I was overcome with the desire to hold a crusade on *100 Huntley Street.* I prayed about this prospect daily. Then the opportunity arose, and David Mainse agreed to hold a one-day Billy Graham crusade in microcosm. The format of this program dictated that I speak for eighteen minutes and then give the invitation directly to the studio audience. This day of Christian testimony featured the famous Montreal Canadien hockey star Doug Jarvis. In 1999, Doug was the assistant coach of the Dallas Stars. The Stars won the prized Stanley Cup that year. Doug offered his testimony across North America. He informed the North American continent that he had been born again.

The success of this one-day mini-crusade led David to prayer. He returned to me, declaring that we should hold a five-day crusade on *100 Huntley Street* in 1994. Dan Southern, a coordinator with Billy Graham, was approached about taking on the job. He agreed, and we then set about organizing a crusade in the studio of *100 Huntley Street* in Burlington, Ontario. This television event was another microcosm of a Billy Graham Crusade. We prepared many counselors for those who might come forward giving their lives to Jesus Christ. My messages

Agape

were again eighteen minutes in length, with an invitation at the end. We brought in James Reese, a dynamic choir leader from Kitchener, Ontario, whose inspired singers brought the Lord to Huntley Street in song.

There were five testimonies given during this mini crusade, and seven percent of the studio audience made decisions for Christ that week. David Cox, who later became an elder with The Peoples Church, was one who made his decision for Christ at that time. In September 2000, David spoke to me personally about the great change the Lord had brought upon his life as a result of attending that 1994 Huntley Street crusade.

The idea for the Huntley Street Crusade was initiated in November 1993, when I suggested to David Mainse that one evangelist appear on his program in each of the twelve months over the next year, beginning in January. This was an exciting time. It was decided that four of Billy Graham's evangelists would make appearances. They were Dr. Akbar Abdul-Haqq, Dr. Ralph Bell, Dr. Howard Jones, Dr. Barry Moore, an evangelist I had known for sixty years, and me—I was the first. Brutally stormy weather that week helped to ensure us a large viewership across North America as people stayed indoors and watched the program.

As a biblical scholar I have always kept a keen eye on world events in light of biblical prophecy and in view of Armageddon. Armageddon was our theme of the 1980s. *Arming for Armageddon* was a book that I published during the Reagan years. Its content dealt with the stark and often terrifying realities of the nuclear arms race between the USA and the USSR. The crisis was making media headlines everywhere. The world was again holding its collective breath, awaiting any news that would stay the hand wielding the hammer and sickle.

Debates were an ongoing part of my life as a Billy Graham evangelist. I was invited to join a lively debating panel on the Canadian Broadcasting Corporation in the early 1980s. The topic before us was "Examination of Armageddon Theology." The panel included the celebrated Canadian author and CBC program host Peter Gzowski and the newspaper columnist Tom Harpur. Another prominent Canadian on the panel was an intellectually astute professor from Montreal, the distinguished Muslim woman Dr. Alvi. The Islam religion holds the belief in the coming of the Antichrist, and Dr. Alvi was an authority on this evil figure. Dr. Alvi wove brilliant postulations concerning the future and destiny of man on earth. The Muslim faith parallels the Christian faith in that it portends that there will be pestilences, earthquakes and famines. A special appearance is promised of the most demon-possessed man in all history, the Antichrist. This latter theme dominated our discussion. The world would culminate in the war to end all wars, which Dr. Alvi said could be called Armageddon.

In the 1980s another program invited me to be a panelist. This program dealt with the most controversial issues. *The Shulman Files* captivated a broad-based audience and featured the Jewish Dr. Morton Shulman, who always presented the secular point of view with alacrity. He was feisty with a sarcastic twist. He had a way of keeping viewers on the edges of their seats, wondering what he would say or perhaps even do next. On one particular panel of which I was a member was the man who flew the infamous aircraft over Hiroshima, Japan, in August 1945. He was the individual who dropped the A-bomb. You want controversy? You've got it. Our panel and the audience became inflamed at the invitation to join the pilot in the cockpit as he wrestled with the moral question of whether to actually drop the bomb, in light of its certain power to annihilate millions of unaware souls.

Then arose a moment in time when I fell under enormous personal pressure. And it was to take place on television. TVOntario invited me to a debate with the genius Dr. Linus Pauling. Dr. Pauling won the Nobel Prize in Chemistry in 1954. In 1962, he won the Nobel again, this time for his role in bringing the Nuclear Test Ban Treaty to the table. Dr. Pauling won another one for peace. I was more than slightly intimidated.

When the moment came to begin the live debate, Linus Pauling, the Jewish gentleman, entered the studio. With sweaty hands and straining eyes, I beheld the countenance of the great debater. To my great surprise and relief I found myself sitting face-to-face with and confronting a dignified elder of unquestionably soft demeanor. Amazed, I immediately detected that he effused a personal sense of grace and radiated a gentle intelligence. A pleasant discussion on the probability and effects of nuclear war ensued.

My evangelism was always on the move. Flashback to 1976 when our son Wes developed a new technique for delivering messages at the

Agape

crusades. The idea had evolved from Bill Fasig's idea. Our technique involved using a 300-slide carousel and an 8x12' movie screen stationed at the rear of the platform. The trick was to coordinate with exact precision the visual images of my slide presentation with the script that I was listening to in my ear. This was no easy feat. Either the buildings in which we held our sermons were so dark that I could not see the slides, or, conversely, too much ambient light flooded into the crusade arena, diffusing the slide images, so as to make their identification impossible.

Wes had developed split-second timing. This picked up the slack. I was able to listen to my sermon while Wes followed along, reading the script and punctuating it with the images he flashed on the screen. I was free to expound the Word of God as we again assailed the masses with our audio and visual presentations. Then Wes and I held meetings to plan our tours. Many times over the next two years we would use our technique that stemmed from Bill Fasig's original idea.

On one tour, Wes flew us in his leased Cessna 180 from Vancouver to California. From there we traveled to Toronto, then out to Jamaica, then to Georgia, and back to Toronto. We went out east to the Maritimes and finally came home again to Toronto. For two years it went on like this. We held over fifty meetings altogether.

My sermons during this time dealt with various subjects, again notably "The Signs of the Times: The Second Coming of Jesus Christ." The slides shown were dramatic. They visually illustrated the many catastrophes that were erupting around the world. There were slides of earthquakes, famines, pestilences, atrocities of all kinds, and the H-bomb. Audiences sat spellbound as Wes and I presented a pictorial showcase of what Jesus had made known in the book of The Revelation.

At "Youth Night" we provided a modern-day presentation of the story of the prodigal son. We showed slides of Yorkville in Toronto, Greenwich Village in New York, Haight Ashbury in San Francisco and Soho in London. Then we contrasted today's hedonism with Christ's ultimate sacrifice on the cross. At the invitation young people streamed to the front to give their lives to Jesus.

We tried this new approach in The Peoples Church. It was spectacular. When the headquarters of the BGEA in Minneapolis got wind of our technique they heralded it as God-given. I took our system with the

Suddenly Silenced

Billy Graham team of 400 people on a crusade to Jamaica. Again, the results were most encouraging. Wes and I discussed the recent events on our plane trips. It seemed that we were equally pleased with the results of our technological implementation.

One Sunday morning Jimmy Pattison, the third wealthiest man in Canada in the 1990s, caught a demonstration of our system in a large church in a Vancouver suburb. Wes and I had dinner with Jimmy. He was positively impressed with our method. Wes and I then flew to Fairfield, California. En route to our crusade, Wes and I almost went to heaven together. Near Eureka, California, a sudden, blinding fog engulfed us. Since Wes did not yet have his instrument rating, it seemed to me a miracle that we didn't crash. It was the Lord's will and Wes's innate "fly by intuition" skill that saved us.

Allan Trott was the commander of America's largest air force base at Fairfield. Under instructions from the Pentagon and the White House, Allan returned that week from the crisis in the Middle East. He had been aboard the world's largest airplane, the C-5. Allan relayed the terrifying story of the C-5's wheels seizing up in mid-flight and how his pilots circled for eleven hours, including an in-air refueling exercise, while waiting to land. Allan later wrote a letter to me outlining how, in desperation, he got down on his knees aboard that military mega-plane and prayed, "Father God, if there is a God and You will let me have my feet safe on mother earth again, I will respond to Your call, whatever it may be."

The next Sunday night, with Wes handling the audiovisual presentation on "The Second Coming of Jesus Christ," Allan and his family were at the crusade and in the front row. At the invitation, Allan and his family came forward and gave their lives to the Lord. Of the hundreds of decisions rendered for Christ at these meetings, Allan's was the most moving. When in Brazil, I received a beautiful letter of testimony from him. He was beginning his staff meetings each morning with prayer, because he reasoned that in such trying times as those, only the Lord could keep us on the path of His will.

In Fairfield, Wes and I had the opportunity to preach to the prison inmates at the maximum security prison where Charles Manson was incarcerated. Wes later flew us to Minneapolis in his Cessna 180. We checked into the Billy Graham headquarters chapel, where 400 workers and leaders were assembled to witness our new method of presenting the gospel.

In Mason City, Iowa, we held another of our Mid-Western crusades. Cathy Wood, secretary to Sterling Huston of the BGEA, told me that this crusade featured the distinguished Mike Fischer, who was converted at one of our previous John Wesley White crusades in Mason City. Mike was described as the finest evangelical musician in the upper midwest. He then went to Drake University and the Boston Conservatory of Music. In 1995, I had lunch with Mike. He talked to me about his personal testimony. It was so interesting and poignant that I used it at the Promise Keeper's rally in Minneapolis.

Billy Graham had appointed me to speak annually on his *Hour of Decision* radio program. In the 1970s, the *Hour of Decision* reached its peak listening audience. Five million radios worldwide were tuning in each week. This unique Christian radio program began airing in 1967. A typical outline for the *Hour of Decision* program was the Philippians 1:21 text *"For to me, to live is Christ, and to die is gain."* In creating outlines for our programs we would simplify biblical concepts into clearly identifiable points and relate them to modern-day living. An example of our outline: point one: *loving;* point two: *living;* point three: *leaving;* and point four: *levying.* The introductory fifteen minutes of each half-hour program were dedicated to setting the stage with current world events: an introduction. The remaining minutes were dedicated to the gospel response to those events. We attempted to carry the gospel messages clearly so that the listeners could easily relate the gospel's significance in their lives. It worked!

The baseball diamond outline was: first base: *hope;* second base: *holding;* third base: *whole;* and then at the plate: *home!* But this historic World Series was actually eclipsed. It was eclipsed by the single most profound testimony delivered in a decade. I present an excerpt from John Pollock's book entitled *Crusades: 20 Years with Billy Graham (1949–1969):*

> Billy took special pleasure also in the remarkable impression made at Anaheim by his brother Melvin, who spoke at a crusade for the first time. Associate evangelist John Wesley White described the occasion on the *Hour of Decision* broadcast the

following Sunday: "The most moving moment in the whole crusade for thousands, including yours truly, occurred when Billy Graham's only brother Melvin, a man of monumental modesty, younger by six years than the evangelist, took the podium, which was located directly over second base.

"He is a farmer from North Carolina. He had never been to Southern California before. He had never spoken on his world-renowned brother's platform before. As he told it, while Melvin was emerging from his teens, his elder brother was emerging as a prophet to the nation, a friend of sovereigns and presidents. Melvin felt, in his words, 'squashed and pressed down.' He avoided the public for years. But recently he had been reading in the Bible about Moses, who complained to the Lord that he had a 'slow mind and a slow tongue.' He read what the Lord said to Moses.

"The fire began to burn. He knew that he must share with others what Jesus meant to him. When he first stood to his feet at Anaheim he seemed short of breath, and some of us suspected that his knees were knocking. But when he got out the first utterances, a hush swept over that vast stadium, and many a person could not hold back the tears. How the Risen Christ spoke through this man! Some of us felt, 'If our Lord has this Spirit-filled man on the farm, whatever are we doing out preaching the gospel with such a gifted speaker around?' But many others felt, 'He's just like me.'"

Many made decisions for Christ then and there, as we learned the next day at the School of Evangelism (I was speaking at Bob Schuller's church that day). Even when his celebrated brother was preaching, some of us were still hearing the reverberations of Melvin Graham, the farmer. We identified with the saintly man and gave ourselves anew to Christ.

I invited Melvin Graham to give his moving testimony many times over the years in Canada and the U.S. Melvin Graham became the example incarnate who illustrated the reason we were preaching. He was always human and humorous. As mentioned, this was the most moving moment in the Anaheim crusade for thousands, including yours truly.

Agape

Of those twenty-nine broadcasts I made on the *Hour of Decision*, many were out-of-country programs, including those in Germany, Japan, Korea, Australia and England. Turn with me to the words of the apostle Paul, in Romans 9:1–3:

> *I say [that's verbal] the truth in Christ [that's academic], I lie not [that's moral], my conscience also bearing me witness [that's his conscience] in the Holy Ghost [that's His Spirit], That I have great heaviness [that's physical] and continual sorrow in my heart [that's emotional]. For I could wish [that's His Will] that myself [that's the entire man] were accursed [that's his eternal destiny] from Christ for my brethren.*

One of the *Hour of Decision* radio broadcast outlines was titled "Prepositions and Propositions, The Passion of Souls":

1. Above: On the Damascus Road the Spirit appeared to the apostle Paul from above.
2. About: Paul then went about taking the Word horizontally to all people.
3. Abyss: *"Knowing, therefore, the terror [the abyss] of the Lord, we persuade men* (2 Corinthians 5:11).
4. Aback: *"For the love of Christ constraineth us [aback on the cross]...he died for all"* (2 Corinthians 5:14,15).
5. Ahead: *"We are always confident, knowing that [the Second Coming is ahead] while we are at home in the body we are absent from the Lord"* (2 Corinthians 5:6).
6. Upon: Jesus said, *"But ye shall receive power, after that the Holy Ghost is come upon you: and ye shall be witnesses unto me...unto the uttermost part of the earth"* (Acts 1:8).

July 1995 was the last time that I had the honor of being featured on the *Hour of Decision*. The topic was "The Harvest." The text was based on John 4:35, *"Say not ye, There are yet four months, and then cometh harvest? behold, I say unto you, Lift up your eyes, and look on the fields; for they are white already to harvest"* (KJV).

Interminably busy, I managed to write twenty-three books during our years of continual crusading. My most popular books were: *Mission Control; Re-entry; Future Hope; Born Again; Arming for*

Suddenly Silenced

Armageddon; The Man From Krypton; The Survivors; The Mysteries of the Kingdom; Thinking The Unthinkable; Twelve Basketsful; Of Wings and Wheels; and *Where Is Wes?*

The text of my books *The Runaway* and *The Devil* were typed by Billy Graham's secretary Stephanie Wills. Stephanie is English. For thirty-five years she has worked with the Billy Graham team. In 1972 Martha Warkentin, Billy Graham's former secretary, got married. I suggested that Stephanie Wills step up to the plate. The suggestion was passed, and for the last thirty years Stephanie has proven that she is up to the task of being the personal secretary to the world's greatest evangelist. She is not only singularly dedicated to her Lord Jesus Christ, but she is the right hand to her employer Billy Graham. She consistently demonstrates brilliance and creativity. Stephanie's competence is beyond question as she brings the highest standard of proficiency to her tasks, whether great or small. I have had a great deal of contact with Stephanie. Over one-quarter of a century, my relationship with her existed through my illustrations for Billy. I have found her to be a secretary of the first order.

The Runaway was based on the life of Jesus and the best-known story in history, The Prodigal Son. I had our boys in mind as I wrote this book. The table of contents included: Squaredom; Bugged with the Straight Life; Splitting; Out of Sight; Getting with It; Hitting the Green; Almost Blowing It; Busted and Twisted; Goin' to the Devil; Coming Around; and Round Trip.

Chapters in *The Devil* are The Devil in Big Red Headlines; Before There Was a Devil; Meet Your Enemy; Tragedy in Paradise; Why Jesus Came; The Devil on Main Street; The Devil and His War Effort; The Devil's Devices; Dare to Confront the Devil; How to Checkmate the Devil; and When the Winning Begins.

Billy Graham held a crusade in Seattle, Washington, in the spring of 1976. The Agajanian brothers assisted Billy. Dennis and Danny Agajanian then joined me as I preached at a prison off the stormy coast of Washington State. I stood in for Ralph Bell. The inmates were exiled on the isolated island of Puget Sound. On this out of the way little island stood one of the two or three toughest maximum-security prisons in the United States. Even as visiting evangelists, we felt like we were in chains as we passed through the ominous blue steel gates at the entrance to the stone prison. The instructions to us were immediate. "Empty your pockets, keep only your black Bible, and enter with caution," the security guard ordered. I was a Canadian and was therefore already suspect.

The gloom of the place was smothering. Yet, as is often the case in these trying circumstances, I could feel the Holy Spirit wash over me as I ascended the platform. I stood before a crowd of 800 male prisoners, many of whom came seeking a way out of their lives of condemnation with no hope of reprieve. I sensed the wind and the fire whirling around me. My lungs expanded, my eyes focused, and my spine straightened.

It was Pentecost. Danny and Dennis Agajanian picked their guitars, perceptively softening the atmosphere. Jesus stepped in, and 200 hardcore criminals gave it up that day. These men were collared, but freed by Christ.

One prisoner, identified as Jim Bloodgood, was originally from a Chicago suburb. He was incarcerated for the heinous crime of committing multiple murders. Amazingly, Jim Bloodgood's father had been a wealthy businessman on Billy Graham's board within the little church in Garden City, Illinois; he was also on the board of Chicago's Sunshine Mission. As a baby in 1942, big Jim Bloodgood had been dedicated to Christ while resting in the arms of Billy Graham. Jim was pastored by Billy for two years.

As a teenager Jim had wandered the West Coast. He murdered one man, and then he began his killing spree. He was busted and sent into exile on the remote island of Puget Sound and condemned to forced solitude. For years Jim sat in a lonely cell and watched the hands of time slowly wind his life away.

But that day Jim watched and listened as I preached. Then, the miraculous happened. The invisible storm of the Holy Spirit stole Jim's soul, and big Jim tumbled under the spirit of conviction. He repented and believed. He prayed the sinner's prayer with me and became new. To this killer was returned his life. That's the love of Jesus.

Big Jim Bloodgood shook my hand after the service. His hand contained a filthy scrap of paper, which he handed to me in the shake. I was astounded to see that on it was a paragraph written to Billy Graham. Jim asked me if I would give it to Billy personally. The paragraph outlined how a generation ago Billy had pastored his family and

Suddenly Silenced

how today Jim had come to the Lord. I assured him that I would give Billy the note. I could feel the wetness of tears streaming down my solemn face as I turned and walked away, a free man.

After leaving the prison I met up with Billy at the hotel, where I dug the scrap of paper out of my pocket and revealed its contents. Billy stood motionless as he recalled that moment in time so long ago that he'd carried God's message to the Bloodgood family of Chicago.

In Washington State another miracle took place in the '80s. This vivid image was broadcast on every television network around the globe. In the 1980s, I held a crusade in Columbus, Georgia. Of the hundreds of decisions made, one stands out, Bruce Ellerbie's; he was a direct descendant of Charles Wesley. Later I learned that Ellerbie had lived a flagrantly unholy life. Turning forty, spiritual life had not yet begun for Bruce.

Bruce was one of the judges on the panel that decided each year's Miss America contest. His time was occupied with his many sports cars. He was a successful entrepreneur, and he would take whole pages to advertise his enterprises in national magazines, yet he was completely unfulfilled. Evenings were spent perched on a barstool, downing oysters and whiskey. He would try desperately to while away the evening, then wobble home and gulp pills in order to get through the night.

Shortly before a crusade in his city, two of Bruce's closest friends committed suicide. When one of my tracts was left at his home, Bruce read it, then took a shower and tried vicariously to wash his guilt down the drain, but to no avail. He anguished for three days and then came to the crusade.

I sensed an unusually great need of the crowd to hear the Word of salvation. I spoke from the Bible, quoting verse after verse on everyone's need to be saved. At the invitation, Bruce and his wife, Agnes, came to give their lives to Christ. It was a passionate surrender.

I ate breakfast with Bruce on succeeding mornings that week. Though he had wasted forty years of his life, Bruce was determined to invest the remainder of his days as his celebrated ancestor Charles Wesley had done, in making Christ known to others. Bruce calls me sometimes, telling me how he had heard the Word of God and was saved.

In November 1979 Dan Southern had coordinated a crusade where I preached. Hollywood movie star Steve McQueen, famous for *The*

Agape

Great Escape among other films, and his wife, Barbara, attended the crusade. Just days earlier, Steve and Barbara had privately given themselves to the faith under the counsel of a pastor on the committee of our crusade. On Sunday Steve secretly told me that he had cancer. I offered Steve Billy Graham's private phone number. Billy went to Los Angeles and while there visited Steve at his home.

When Billy and Steve met at the Los Angeles airport, Steve got into Billy's limousine. Billy told me that Steve confessed his checkered life to him. Billy gave his Bible to Steve. Led by the Holy Spirit, Billy directed Steve to Titus 1:2: *"In hope of eternal life, which God, that cannot lie, promised before the world began."* Billy double-underlined this verse.

Later that afternoon, in Ciudad Juárez, Mexico, Steve went to the hospital. He died the next day. *The Great Escape* lay in the fact that Billy's Bible lay open on Steve's chest at Titus 1:2, *"In hope of eternal life, which God, that cannot lie, promised before the world began."*

CHAPTER XIV

Richmond College

In Canada's centennial year, 1967, we began the first season of fall classes at Richmond College. Richmond College operated as a liberal arts degree-granting institution based on a document issued by the Province of Manitoba to the Association for Education and Evangelism in 1963. Billy Graham and the team visited our home for the first time, and he was convinced that it was God's will that Richmond College be constructed. In fact, the BGEA was generous and presented the $10,000 required for the down payment on the building.

In the Old Testament Elijah was the major and fiery prophet of his era. To the wicked King Ahab and from high atop Mt. Carmel he assailed the assembled masses, proclaiming the Word of the Lord: *"How long will you falter between two opinions? If the LORD is God, follow Him; but if Baal, follow him"* (1 Kings 18:21). A school of 450 prophets was established in Israel.

In the preface of my Oxford doctoral thesis I identified the first evangelists, Matthew, Mark, Luke and John, who are known as the authors of the Gospels of the first century. Jesus appointed twelve among His followers to go into all the world, and when He had called His twelve disciples to Him, He gave them the power of the gospel. The names of the twelve apostles are Peter, Andrew, James, John, James the Less, Lebbaeus, Simon, Judas, Philip, Bartholomew, Matthew, and Thomas (Matthew 10:3,4; Luke 6:14). Jesus said to His disciples, *"Go into all the world and preach the gospel to every creature"* (Mark 16:15). And they did so for the three years before the resurrection.

Suddenly Silenced

Peter from the West was a martyr and was crucified upside down. Thomas from the East was a martyr.

For historical clarification, it needs to be pointed out that one of the most enlightened evangelists and scholars of all time was Master John Wycliffe, who lived in the 14th century and was a leader of Oxford University, the primary English-speaking university in the world. He took the gospel to most of England—on foot! Wycliffe was the leader of the Lollards, who were likewise pedestrian evangelists. The Lollards were notably poor and persecuted people whose brilliant scholasticism effectually enabled them to translate the Bible from its original Hebrew, Greek and Latin into the English language of the day—an amazing accomplishment in any age.

John Harvard was an Englishman who traveled to New England in 1636. He was a Puritan, an evangelical. He was a preacher who accomplished an astounding amount of work in the Lord's service in his short thirty-one years of life. Not the least of these accomplishments was the founding of Harvard University at Cambridge, Massachusetts, when he was twenty-nine years old. Harvard was known by his slogan: "Preach the Word of God."

The second oldest university in the new world is Yale University in New Haven, Connecticut. Cotton Mather hailed from a devoutly Puritan lineage and was a preacher and scientist. He was a founder of this institution of advanced learning.

Then, in the 1730s, Tennents and Jonathan Edwards, two brothers from an evangelistic family founded a log cabin college that almost incredibly evolved into the prestigious Princeton University.

Jonathan Edwards was an accomplished scholar of twin subjects, theology and philosophy. His charisma was a catalyst to the dramatic "Great Spiritual Awakening" in those burgeoning little and independent thirteen colonies prior to the formation of the United States. Jonathan Edwards became the President of Princeton in the 1750s. In 1758, he died of small pox, a particularly disabling and painful ailment.

It was George Whitefield, a charismatic revivalist in the 1730s, whose lofty scholastic influence extended over the three prominent universities: Harvard, Yale and Princeton. No less than thirteen times did Whitefield cross the Atlantic from America to Great Britain and back again for a generation in his effort both to evangelize and to educate.

Richmond College

He propounded the Word of God with a distinctly theatrical style. History records that close friends of Whitefield's were none other than John and Charles Wesley. Interestingly, centuries ago at Oxford University there was a well-known religious fraternity who called themselves the "Holy Club," of which these men were members. Whitefield triggered the "Great Spiritual Awakening" in New England's middle colonies and in the southern colonies.

Francis Asbury was born in Birmingham, England, in 1745. He was employed as a blacksmith from 1759 to 1771. In 1759, Asbury had a dramatic conversion to Jesus Christ while under the influence of John Wesley. John Wesley suggested that Francis Asbury sail to America and journey by road to America's new frontier—the southwest—in 1771. He would evangelize and found a college under his own name. Asbury College became one of the most successful evangelical colleges in the United States. The Lord presented me with the glorious opportunity of spending during a week of revival at Asbury College in the 1960s.

Charles Finney began his work in the 1820s. This was the "Second Great Spiritual Awakening." His work and influence were so profound that he would remain the best-known evangelist in America in its first century of evangelism. Finney's classic book *Lectures on Revival* remains a must-read to this day. It was and continues to be used as an evangelistic preaching manual. Finney was the president of Oberlin College in Ohio. Interestingly, Lyman Beecher was a revivalist who founded Lane University in Cincinnati, Ohio.

William Booth was the evangelist who founded a chain of evangelistic colleges and, most recognizably, the Salvation Army. He emerged in the latter half of the 19th century and will not be written out of the pages of history. His name is spoken daily in the civilized nations of the world.

In the second half of the 19th century, it was an undeniable fact that America's greatest evangelist was uneducated in the formal sense. D.L. Moody from New England became a household name in evangelism throughout America and, of course, Great Britain. By the 1870s he had spent a third of a generation on the evangelistic campaign trail. D.L. Moody founded Chicago's Moody Bible Institute in 1886. In 1948 I enrolled at Moody Bible Institute in Chicago, and I graduated in 1950.

Terms representing Christian gatherings have evolved four times over the past 300 years. First, there was the *revival*. Then followed the *campaign* of the Civil War era. This term was used right into the second half of the 20th century. Next came Billy Graham's *crusades*. Franklin Graham has introduced a new term, *festivals*. The Moody team would hold citywide interdenominational "campaigns" throughout Britain and North America.

The brilliant evangelical scholar R.A. Torrey attended Yale University and went to Chicago to become the successor to D.L. Moody. For ten years Torrey was the foremost English-speaking evangelist in America. After his memorable reign at Moody Bible Institute, he moved to southern California to found a sister Bible school to Moody Bible Institute. This academic institution later evolved into the well-known Biola University.

By the 20th century, evangelical churches were proliferating throughout America. Yes, evangelical colleges were spawning thousands of evangelical students, which resulted in a resurgence of God's Spirit in North America.

There were hundreds of evangelicals in America who were founding colleges. Three of the best known colleges are Bob Jones University in Tennessee, John Brown University in Arkansas, and Northwestern College, founded by W.B. Riley in Minneapolis. In 1948 Riley died, and Billy Graham succeeded him as Northwestern's president from 1948 to 1951.

Six Notable Canadian Evangelists

There are six Canadian evangelists who have made an everlasting mark on the pages of history. The first is Albert Benjamin Simpson. He was born in Cavendish, Prince Edward Island. During Albert's youth, his father moved the family to Chatham, in Southwestern Ontario. Later, A.B. Simpson enrolled in Knox Presbyterian Church in Toronto prior to accepting his role of pastor at Knox Presbyterian Church in Hamilton, Ontario. In 1873, Simpson's calling took him to the largest Presbyterian Church in North America, the Louisville, Kentucky Presbyterian Church where he became the church's unforgettable pastor. His career climaxed as eight years later, he accepted his post at the Thirteenth Street Presbyterian Church in New York City. His flagship Alliance Missionary College and Seminary headquarters was in Nyack,

Richmond College

New York. But his name and his "Full Gospel" approach lives on as Simpson created a worldwide Evangelical Missionary Alliance and the Christian Alliance churches. It should be noted that Canada's Prime Minister, Stephen Harper, is a longstanding member of the Alliance in Calgary and now in Ottawa.

In 1881, A.B. Simpson developed the "Full Gospel" approach to the Scriptures. In his time of preaching Simpson wrote a prolific 70 books and the *Alliance Witness* magazine, while holding hundreds of healing services. He became a father of the Charismatic movement. Simpson preached that the gifts of the Spirit were fully operational. As a basis for his proposition he referred to Acts 1:8 which illustrates the power of God that works in the human life and the conversion experience.

The second of the great Canadian evangelists was Aimee Semple McPherson who followed A.B. Simpson's "Full Gospel" approach with her "Four Square Gospel." Oswald J. Smith spent an entire year with Aimee McPherson. That was 1928. McPherson was famous for proclaiming: Jesus Saves. Jesus heals. Jesus baptizes in the Spirit. Jesus is coming again. this was foursquare. It stuck in the minds of millions.

McPherson was born in the rural Ontario farming town of Ingersoll. The *National Post* posts: "The most influential Canadians of the 20th century (like) Tommy Douglas, and Pierre Trudeau (are memorable). Yet there was a woman who eclipsed all of these men: a Canadian preacher who reinvented American Protestantism" (*National Post*, July 24, 2007).

Aimee McPherson was decidedly a social conservative. She possessed a dynamic flare for dramatic oratory. She had the captivating combination of an angelic quality and a dramatic oratorical presence. She embodied Hollywood, before there was a Hollywood. Hollywood was Jewish. McPherson was Christian. In the 1920s she took to the radio. Her plan was to move up the radio dial captivating people for Jesus as she went. McPherson advanced fundamental Christianity wherever she could. She criss-crossed North American in her "Gospel Car", the doors of which the words "Where are you going to spend eternity?" where emblazoned.

Interestingly, when she spoke at Paul Radar's temple a thirteen-year-old Richard Milhous Nixon was in attendance. He experienced a spiritual reawakening and was converted to Jesus Christ. Nixon continued listening to McPherson on the radio and attended her services over a significant period of time. Astoundingly, those who followed the foursquare principle became a Christian denomination. McPherson's combination of the Lord's physical healing and His power of salvation brought people to her in droves. She founded the Lighthouse of International Foursquare Evangelism Bible College as well as her 5,000-seat Angeles Temples in Los Angeles.

Her Temple Bible School trained pastors, evangelists and missionairies. The college's pianist was the renowned Howard Gay. In the '30s Howard was a mentor to my brother Hugh at Trossach's Camp, inspiring Hugh to play the piano. Hugh graduated from the Royal Conservatory of Music.

The third great Canadian evangelist was Tommy Douglas. His was the "Social Gospel" In 2004, a powerful documentary on the life of Tommy Douglas aired on the Canadian Broadcasting Corporation. This enlightening program pointed out that Douglas' political stance was left-leaning, as he moved to advance socialized programs such as his famous "Medical Services for All" plan. He was really the father of Canadian socialized medicine. Yes, his was the "gospel of socialism."

In rural Saskatchewan, Premier, the Reverend Tommy Douglas had been a Member of Parliament in our riding when I was twelve years old. I remember that Douglas had the fiery oratory skill of the Baptist preacher Charles Spurgeon. My father and I would see Douglas speak in Pangman and he had us in laughter and tears.

The fourth great Canadian evangelist was Percy Crawford. Crawford was born in the 1880s. he hailed from Manitoba, not far from the birthplace of my mother, int he southwestern corner of that province. His conversion experience took place in R.A. Torey's church in Los Angeles. Motivated to bring the Word of God to his country, Crawford moved and made his sojourn to Philadelphia where he became an itinerant preacher. After graduating and establishing himself as a first-rate evangelist, he founded and was the President of King's College in Nyack, New York. In the 1960s I had a week of revival, which saw both faculty and students of King's College come to Christ.

Of interest to Kathleen and I was the curious fact that Percy Crawford had four sons. Like our sons a few years later, Percy's boys trumpeted and sang in a gospel quartet on television in 1948 during the glory days of black and white television and the pioneering days of televangelism. Their program ran coast-to-coast in America. Percy Crawford has gone to heaven now and was succeeded by the founder and President of Youth for Christ in the world, Bob Cook. Bob later became President of King's College. The Lord blessed me with the further opportunity of holding a week of meetings in the 1970s at that distinguished college.

The fifth great Canadian evangelist was Premier Bill Aberhart, who constructed his Prophetic Bible Institute for school evangelicals in the 1930s. Ernest Manning the preacher, prior to becoming Premier, headed the school for a generation. Upon Aberhart's death, Ernest Manning took over the reins of both the Alberta government and Aberhart's *National Bible Hour*, which, at its peak, had a weekly Canadian audience of 600,000.

The sixth great Canadian evangelist was Charles E. Fuller. He hailed from the Maritimes. Fuller made a monumental decision to move to California. He had a syndicated program throughout America that aired from the 1930s to the 1960s when radio was king. Charles Fuller reached millions of listeners across the country. At a time of spiritual fervor, he founded the Fuller Seminary in Pasadena, California. Fuller Seminary has graduated tens of thousands of ordained ministers and missionaries.

In the 1930s and the 1940s, "The Lutheran Hour" reached tens of thousands of homes across America. This spirit-filled radio program was the brainchild of Dr. Walter A. Maier, the great Lutheran theologian and evangelist from the St. Louis, Missouri Lutheran Synod. Maier received his Ph. D. from Harvard University and resided at Concordia University in St. Louis. Maier had cottoned on to the idea of combining scholasticism with evangelism. This one-two punch had a great appeal to young ordinants. Maier's intellectual skills were many, but he was especially gifted in preaching to the multitudes, even the nonbelievers, across America. In 1950, Dr. Walter A. Maier died of a heart attack. America mourned.

During the mid twentieth century Jerry Falwell gave his life to Christ under the preaching of Charles Fuller. Falwell's vocation lay before him like a shining light—it was evangelism. Led by the Spirit of

Suddenly Silenced

Jesus, Jerry Falwell founded a small evangelical school in Virginia that eventually grew to proportions that would make itself recognized worldwide. By the turn of the millennium Liberty University's enrollment reached 10,000 full-time students and 17,000 part-time students. Franklin Graham's two sons attended Liberty University. We were greatly blessed to have Jerry speak at Richmond College to one year's graduating class. I was doubly blessed to have had the opportunity of handing our own sons Bill and Wes their BAs following Jerry's talk. In May 2007 Jerry Falwell succumbed to congestive heart failure and lost consciousness at his desk. Later, he was pronounced dead at the hospital. Franklin Graham eloquently and passionately presided over his funeral. CNN and the Fox News Network covered this momentous event and broadcast it to the world.

Oral Roberts, the strict Pentecostal evangelist, had a television program that has run across North America each week for a generation. Oral founded Oral Roberts University in Tulsa, Oklahoma, in 1967. Today this university attracts students from all over the globe. Among the university's graduates is the TV celebrity Kathie Lee Gifford.

On March 28, 1984, Ted Cornell joined us as we flew in a private plane from Great Bend, Kansas, to Oral Roberts University in Tulsa, Oklahoma. Oral Roberts presided over a chapel of 4,800 faculty and students. He spoke on Matthew 9:35–38. Roberts was aflame—blazing in the Spirit. Ted was a classical pianist, trained at none other than New York's Julliard Conservatory of Music. Ted played the emotionally moving favorite. The students caught a buzz and gave Ted a rousing standing ovation.

After the service Ted Cornell and I ascended into President Oral Roberts' great prayer tower. It jutted from the ground, extending 300 feet into the air. It was the centerpiece of the campus. Be it known that Ted Cornell was a stoic Baptist who rarely wore his emotions on his face. But this time Ted was overcome in the Spirit. President Roberts laid hands on Ted's six foot six inch frame, and Ted fell to his knees in spiritual ecstasy. Suddenly, President Roberts laid a hand on me. For the past fifteen years, the memory of this has lingered.

Being asked to join Pat Robertson at his Regents College as dean was a distinct honor. Pat was campaigning for the presidency of the

Richmond College

United States, yet he flew me from Toronto to his college in Virginia Beach, Virginia. Pat's college was in the limelight of Christian colleges in America, and all the prospects for the school's survival and growth were most promising. Pat Robertson's CBN television network carried our *John Wesley White Program* to the United States free of charge for two years. Pat is a Solomon on his *700 Club* news program, which airs from 9 a.m. to 10 a.m. weekdays. I seldom miss Robertson's program, which deals with Christian issues from a conservative perspective.

Billy held another personal meeting with me and suggested that I become the president of Westmont College in California. Billy's board recommended Westmont College for me. It was the twin college of Wheaton in Illinois. The college's active president, Roger Voskuyl, was retiring. He was one of the team that developed the atomic bomb that ended WWII. I considered Billy's and the board members' recommendation carefully.

I thanked them all for their thoughtful and best wishes for me, but I explained that I was called to evangelism. I have been offered the presidency of many colleges over the years, yet I have always declined, based on my calling to be an evangelist. At the time each of these offers was made, the decision to turn it down was heart-rending. However, I was deeply involved in my life's work with the Billy Graham Evangelistic Association, and I felt very much a part of the team. So, in at least one sense, the offers were easy to turn down. I would accept the avocation of chancellor of Richmond College. This would not stand in the way of my God-ordained vocation as an associate evangelist with Billy Graham.

My appointment as chancellor of Richmond College began in England. During the 1950s and the 1960s I had been praying and studying. I asked God whether He was leading me to become the chancellor of Richmond College.

Elmer McVety was the first president. My brother Hugh was the second president. Following a decision to establish the college in Toronto, an extra-provincial license was obtained from the Province of Ontario in 1967. Richmond College's position was conservative evangelical. The founders of the college envisaged Richmond becoming the Canadian equivalent of Wheaton College in Chicago.

The affairs of the college were under the jurisdiction of the board of governors, a group of competent business and professional men from

Suddenly Silenced

various parts of Canada. Among these men were Chairman James Clemenger, who had been the treasurer of the Social Credit Party of Canada; Russell Wells, treasurer; Dr. Robert Thompson, M.P., Progressive Conservative Party; Hon. Walter Dinsdale, M.P., Diefenbaker Cabinet; Dr. Paul Smith, pastor, Peoples Church; Donald Reimer, trucking entrepreneur; Douglas Judson, aide to Billy Graham; Professor Rolland K. Harrison, Wycliffe College, University of Toronto; Morris Farquharson, Realtor; Allan Goheen, Realtor; Dr. James Wetheral, United Church of Canada; Reverend Marwood Patterson, Anglican evangelist; and Dr. William Virgin, physician.

The courses and programs included Division of Humanities and Languages; Division of Natural Sciences and Mathematics; and Division of Social Sciences. At convocation in 1970 there were thirty-seven graduates from Richmond College.

The Zacharias family emigrated from India to Toronto in the 1960s. The academically brilliant Zacharias sisters enrolled in Richmond College in the 1970s. Evangelist Ravi Zacharias, the world's leading apologist for evangelism, was a student at Alliance College in Nyack, New York, prior to moving to Toronto. Dr. Zacharias was featured at the Billy Graham congresses of 1983 and 1986 and most recently the Congress for Ten Thousand Evangelists in Amsterdam in July of 2000. For a third of a century, C.S. Lewis debated in the greatest debates at Oxford University. In the summer of 2000, Dr. Zacharias was involved in one of the most intense debates of the latter third of the 20th century at Oxford. The debate was a classic one on Christianity versus agnosticism.

Hugh White was the president of Richmond College in Toronto in the 1960s and 1970s. In the 1970s, Richmond College conferred honorary doctorates on many distinguished men. Included among their numbers were Sterling Huston and Ralph Bell of the Billy Graham Evangelistic Association. Leaving us in great loss, my brother-in-law and life-long friend Elmer died in 1992. I spoke at his funeral. Aside from being beloved brothers-in-law, Elmer McVety and I founded Richmond College in the 1960s.

It need hardly be said that a very emotional funeral for me was that of my eldest brother, Hugh, following his death on January 5, 2004. We were grateful that Canada's most prominent evangelist, David Mainse,

Richmond College

spoke at Hugh's funeral in Ottawa. David honored us in an acknowledgment that Elmer, Hugh and I were the three founders of Richmond College. In this regard, he announced that we had been "the roots of four notable evangelical Canadian universities."

It was at this time that after much consideration and prayer, I made the suggestion that Elmer's son Charles McVety take over the presidency of Canada Christian College, the extension of Richmond College. The presidency of Canada Christian College was then given to him. Charles obtained his PhD in St. Petersburg, Russia. I am joyful that the Lord led me to make that suggestion, for today Canada Christian College continues to expand its 1,200-person enrollment.

Recently, at an assessed cost of $10 million, the college was housed in a large and attractive building in downtown Toronto. Almost incredible to me is the fact that what took $10,000 in 1967 to establish now takes $10 million. In 2003 my facilitator, Stephen Edward Trelford, a professor of communications, was conferred a doctor of literature degree from Canada Christian College. Other recipients that year included perhaps Canada's most historic hockey icon, Paul Henderson, and the Princeton educated James Flaherty, Canada's finance minister. Likewise the Honorable David Onley, who in July was appointed by the Stephen Harper government as the new lieutenant governor of Ontario, received an honorary doctorate from Canada Christian College.

Today, Canada Christian College has evolved into a spiritual and academic degree-granting institution. It hires only evangelical and highly trained faculty. The college has graduated hundreds of students, who go into the world spreading the gospel of our Lord Jesus Christ.

For over forty years, I have spoken about Jesus Christ our Lord and Savior to hundreds of colleges and universities around the world in the clearest and most definite way that I know how. In 1964, in my first month with Billy Graham, I was invited to speak with him and T.W. Wilson at the prestigious Harvard University. After Billy had spoken on Christianity, he left the room.

A mammoth six foot six inch Muslim cornered Billy against the wall. It was Muslim against Christian. Billy's bodyguard, the powerfully built T.W. Wilson, rushed to the scene and squeezed between the two men. T.W. would call the Muslim's bluff this day as he discreetly fidgeted around in his jacket as if fondling a revolver. Now the Muslim

Suddenly Silenced

had to ask himself only one question: "Is T.W. trigger-happy?" Then T.W., in an even but easily discernable voice, said, "Take it outside, mister." T.W. had earned his salary that day.

We were in London at Gray's Inn in 1967 when Billy Graham appointed Akbar Abdul-Haqq, PhD, to team with me in a debate. The subject was Christianity versus agnosticism. The agnostics were haughty bigwigs, and we had our hands full with their attitudes. It reminded me of being at the House of Lords at Oxford. The debates there often involved faith versus rationalism.

One agnostic piped up sarcastically, referring to the distinguished scholar as "Akbar Abdul-Hack." This really ticked Abdul off. From that moment on neither I nor the less-than-dignified men of logic who were looking for time to voice their polished Oxford accents could get in a single word.

Then the time clock stopped. The debate, however one-sided it was, was over. The vote was put to the audience, and a full two-thirds applauded Dr. Akbar Abdul-Haqq. The agnostics' faces fell to the floor. They voted with their feet and left the hall. Back at the hotel when I repeated the story to Billy and the team, they erupted into volleys of laughter.

In 1968 at the University of Sydney in Australia, after two years of international flower power, the students were in a revolt, as it seemed they were everywhere. I lectured before Sydney's rebellious clan of hippies. I felt like the apostle Paul in the book of Acts, who was ignored in Athens, Greece, as he might as well have professed the Lord—mute! Sydney was a din of noise. I was heckled and ridiculed. The crowd was raucous and didn't listen to a word I said. The racket was so bad that I didn't know whether I could continue with my talk. Later, in a moment of serious inquiry, Billy asked about my meeting at the university. I just mentioned something briefly, hung my head dejectedly and flew off to my room in our hotel.

We were at the Roman Catholic University of Notre Dame in 1976. In contrast to the Sydney fiasco, I found the students there listening acutely to my lecture, which was followed by a crisp question-and-answer period. The chancellor of Notre Dame was Dr. Theodore Hesburgh. He summed up my lecture respectfully.

We were crusading at the University of Calgary in 1981 when we teamed with the popular Christian rock icon Amy Grant. I spoke to the faculty and students of the university. It was the first time that I can remember speaking to a crowd of people when not one eye was cast in my direction. You see, Amy was on stage beside me.

In 1982, I substituted for Billy Graham and addressed the faculty at Oxford University. Prior to my speaking that day, I had had an hour-long chat with the grandson of Sir Winston Churchill. I also had the most welcome opportunity of reacquainting myself with my tutor, who I had not seen in eighteen years—John Walsh.

In October 1995 I preached at a Billy and Franklin Graham crusade at Saskatchewan Place. That Friday at noon, I spoke to the faculty of the University of Saskatchewan. The topic of the day was "A Canada Divided." That weekend Canada was facing its most difficult considerations in over a century. The Francophones, it seemed, had had enough. And so had the Anglophones. It was at this time that Quebec was split right down the middle on the separatist issue. Four days later the Quebec referendum returned a squeaker vote, extolling Canada as a united nation in a 51 percent to 49 percent decision.

Of the decisions rendered for Christ at the meeting was that of professor Alan Reese. He testified it all when he stated, "I have accepted Jesus Christ personally as my Lord and Savior before, but I have not been living for Him. I want to rededicate my life to Christ—and to Canada."

I deem that my most enjoyable appearances over thirty-five years were those 477 luncheon meetings held at Rotary, Lions and Kiwanis clubs throughout Great Britain, New Zealand, Australia, South Africa, Canada, the U.S., and numerous other countries. The meetings were always attended by the cream of the crop—successful professionals and businessmen.

The meetings stand out in sharp contrast against the university lectures to sophomoric know-it-alls. The students, as would be expected, were immature liberals for the most part. The professionals and businessmen were mostly conservative. At each of the luncheons we would take the newspaper headlines of the day and marry them with the gospel of Christ in a relevant and practical way. I always loved this challenge and saw its immediate significance to the community at large.

Suddenly Silenced

I felt as though the Lord was affording me the opportunity to reach deep into the professional and business world. In this way Jesus became meaningful to men in every walk of life. Tom Bledsoe and Ted Cornell performed at the luncheons as well as at evening crusades. Other talented musicians performed at these luncheons as well.

One might imagine an academic preacher living a cloistered existence entirely removed from what we refer to as "the world." However, ever since I was a boy I had a burning passion for sports, particularly hockey, baseball, football, basketball, and track and field.

I was not only the chancellor but also the coach of Richmond College's hockey team. Three of our boys skated for Richmond team, which was part of the Evangelical Hockey League, and we traveled to Chicago and Boston for exciting games that united the White family—on ice. I drew upon my hockey experience. And as mentioned, at eighteen years of age I had been appointed vice-principal of Preeceville High School in Saskatchewan. I coached the high school hockey team there, and we won the provincial championship.

In 1974 our four boys and their cousins Don White and Doug and Charles McVety formed half of our team. We only had twelve hockey players one night. Many of our regular players had jobs and could not play. We drove together all day to Wheaton College, my alma mater, in Illinois for a big game. I had the sporting highlight of my lifetime that night. Billy Graham's eldest daughter, Gigi, and her husband, Stephan, had come to Wheaton from Milwaukee. They were sitting with the boys' proud mother, Kathleen, her three poodles, which were barking up a storm, and the Irish psychiatrist Basil Jackson. They were all beside themselves with the anxious knowledge that our boys were actually going to play in the game.

Harv Crouser, a colleague of mine, approached me just prior to the game. He was grimacing at me and said, glancing across the rink at his bench, "Are these college students, John? They're the smallest college students I've ever seen." He was seriously worried for my small son Randy and his two little cousins who were dressed to play. Harv was compelled to ask me not to play them at all.

I started to reconsider the whole thing myself. What had I gotten the boys into? Maybe Harv was right. Expressionless, I looked over to the Wheaton bench. There was Harv. He was obviously concerned.

Richmond College

With increasing nervousness, I reflected on the Wheaton alumnus, Gill Dodds, who had been a world champion indoor miler and my track coach. The college was famous for, among other things, producing fantastic athletes. The hockey team was surely no different. It was a hockey game, but I thought that I could feel an inflating football in my stomach.

That night Wheaton had some very tough-looking big guys dressed to play on their team, and I almost couldn't watch. I suspected that whatever the outcome, this would be a game that we'd always remember. I gathered up all the courage I had and shouted to Harv Crouser that we'd be all right.

He responded across the gleaming ice, "Okay, then—you'll play at your own risk." When the jeering crowd got a first look at our team their boos turned to snickers. I felt like burying my head in my hands and just going home. My heart beat like a tribal drum as it did when I was a boy riding my Royal Enfield in Pangman.

The whistle blew. It was the first face-off. The referee seemed to suspend the puck over center ice for an eternity before finally deciding to drop it. The game began.

The first shift didn't see any of our boys on the ice. I wanted to get a good look at Wheaton's team before I led my own sons to the slaughter. They sported jerseys that featured their names on the back. Kathleen had carefully stitched their names in big letters so we knew exactly who was on the ice. I winced as the first shift came back to the bench having trapped themselves in their own end.

I prayed and sent the second shift out onto the ice. This time our boys went in. Wes was at right wing; he was a comic and a laugher. Paul was at center. He had played for the junior nationals the same season that Wayne Gretzky did. Later, Paul won the scoring championship for the All-England Hockey League while working on his PhD. Little Randy was on left wing; Bill and his little cousin Donald White were on defense.

The puck was dropped again. Paul won the face-off and snapped the puck through his legs to Randy behind him. He backhanded a pass around the backboards to cousin Donald. Donald head-manned it through a Wheaton defenseman's legs to Bill, who one-handed a pinpoint pass to Wes. Wes reached behind and pulled the puck forward in

Suddenly Silenced

his skates, barely onside, and streaking like greased lightning over Wheaton's blue line, he was in full flight.

My stomach lurched as I watched Wes fly. I could barely believe what I was seeing. Wes wove in and out of the huge Wheaton wall of defense. He deked right, then left, and moved in toward the goalie.

The sound of the large Wheaton crowd rose as they stood on their feet. Wes bore down on the net. He faked a wrist shot to the roof of the net. Then, as the goalie lunged sideways, Wes let go a bullet toward the upper right-hand corner of the net. He shot! He scored! The red light flashed. So did my memories of the Toronto Maple Leafs and the unforgettable voice of Foster Hewitt.

Our bench went wild. With arms flailing around and leaping up and down, the bench hurrahed their approval to Wes. The vast Wheaton crowd fell into a muted disbelief; they were suddenly silenced. The great Wheaton team had just fallen to the White boys, their two McVety cousins and five other players.

I do not know when I have felt so proud. It was a David-and-Goliath story that played itself out through three thrilling periods that saw a final victory of our Richmond team over Wheaton by a score of 11 to 6. When the fog settled, Wes had scored five times. His speed-demon tendencies and his strong weight-trained body led the boys that day—the day the White family will never forget. This victory could not have happened at a better place or at a better time as far as I was concerned. We left Wheaton on top of the world!

That February 6, 1974, I was speaking at the chapel at Wheaton College. President Hudson Armerding introduced me to the assemblage of 2,000 faculty and students. I opened with two or three poignant jokes. Then I delved into a most sobering topic.

All at once, I heard an incredible commotion coming from the organ loft. I wondered what it was; I was in the middle of my message. The whole place had gone from being deathly silent to reverberating in a mysterious cacophony of disharmonious noise. What was going on?

The entire chapel service glanced up from their pews to the organ loft. I looked down at President Hudson Armerding. His face was as red as a beet. I guessed that he knew what was going on. It was four or five of the tough hockey players from the Wheaton team up there. They

Richmond College

were booing Richmond's coach. They were paying me back for beating them.

My message from Wheaton was being broadcast on the radio, and much of West Chicago was listening. George Beverly Shea met up with me later at the crusade, announcing that he had been listening to the chapel broadcast and had wondered what the racket was. Now I had the red face as I explained my predicament. Bev chuckled.

Later at a meal in Florida with President Armerding and Billy Graham's team at the head table, I learned that President Armerding had been in the crowd that night we had so handily defeated Wheaton. I told the story of the game. Billy was thrilled, but Dr. Armerding hated hearing it. He was a saint and a scholar, but, like Harv Crouser, he had a passion against Wheaton losing at anything. Victory was sweet.

While I'm on the topic of hockey, Mark Osborne was a Toronto Maple Leaf icon. Mark was a teenager in 1975, and his dream was to become a NHL hockey player. One day he came to one of our meetings in West Toronto. He was in tears as he listened to me speak on the topic "Life and Death." His uncle, a Presbyterian minister, had died that week. Mark came to the front and offered his life to Jesus Christ. Then his dream came true. He was selected in the first draft and was called up to the Detroit Red Wings in the National Hockey League. He was eventually traded to the New York Rangers and finally to his beloved Toronto Maple Leafs. It's amazing what Christ can do in a young man's life. Today, Mark gives back to Jesus as he joins crusades to give his testimony across North America.

Mark married a Hollywood actress named Madolyn Smith. These days, Mark, Madolyn and their children live happily in West Toronto. I pray for the Osbornes morning and night. In 1994, Mark spoke to North America when he offered his testimony on David Mainse's *100 Huntley Street*. Mark and I twinned. Mark spoke and I preached that day. The Osborne family attends our nephew Roy Sommerville's Queensway Baptist Church in Islington, Ontario. Mark is a soul winner.

I was preaching in a chapel in downtown Toronto in January 1981 to a number of professional hockey players. Among them was Ryan Walter, who was converted to Jesus Christ. Then Leighton Ford, Billy Graham's brother-in-law, stood in for Billy, who was ill at the time. Leighton preached a crusade at the Forum in Montreal that June. I traveled to Montreal to meet up with Leighton. At the crusade on Sunday morning in West Montreal I preached, and, much to my surprise, Ryan Walter of the NHL came forward to rededicate himself to Jesus Christ and to dedicate his children to the Lord. He had ensured eternal life for his family.

Interestingly, a year ago, I tuned in to the radio to hear Ryan give his testimony around the world on the Focus on the Family program. I warmed as I listened to Ryan speak of my preaching as the turning point of his life in 1981. I recalled that it was all-star Ryan Walter who scored the game-winning goal for the Montreal Canadiens over the Calgary Flames in the 1986 Stanley Cup finals. It was heaven and hockey for Ryan.

In 2006 the same Ryan Walter spoke to 6,000 men in a hockey arena at a Promise Keeper's rally in West Toronto. Ryan is now a hockey broadcaster in Vancouver. Yes, hockey has been a favorite of mine since almost as early in life as I can remember.

But another sport also enthralled me—baseball.

It was earlier in 1981. I was preaching in Florida when the former first baseman for the Philadelphia Phillies, Cal Emery, gave his life to Christ. He was brought to the service by Watson Spoelstra, the man who originated the ministry to baseball players called Baseball Chapel. I was speaking on the signs of the second coming of Christ.

In Montreal, Watson Spoelstra invited me to address the players before the all star game on July 13, 1981, in a packed chapel. Again I spoke on the signs of the second coming of Christ and on my new book, *Arming for Armageddon*. In the chapel, managers, players and assistants lined the room. The cold war was heating up again. The tensions between the U.S.A and the U.S.S.R were escalating at an alarming rate. President Ronald Reagan was coming down hard on communism.

Pierre Elliott Trudeau appeared in the doorway with Howard Cosell. They watched in silence as I, anointed and fiery, expounded at the front of the chapel. Many men were making decisions for and rededicating themselves to Jesus.

That same July, Britt Burns, the all-star pitcher for the Chicago White Sox, was in tears at our chapel at Exhibition Stadium in Toronto. He made his decision for Christ that day. His father had died of a heart attack that week. Two months later, Britt gave his personal testimony

Richmond College

at Atlanta's airport. I happened to pick up a copy of an Atlanta newspaper and turned to the sports section. I read that Britt had given a public testimony for Christ at Atlanta's International Airport.

Further on the baseball beat, at a crusade in Hastings, Nebraska, a year later in November 1982, Johnny Hopp, the famous St. Louis Cardinal first baseman during the Stan the Man Musial era, made a personal decision for the Lord as I preached.

I have ventured extensively throughout America and its ballparks and have had the privilege of hearing many great baseball broadcasters. As exciting as other baseball broadcasters may be, in my books Jerry Howarth is the best broadcaster in the game. The October 2, 2006, issue of *Maclean's* headlines supports my feelings about Jerry: "The Best Announcer in Baseball." *Maclean's* went on to say, "He [Jerry Howarth] is extremely knowledgeable about his favorite game, America's pastime—baseball." Furthermore, in August 2006 the *Toronto Star* announced that, over a generation of all sporting broadcasters—hockey, football, basketball, tennis, golf, soccer, swimming and track and field—across Canada, baseball's Jerry Howarth is the greatest. Foster Hewitt was the best of the previous generation.

Jerry and Mary Howarth have become close friends to Kathleen and me, particularly since my stroke. Jerry is a dedicated and thoughtful Christian who has visited us in our home, offering his camaraderie and conversation. Each year on my birthday, September 15, Jerry opens the broadcast across Canada with the announcement of my birthday.

When my heart stopped in March 1992, Jerry came to support me on what happened to be Kathleen's birthday, April 26. Kathleen was worried. I was told that I needed six weeks of convalescence. After those seemingly long six weeks, I held two back-to-back services in the Blue Jay chapel in the SkyDome. The first service was to the visiting Kansas City Royals. I was visited by five Kansas City Royal players. Among them was the dashing icon George Brett. He turned a ball bucket upside down and squatting on it listened as I spoke. He gazed up at me, but remained silent.

However, Tom Gordon, the rookie pitcher for the Royals, listened attentively. Then he broke into tears and made his decision for Jesus Christ. Tom had traveled from Kansas City to the Yankees, then on to

Suddenly Silenced

Philadelphia, where in 2006 he was fourth best closer in all of baseball, with thirty-four saves. The text was taken from Romans 10:9–13:

> *If you confess with your mouth the Lord Jesus and believe in your heart that God has raised Him from the dead, you will be saved. For with the heart one believes unto righteousness, and with the mouth confession is made unto salvation...For "whoever calls on the name of the LORD shall be saved."*

The second service in the chapel was to the Toronto Blue Jays. The hardball hurling Mike Timlin was converted. Outside, after I had spoken, I was approached by a big-boned, burley redhead. She strode right up to me and announced, "I'm Mike Timlin's mama. My son was converted as you preached today." Mike Timlin, from Midland, Texas, has won hundreds of games in baseball's major leagues. In Toronto on April 26, 1992, I was in the Blue Jays chapel when Joe Carter, a fervent Christian, led the ball players in for the service. I was preaching my sermon on "spiritual heart trouble."

Ten years ago, Mike delivered the mighty pitch that clinched the World Series over the Atlanta Braves. It was a moment of great suspense when the Toronto Blue Jays eclipsed the Atlanta Braves at Fulton County Stadium. The Toronto Blue Jays were elevated to that most prestigious place in baseball history. They became baseball's world champions. Mike Timlin had closed the deal, but under the prevailing pressure, that closure didn't come easily. "'When he [Mike Timlin] picked up the bunt,' said [Toronto's] manager, 'I had to wonder if Mike [Timlin, the seventh and final Toronto pitcher that fabulous night] was ever going to throw that ball'" (*Toronto Star*, October 22, 2002).

History has recorded that Mike Timlin did throw the ball, putting the wheels in motion for the much-coveted World Series trophy to traverse the international border, leaving the United States to reside in Canada. This was the toss to first that was grabbed by the same Christ-centered Joe Carter for the final out. History would also record that the very next year Joe's homerun blast in the final inning of the final game at Toronto's high flying SkyDome would send a concussion resounding around the globe, signaling a second consecutive World Series championship for the Blue Jays and for a nation of baseball fans. These patient fans, who had waited for decades, erupted into a fevered frenzy for the American pastime.

Richmond College

Mike Timlin has established himself as a fine pitcher with the division-winning St. Louis Cardinals in baseball's senior circuit—the National League. Mike was a part of three World Series winning teams: the Toronto Blue Jays, the St. Louis Cardinals and the Boston Red Sox. In 2007 Mike was still pitching for the league-leading Boston Red Sox. Yes, baseball is quite a sport.

Then there is basketball. In 1967 a pair of teenage twins made decisions for Jesus Christ while I preached a John Wesley White crusade in the Bahamas. One of the twins, Mychal Thompson, went on to be a professional basketball player. Mychal played on the Portland Blazers of the NBA and then was traded to the champion Los Angeles Lakers. Mychal took the opportunity to witness to one of the greatest basketball players of all time, Magic Johnson. Johnson tested HIV positive, and his faith no doubt has been a source of comfort to him. Mychal went on to dazzle the sports world as an all-star Christian basketball player. During television, newspaper and radio interviews he has broadcasted his love of Jesus to sports fans everywhere. Yes, basketball has held its fascinations for me.

Then there is football. In 1975, we held a John Wesley White crusade in a 12,000 seat auditorium at Notre Dame in South Bend, Indiana. There were hundreds of decisions rendered for Christ at this crusade. The chancellor, Dr. Theodore Hesburgh of Notre Dame, joined us at our prayer breakfast. Mike McMahon, the all-star quarterback and football icon from Notre Dame in the 1960s, gave his testimony at our crusade. Mike was later with the NFL's Green Bay Packers and was a hero to many.

At the invitation, Mike spotted his father coming forward. Suddenly Mike grabbed my arm. I felt like I had been hit by a big "Cat" bulldozer. Mike burst into tears and cried, "My dad is in the crowd, and he's coming up here. My dad is an alcoholic, and he's coming." Mike's dad did come forward of his own free will to the altar. This was the moment when Mike McMahon's father found Jesus. He was born again!

Five years later Mike again inspired the crowd with his testimony in Pennsylvania. This time his daughter came forward.

During the 1990s Mike was the chaplain to the championship Atlanta Braves baseball club. In 1999, Mike's son was a quarterback for the Calgary Stampeder's football club in the Canadian Football

League. His name is known across North America. That made three generations of McMahons for Christ. On June 9, 2007, with McMahon as quarterback, Mike's Toronto Argonauts defeated the Montreal Alouettes 27–13. Yes, football is a tough and interesting gridiron challenge.

Then there is water skiing. In November 1981, I was preaching in Markham, Ontario. The twenty-one-year-old world champion water skier Joel McLintock made his decision for Christ. His grandfather, who gave his life to Jesus, was a land developer who built Tyndale University just around the corner from our house in North York, Ontario.

And there is track and field. Another important sporting story sprints to mind. Long before there was any question of drug use, our son Wesley flew Ben Johnson to Montreal in the Dash 8 to perform running heats before the crowds at Olympic Stadium. A nation marveled at its upstart Olympian hopeful. On September 24, 1988, Ben Johnson had his weekend in the sun. He was proclaimed the world's fastest runner in his event, the 100-meter dash. Yes, he was king for a day. He had run in the Olympics in Seoul, Korea, and he had outrun his competition, in particular his American counterpart Carl Lewis, by an astounding margin.

Seoul's Olympic Stadium roared as Johnson's time flashed on the Jumbotron: 9.79 seconds, beating the old record of 9.83 seconds. Johnson threw up his arms as he exploded into the record books. A world's record had been set, and an icon had been raised.

Headlines on television, radio, newspapers and magazines around the world proclaimed the name of Ben Johnson. The great runner soared to become the most famous man on earth. His country, Canada, flared into celebration as Ben Johnson was decorated the fastest man alive.

Then Ben Johnson fell farther from grace, it seemed, than the Roman Empire had fallen centuries ago. There was trouble in paradise. An investigation was underway into allegations that the hero of a nation was on drugs.

The night fell on the nation as it was discovered that Ben Johnson had used an illegal performance-enhancing substance, an anabolic steroid called stanozolol, to win the race. Canada's champion racer had dashed the dreams of a country of 25 million people. It was a nation embarrassed. Sports minister Jean Charest vowed that Johnson would never again compete for Canada.

Our youngest son, Randy, and I visited the Johnson home in the east end of Toronto. We were calling on the family to offer them our reassurance and Christian comfort. We found the Johnsons glum. They were reviving themselves from the shock of what had happened. The Johnsons were perpetually inundated by the news media. Reporters swarmed their home like bees to a honeycomb. Ben's mother, Gloria, was a Jamaican Christian who loved the Lord and was in her deepest sincerity seeking the guidance of God, desperately looking for a sign. What should she do? Her son had been disgraced! She courageously accepted our comforting.

Ben's sister Dezrene was in the congregation of Peoples Church as I preached the week following Ben's infamous race. She rushed to the altar in tears. She knelt with her head back and her arms open wide as she gave herself to her Lord Jesus Christ.

That month I again spoke at the large Pentecostal church in Agincourt, Ontario. Dezrene, the spokesperson for the family, testified to "My Lord Jesus Christ." Her five-minute testimony was moving as she let out the anguish of a time and a torment that she would never forget.

In 1993, after again testing positive for steroids, Johnson was handed a lifetime suspension from track competition. It was a dismal end to an illustrious career. It would be "Big Ben" no more. In 1998, in Charlottetown, Prince Edward Island, the great speedster Ben Johnson pulled a publicity stunt. He ran against two racehorses and crossed the finish line behind his four-legged counterparts. The horse won—by about a second.

The name of the spiritually unrepentant and once renowned sprinter Ben Johnson shall surely fade in the memory of men, while the name of his converted sister Dezrene Johnson shall appear in the Book of Life as she revels in the eternal fellowship of Jesus Christ.

CHAPTER XV

Near Death

John Dillon was the coordinator for the "associate evangelist crusades" for over twenty years. Then in 1984 Grover Maughon took over as the coordinator of the associate evangelist crusades, until his death in 1999. He, a veteran coordinator, was intimately familiar with the specific requirements of the Billy Graham associate crusades over sixteen years.

In March 1992 we flew to Atlanta and then traveled over land to Newnan, Georgia, to attend Grover Maughon's wife's funeral. She had been laboring with cancer for some time and succumbed earlier that week. Martha had been an elegant woman and an author who had written bestsellers. She would be sadly missed by the at least 800 people who found their way to the First Baptist Church and her funeral. Grover did me the distinct honor of selecting me to preach at this solemn affair.

In August 1992, I flew from Toronto to Eugene, Oregon, for Grover's second wedding. His new wife was a sophisticated woman named Marcie who had lived in the fast lane until her conversion to Jesus Christ. A remarkably dedicated Christian woman, Marcie wanted all her friends and family to know the love she had for Jesus. I presided over the wedding with the parish pastor as the two, very much in love, delivered their vows. Marcie asked me to tell the gospel message to those at her wedding.

One of the twenty-five people who responded to Christ's call at the wedding was Grover's brother Robert Maughon, who was a prominent psychiatrist. As an indication of Robert's professionalism and skill, one of his patients at the time was former president Jimmy Carter. Robert had been married and divorced four times, and his family was large and scattered.

In the last year of his life Robert lived a dedicated Christian life. Just prior to his death he asked Grover if he would ask me to preach his funeral sermon. He asked also if I would explain the gospel the way I had at Grover's wedding and give an invitation call. I gratefully accepted Grover's kind invitation. Following my message seventeen people came forward, making their decisions for Christ. Among them were two of Robert's daughters, who spread themselves over the coffin, wailing prayers.

But we were all in for a shock and another service, presided over by Franklin Graham. Sadly, in 1999 Grover was instantly killed when his large vehicle suddenly spun out of control on an invisible patch of black ice. The car slid uncontrollably into oncoming traffic. Grover Maughon, our friend for a quarter of a century, was dead.

During the five years between 1984 and 1989 I held ten crusades in Alaska. Alaska has a population of only one-half million people. Yet it is geographically the largest of the fifty states.

Grover Maughon was the coordinator of our northernmost series of John Wesley White crusades. He coordinated three John Wesley White crusades. We held two of the crusades in Juneau, Alaska, in 1984 and in 1989.

At the first crusade in 1984 Mayor Joe Ceraula and his wife, Marlene, made decisions for Christ. *Decision* ran a man's testimony concerning his decision for Christ of eleven years earlier in its March 1995 issue:

> I felt as depressed as the dismal weather on the cold, gray, rainy day in Juneau, Alaska. While working as a carpenter at the peak of a wet metal roof, my feet slipped, and I sat down in full rain gear and began sliding, faster and faster, until I went over the edge and slammed onto the driveway below. I lay gasping for breath. Oliver, our golden Labrador retriever, jumped out of the pickup truck, lay down beside my head and started to lick my face. My son Shawn, who had heard the dull thud on the ground, was at my side in moments. Soon I could breathe and

Near Death

was able to sit up...[I] snapped my left elbow, split my right knee cap and stabbed hammer claws into my forehead one-quarter-inch from my right eye...One day a friend encouraged me to attend an evangelistic crusade in Juneau. I attended four of the five evening meetings of the John Wesley White crusade...I listened as Dr. White...explained truths that I had never heard. I was impressed with the man and was overwhelmed with the message of salvation that he preached. With a broken heart I walked forward on one of those evenings and asked Jesus Christ to take charge of my life. By then it was clear that my own methods for living had produced only pain, suffering, guilt, anguish, shame and rejection. My crusade counselor, a man for whom I had once worked, told me that he and his wife had been praying for me for a period of time. I cried tears of happiness and gratitude. Since becoming a Christian, I have taken another dive. This time into God's Word, and I have immersed myself in it. One of my favorite verses is *"Seek ye first the kingdom of God, and his righteousness; and all these things shall be added unto you"* (Matthew 6:33). I started attending...a Bible church...[I] became interested in Bible study. I met people who were different from those I had known before, people who cared about their fellow humans and who took the time to show it. My learning and studies led to a new awareness of who I am and who God is. I moved to the Puget Sound area [Seattle] and soon become interested in prison ministry. I found that I could relate to people who know rejection and feel as if they are outcast, because I myself have experienced it. We hold church services and bring them God's Word. I have shared my testimony many times with men and women behind bars and have shown them that there is hope when we put our trust in Jesus Christ.

We had held our Billy Graham crusade to Anchorage, Alaska, at the Sullivan Arena. With regard to my work with Billy, I was called on to perform suddenly and unexpectedly. The March 17, 1984, issue of *Christianity Today* relayed the story of one of the messages from Anchorage, Alaska, that did not go smoothly. Billy was about a quarter

Suddenly Silenced

of the way through his message when he was struck with laryngitis. He stopped, wheeled around and said, "John Wesley White will deliver the rest of the message tonight." Yes, the Lord calls us to be ready to serve.

The message was on Samson. What was I to say?

At that moment God spoke to me. My friend Glen Greenwood from the Moody Bible Institute had supplied me with an outline on the story of Samson: 1. Blinding. 2. Grinding. 3. Finding. He had prepared this outline in 1949. I told the crowd that 2,000 years ago JC died. In my message I said in a pronounced voice, "JC—Julius Caesar—died. Who cares!" Then I took a five second pause. "But, JC—Jesus Christ—died and rose again."

Everyone fell silent in a kind of shock. Then they burst out in emotion and started to cheer. I looked over at Billy, and he was signaling people to come forward at the invitation, and I spoke the words. The crowd flooded into the aisles. More were saved that night than any other night from Monday to Thursday. Later, I saw our photographs in *Christianity Today*. Billy was signaling and I was speaking.

In 1989 in Fairbanks, Alaska, as Ted Cornell sang in front of the crowd, he announced that it was brutally cold—a record breaking 71 degrees below zero Fahrenheit had chilled the state to the bone. Of those hundreds of decisions at Fairbanks, a youth came forward. He was David Majors, who was converted. In 2004, I received a letter from his father stating that David is still serving the Lord. Then following Fairbanks we were off to the hockey Arena in Anchorage. I had been in that very building five years earlier with Billy Graham. I had stepped up to the plate for Billy. Amazingly, I was speaking for Billy Graham.

I recall that a man who stood a giant six feet nine inches tall came from Fairbanks to join the crowd. He had been convicted at the Fairbanks crusade, but it wasn't until Anchorage that he made his decision for Christ. Then, in Juneau, it was Franklin's time to step up to the plate. His evangelistic debut had come.

In March 1989 what had been previously unthinkable happened. Franklin Graham, who at all times had rejected the idea of being an evangelist on the grounds that everyone would compare him to his father, finally accepted my suggestion that he make his evangelistic debut in Juneau, Alaska, at my John Wesley White crusade. Cliff Barrows, Billy Graham's partner and lifelong friend, was quoted as saying, "John Wesley White...was directly responsible for Franklin Graham's decision to take up preaching, persisting in talking to Franklin about his calling even when Franklin wasn't interested" (*Decision,* January 2006).

Who could really blame Franklin for his reluctance to preach? After all, he held the consuming notion that he must become another Billy Graham. However, the die was cast, and Grover Maughon coordinated the Juneau, Alaska, crusade in March 1989.

As it happened, Alaska's governor, the Honorable Stephen Cooper, was originally from North Carolina. On Saturday morning, March 4, Franklin's crucial moment came. He held a governor's breakfast, at which I spoke.

Dennis and Danny Agajanian were minstrel geniuses from southern California. In fact, Johnny Cash described Dennis Agajanian as the "fastest flat picking guitarist in the world." The brothers Agajanian are of Armenian descent. The youngest Agajanian brother is a successful attorney in Los Angeles, and their uncle was the kicker for the Dallas Cowboys. Another uncle was a famous Indianapolis 500 race car driver. Quite the family, wouldn't you say?

In the fall of 1975, Franklin was introduced to the affable Dennis Agajanian, and for thirty years Dennis has been Franklin's closest friend. Actually, Dennis is like a brother to Franklin.

It was John Dillon, the director of the associate evangelist crusades, who featured Dennis and Danny Agajanian. And it was John Dillon who invited the Agajanians to join the John Wesley White crusade at the baseball stadium in Tiffon, Ohio, in August 1973. Fresh in our minds was our disappointing crusade from October 22–29, 1972, in Wasco, California. So few made their ways down the aisles at our invitation that I was discouraged.

John Dillon was a master at reading people. Concerning the crusade he gingerly approached me with a hopeful word. He explained that in California the rebellious hippies were now becoming the "Jesus Movement." There was no question; John's words had the effect of comforting me. I had often prayed for the young people.

By the time we made it to Tiffon, the John Wesley White team was featuring the Agajanian brothers regularly in the crusades. They were already being featured at high school assemblies and on college campuses. These were immensely versatile musicians and brilliant songwriters. People would come in droves to hear Dennis and Danny play.

One day at noon we visited an old folks home in Tiffon. Dennis and Danny started a pickin' and a singin' that old favorite "We Don't Smoke No Marijuana in Muskokie." Those gray-haired old folk, aged now and restricted to wheelchairs, cranked up their hearing aids and pasted coke-bottle thick bifocal lenses to beady eyes. During the melody many found themselves wryly smiling and tapping out the beat with their canes and trying to clack out the words through varieties of ill-fitting false teeth. We broke up belly laughing.

The second of the Agajanians' John Wesley White crusades was in June 1974 at the university's football stadium in Modesto, California. The brothers nailed down a regular spot on the crusade team. They had dual responsibilities: a pickin' and a singin' on the crusade platform, and going around to the high schools talking about the perils of drinking and drug abuse. Interestingly, Cliff Barrows, Billy's right-hand man, is a native of Modesto, and over a quarter of a century earlier Billy had held a crusade there.

That September we were euphoric when at Santa Rosa, California, hundreds came forward at the invitation to receive the Lord Jesus Christ. Where there had been hippies, jus' truckin' along, sporting waist-long hair, roach clip hats and hookah pipes, they were now being transformed from meaningless existences into "Jesus People" whose lives had found purpose. Dennis and Danny were ideal. So we incorporated them into the John Wesley White crusades.

In 1989, Franklin had agreed to place both his feet in the preaching pool. On that Sunday in 1989, Dennis co-operated with an idea I had. We needed to increase the numbers that would attend our crusade in the arena that evening. So it came to me that if we ran a contest to win Dennis' $300 Johnny Cash-style hat, the people out there might bite. Well, the announcement about winning that hat was made, and folks lined up and then packed the place. Dennis had indeed lost his hat.

On Monday afternoon I pointed out the following Scripture to Franklin. Jesus taught His disciples at the Last Supper,

> "*I am the vine, you are the branches. He who abides in Me, and I in him, bears much fruit; for without Me you can do noth-*

ing...As the Father loved Me, I also have loved you; abide in My love...Greater love has no one than this, than to lay down one's life for his friends...You did not choose Me, but I chose you and appointed you that you should go and bear fruit, and that your fruit should remain, that whatever you ask the Father in My name He may give you. These things I command you, that you love one another" (John 15:5–17).

Recalled is the fact that the apostle Peter denied Jesus three times prior to Pentecost. Then, he was anointed with the power of the Holy Spirit. And when he preached his historic message, 3,000 souls were saved. A generation later after the death of Jesus Christ the apostle Peter explained, *"the things which now have been reported to you through those who have preached the gospel to you by the Holy Spirit sent from heaven—things which angels desire to look into"* (1 Peter 1:12).

I suggested to Franklin that, yes, admittedly after a decade as the CEO of Samaritan's Purse he was a gifted and professional speaker, always motivating people. Of necessity, the instruction was always that they "go, go, go." For a decade with Samaritan's Purse, Franklin Graham had been instructing physicians and surgeons as well as countless others to "go." Now, however, I counseled him to make a 180-degree turn as an evangelist and to always invite people to "come, come, come." Franklin's first message was on the topic "Jesus heals blind Bartimeus" (Mark 10:46–52).

Franklin was now an evangelist, who would repeat time and time again, "My sister Anne is a obstetric teacher, and I am an pediatric preacher." He is the fisherman, and his sister cleans the fish. The prophet Isaiah tells us that *"one cried to another and said: 'Holy, holy, holy is the LORD of hosts; The whole earth is full of His glory!'"* (Isaiah 6:3).

Now, as an evangelist, Franklin was inviting people to "come." He spoke the words of Jesus Christ: *"Come to Me"* (Matthew 11:28). *"Come, for all things are now ready* (Luke 14:17). *"This is the way, walk in it"* (Isaiah 30:21). *"Rise [Bartimeus], He is calling you"* (Mark 10:49). During that first sermon it was imperative that he set the pace and the routine, and so three or four times he boldly spoke the word

Suddenly Silenced

come. I wonder if that evening Franklin thought long and hard about his decision to "come," even though I suspected that he may have wanted to "go." After my hour of prayer I got up from my knees.

It was my privilege to introduce Franklin and his son William Franklin Graham IV to the pulpit that Monday. The teenage Will actually appeared in front of the crowd to offer the prayer before his father came up. He did well. It was his grandfather, then William, then Franklin to the pulpit.

When Franklin got up there he was nervous, but he was anointed. As I looked around, I was apprehensive about the crowd as Franklin spoke. Were they getting the message? It was difficult to read them.

At the invitation, the floodgates opened. They rushed the platform. I looked over and caught a glimpse of Dennis' and Danny's faces. They were beaming.

We thought wisdom the greater part of valor, so we decided to let Franklin adjust to his new role, a role to which he would increasingly adapt. Correspondingly, Juneau's radio station and only television station made the decision to spotlight Franklin. We noted that Franklin's face was starting to be recognized by people.

Once the announcements got out that Billy Graham's son was preaching, the town hall was filled to the brim every night. That Wednesday Franklin's delivery was flowing like a river. And the crowd elbowed each other out of the way to get to the front when the call was made.

Franklin talked about the key to his decision for Jesus Christ:

> "The old days, the days of drinking, smoking, and driving in the fast lane. I got sick and tired of being sick and tired. One night, in a small hotel in Jerusalem, I knelt beside my bed and asked Jesus Christ to come into my heart and to forgive me and to make me the man I ought to be."

The climax on the final evening during the crusade saw Franklin repeating his testimony of his "born again" experience in Jerusalem. The apostle Paul gave his testimony three times in the book of Acts, in chapters 9, 22 and 26. Interestingly, Billy had been converted to Christ at the age of sixteen. So Franklin relayed to the crowd the specifics of his testimony of his conversion experience in Jerusalem at the age of twenty-two. The climax of the crusade was Franklin's identification with the young people in the crowd. I recognized the positive effect that Franklin's testimony had on those youth in attendance, so I suggested that this strategy become an adopted pattern for crusades to follow.

Scores were moved to come forward at invitations throughout our crusades. But the fruit of that first crusade in Juneau was the 177 people who came forward for Jesus. Among them was a young man named Jim Livingstone. Jim worked in an office in the city borough in Auk Bay, Alaska.

In the 1950s, Billy completed a sixteen-week back-to-back crusade in New York. Then there were his ten-day crusades. I had set a less grueling pattern so that a Franklin Graham-John Wesley White crusade would be no longer than three to five days. Franklin has kept this pattern for the first seven years of crusades and the next seven years of festivals.

In witnessing the success of the Juneau crusade, I was moved to challenge Franklin Graham to make "crusading" a full 10-percent of his work. A moment came when Franklin and I knelt by the bedside in prayer. When just the right time came, I challenged Franklin. I waited for a second. Then I was ecstatic when Franklin gently turned to me with eyes wide open and simply said, "Yes!"

Away we went. We scheduled nine crusades that year. So, I conferred a plan to Grover. I had been praying day and night about how we could best serve the Lord in our Franklin Graham-John Wesley White crusades in 1989. I then set out to strategically design a crusading plan. Again, Franklin and I went to our knees, and we were answered with the insight of Scripture.

"As they ministered to the Lord, and fasted, the Holy Ghost said, Separate me Barnabas and Saul for the work whereunto I have called them. And when they had fasted and prayed, and laid their hands on them, they sent them away" (Acts 13:2,3). These two spiritual soldiers journeyed throughout Eurasia.

In the wake of all of this planning Franklin and I twinned from 1989 to 1996. *"[The proconsul] called for Barnabas and Saul, and desired to hear the word of God"* (Acts 13:7). And *"Paul and Barnabas, who, speaking to them, persuaded them to continue in the grace of God"* (Acts 13:43).

Suddenly Silenced

Yes, I had been the leader of our team. But I had worked closely with Franklin, and I could clearly see that he had the God-given gift of leadership and the calling. I became his encourager as Barnabas had been to Saul, then Paul to Barnabas. For seven years at stadiums, arenas, meetings, and rallies I would sit directly behind Franklin, gently calling out his name over and over again, "Franklin, Franklin, Franklin, Franklin," a dozen or more times while he preached until, like Barnabas, Franklin would come to realize the support that I extended to him was beneficial.

I had gone from being a wheel to a wheel within a wheel. What had been the John Wesley White crusades became the Franklin Graham-John Wesley White crusades. This was an assertive and positive shift. *"There is a friend who sticks closer than a brother"* (Proverbs 18:24). This is how I felt about Franklin. We were loyal to each other.

For these precious yet demanding times we set a pattern of activity. Seven or eight members of the team, including Tom Bledsoe, Ted Cornell, the Agajanian brothers, Franklin and me, met at 7:00 a.m. for breakfast and shared fellowship and stories. Danny Agajanian would supply a multitude of jokes. We all laughed.

From 8:30 to 9:30 am, thirty or forty of our committee members would form a prayer circle, and on our knees we would take turns offering prayers to the Lord. At 9:30, the Agajanians would visit the prisons and the schools. At noon, Franklin and I would speak at the Rotary Club, the Lions Club, and other clubs, colleges and universities. Upon leaving these locations and returning to the hotels, we'd prepare for the evening crusade. Following the crusade, the team ate and relaxed, prior to going to bed between 10:00 and 11:30 pm.

When we awoke to the next sunny morning, the headlines of Juneau's major newspaper featured Franklin's crusade, and Franklin hurried to send a copy to his mother and father. Franklin was justifiably proud. He was on top of the world—at the top of the world!

Franklin and Will flew back to the lower forty-eight. In the morning there were clear skies, but in the afternoon a sudden and terrible blizzard came up. I had to cancel our Thursday crusade.

On April 28, 1989, during a crusade in Syracuse, New York, I joined Billy for lunch in his room at the Holiday Inn. I reported the news of the Juneau, Alaska and Huron, South Dakota, crusades with enthusiasm.

Near Death

I had met Franklin Graham a few times by the time the Lausanne conference in 1974 came around. In July 1974 Kathleen, Wes, Randy and I flew to Lausanne, Switzerland, to the International Congress of Evangelism. We found ourselves crowded into a dingy, dirty little hotel room. For three nights the four of us were sleepless. Incessant pounding jackhammers broke the day, obliterating the concrete street just outside our room.

Kathleen was coming to her wits' end. She approached Franklin with our concerns. Selflessly, Franklin leapt to our aid. We moved into Palais de Beaulieu. This splendorous hotel really was a palace fit for a king. We can never adequately thank Franklin for this. Billy and Ruth's son was suddenly elevated from an acquaintance to a close friend. Yes, Franklin has remained one of our closest friends for a third of a century.

Once Franklin had had his experience in Jerusalem he was really and truly converted to Jesus Christ. Franklin knew what he must do. He made that long journey back, from doubt to belief, along his Damascus Road—from Jerusalem to Little Piney Cove. Franklin Graham, the son of Billy Graham, was born again. Paul, in 2 Corinthians, said, *"Therefore, if anyone is in Christ, he is a new creation; old things have passed away; behold, all things have become new"* (5:17).

The following summer, in 1975, Franklin introduced his new bride to Dennis and Danny Agajanian. They were to meet at Franklin's father's crusade in Lubbock, Texas. The Agajanians would perform, and Dennis was to give his testimony at this youth rally. All went according to Hoyle. Thus began the closest friendship Franklin had ever known. It's been more than thirty years since that time, and the two men have been inseparable ever since. So, it was like David and Jonathan in the Bible, or perhaps like Billy Graham and Grady Wilson—best friends.

On March 23, 1976, at Wenatchee, Washington, "The Apple Capital of the World," I held a John Wesley White crusade, and Franklin was the first to give his testimony. Franklin and Lowell Jackson drove over 200 miles in a station wagon to get to the meeting at Wenatchee from Seattle. They had to drive through a winding mountainous pass in whiteout conditions. By the time they arrived at the meeting, they were all pumped up. They'd had hours in the car together and talked about being preachers' kids. They were both the sons of evangelists. It isn't very often that one PK has the opportunity to talk to another PK about the realities of life as a preacher's kid.

Lowell Jackson, an attractive man with a distinctive personality and bass voice, graduated from Fuller Seminary before he was offered the job of master of ceremonies on our television program *Agape*. As I preached, Lowell sang with George Beverly Shea and John Innis. For three years we traveled together coast to coast, rallying for *Agape*.

By now Franklin had plenty of personal experience moving around the Third World with Dr. Bob Pierce. So it was appropriate that he give his conversion testimony and an account of his adventures in the Third World. Franklin had been anointed, and his testimony resulted in ninety-nine young people coming forward. One of those was young Billy Joe McGlassan. Billy Joe McGlassan came up to the front of the platform to receive his Lord and Savior.

Two months later I learned that he had suffered a dreadful death. Billy Joe was on a school trip as a science project to Saddle Rock Cliff in the neighboring countryside. At lunchtime Billy Joe joined his friend to eat. All of a sudden his friend's lunch bag slipped out of his hands, and Billy Joe lunged for it. Billy Joe hurtled to his death at the bottom of the cliff, to rise into everlasting life with Jesus.

In 1978 Franklin received his bachelor of arts degree from Appalachian State University, in Boone, North Carolina. Now had come the time for him to go to work. Bob Pierce had already suggested that Franklin succeed him as head of Samaritan's Purse, and Franklin was greatly anointed.

It fell to Dr. Bob Thompson, chairman of the board of Samaritan's Purse, to find the best person to head up this effort. Dr. Thompson had led the Social Credit Party of Canada to its only victory in 1962. The country had been on an electoral teeter-totter, first Liberal, then Conservative. First John Diefenbaker, then Lester Pearson. But Thompson's Social Credit Party marched right up the middle and split the vote. They won thirty seats that year, making Thompson the most powerful political figure in Canada.

In the 1960s Dr. Thompson became a charter board member of Richmond College. We talked regularly and became fast friends.

Near Death

Dr. Thompson had years of experience abroad and knew what it took. At the crucial meeting he looked around the Samaritan's Purse board and one by one eliminated the potential candidates. When he came to Franklin he stopped and said, "I see what Bob [Pierce] saw in Franklin. He's got what it takes." The board members were already applauding, and Franklin was then elected as the chairman of the board of Samaritan's Purse at the still youthful age of twenty-eight.

In 1979 Franklin Graham took his place as president and chairman of Samaritan's Purse and World Medical Mission. The brothers Lowell and Richard Furman, two brilliant, enterprising and spiritual surgeons, were called in to help organize a system whereby physicians could be sent around the world to help those in need.

In December 1979 Franklin joined the Billy Graham team for our annual spiritual renewal meeting in Callaway Gardens in Georgia. Billy asked Franklin to sit on the board of the BGEA. He was honored. Billy talked to me about Franklin's appointment to the board of Samaritan's Purse. In 1981 he asked me to join the board.

On January 10, 1982, Franklin became a minister of Jesus Christ. His father presided over the ordination. That morning I had given a particularly eloquent sermon. You see, I had a particularly warm feeling for Franklin's ordination and for the mission of Samaritan's Purse and World Medical Mission.

Franklin's ordination caught the attention of magazines, newspapers, radio stations and television stations around the world. It had been accomplished: Franklin Graham was an ordained minister of Jesus Christ. Later that day I traveled from Tempe, Arizona, to Chicago's O'Hare airport. I glanced at the front page of the *Chicago Tribune* and was astounded to see that Boone, North Carolina, was experiencing an historic deep freeze. The mercury plummeted to an almost unbelievably bone-chilling 34 degrees below zero!

For ten years Franklin Graham was the president and chairman of Samaritan's Purse, but he was no evangelist. Franklin kindly refers to me as a friend. I prayed daily prior to Franklin's ordination in 1982, *"Let us therefore come boldly to the throne of grace, that we may obtain mercy and find grace to help in time of need"* (Hebrews 4:16). For years I had been telling Franklin that I thought that God was calling him to evangelism, and after careful consideration his father deeply agreed. Billy and I also agreed that I should be the one to deliver the message to Franklin, as there are obvious difficulties when any father attempts to advise his son on an important personal issue of this nature. For a time I felt as though I were in the middle of father and son.

For ten years I had been praying day and night for Franklin. I was mild-mannered and therefore had the temperament by which I could approach Franklin, a commited leader, on such a crucial issue as his calling as an evangelist. Franklin explained again how people would always compare him to his father, and that he never wanted. I suggested that no one was implying that Franklin be a second Billy Graham, instead only that he had his own unique qualities that would serve the Lord well in evangelistic preaching crusades. I told Franklin that he could not ignore this.

I think that at first Franklin took some exception to my inference that God had told me what he should do. I met with Franklin biannually on the Samaritan's Purse board. On those occasions I took the opportunity to take Franklin aside and in private suggest to him again and again that God was calling him to preach.

In 1988 I tried another approach on Franklin. I telephoned him and told him that I would love it if he would join me on my Juneau, Alaska, crusade the following March. I suggested that each of us would preach three times. This time Franklin was convicted in the Spirit and considered my proposal. Billy and Ruth had been praying for this moment since Franklin was born. As he states in his book *Rebel with a Cause*, he would receive the calling to preach. "In the back of my mind I thought, if I do this, Juneau sounds like a good place. It's a long way from home. There's probably not much that happens way up there; the people won't be expecting too much! If I fall flat on my face, who's going to know?" Six months later Franklin got his feet wet in the deep arctic pools of evangelistic preaching.

The first of Franklin's crusades were in Juneau, Huron, and three crusades in Ohio. Bill Butters, who formerly played with the Minnesota North Stars, attended our crusade at Forest Lake, Minnesota, in the summer of 1989. In 1999, Bill was a member of the Stanley Cup champions Dallas Stars when the team moved from Minnesota to Dallas. Formerly he was a goon and a violent drunkard. But Bill was "born again." Bill's mother, their two children Troy and Tony, and his sister

Near Death

Roseanne Strum came forward to give their lives to Jesus while we preached at Forest Lake. Two years later Bill gave his testimony in the Minot Dome at our crusade there. Bill then informed us that Roseanne was overjoyed that her brother was now a wonderful Christian. Today, he is a college coach in Minnesota.

In September at our crusade in Litchfield, Minnesota, the principal of the Litchfield high school, Leo Plate, and Litchfield's pharmacist, Bill Peltier, gave their lives to Christ. Upon reaching his hotel Ted Cornell heard the ear-shattering screeching of sirens racing to the scene of a terrible accident. When he arrived at the meeting Ted informed us that a man had been killed in the accident. He had died instantly. Ironically, the message spelled it out: "Because none of us knows when death will take us!" Back at the hotel after the meeting we learned from one of his relatives that the man who had been killed had gone to the meeting but rejected Christ. On the way home this man met his fate and judgment. *"It is appointed unto men once to die, but after this the judgment"* (Hebrews 9:27).

At the end of September 1989 Billy Graham held a crusade in Little Rock, Arkansas. Here I spoke at the Billy Graham School of Evangelism before 700 ministers each day. In the evening I was seated on the platform with Governor Bill Clinton. He was seated in the front row of the platform. In 1992, Bill Clinton was elected the president of the United States.

In October 1989 the Franklin Graham-John Wesley White crusade headed for my home province. We held a crusade in Moose Jaw, Saskatchewan. Franklin was gaining confidence rapidly. We left Moose Jaw and traveled to Regina, then to Saskatoon.

In November 1989 Franklin and I took the three-hour flight from Saskatoon to Calgary in the Samaritan's Purse plane. After we had landed we rented a car and had another three-hour drive before us to Lake Louise, where Franklin and I would address 800 ministers at the Billy Graham School of Evangelism. We talked about the last nine crusades. This seemed to open lines of thought concerning the big picture—evangelism as a means of salvation for sinful man. So we discussed the biblical text that serves as a foundation for all evangelism. It is found in 2 Timothy 2:1–2: *"Thou therefore, my son, be strong in the grace that is in Christ Jesus. And the things that thou hast heard of me among many witnesses, the same commit thou to faithful men, who shall be able to teach others also."* The apostle Paul reveals God's law in Galatians 3:24: *"The law was our schoolmaster to bring us unto Christ, that we might be justified by faith."*

I told Franklin that his father had learned a great lesson at the 1949 Los Angeles Crusade, exactly forty years before. Moses brought down from the mountain with him the ten commandments of God. They were the Law then, and they are the Law today. In the 1800s John Wesley delivered his primary sermons concerning the ten commandments. Wesley's second part of his sermons concerned the grace of God. I reminded Franklin that his father has upheld those same ten commandments for the past forty years. In the '90s Billy explained, "The mantle falls to you, Franklin, to carry those same ten commandments—the same law to the world."

I brought to Franklin the text concerning the cross in 1 Corinthians 1:18: *"For the preaching of the cross is to them that perish foolishness; but unto us which are saved it is the power of God."* And 1 Corinthians 2:2: *"For I determined not to know anything among you except Jesus Christ and Him crucified."* And Matthew 11:28: *"Come unto Me [Jesus Christ], all you who labor and are heavy laden, and I will give you rest."* Also, Matthew 18:20: *"Where two or three [or one, or a hundred, or a thousand, or ten thousand] are gathered together in My Name, I am there in the midst of them."* This is the substance of the invitation and the essence of evangelism. The basis of good evangelism is broken down into three items: prayer, biblical content within a sermon, and how to receive the invitation.

Franklin and I finally had time alone. Franklin took the opportunity to ask me questions about how he was doing in his budding evangelism. I had been a veteran crusader for forty-four years, but Franklin was still a rookie and was leaning on me for advice and counsel. I encouraged Franklin by telling him that, though there were still rough spots in his preaching, he was definitely maturing and his conviction for Christ was coming through to the crowds. I reinforced this thought by telling him that he was bold in the Holy Spirit and that together he and the Spirit of Christ could one day move mountains. We discussed the details of how he could win more souls for Jesus as a preacher. I came to see that his father's wishes were being fulfilled. This was most gratifying. I could see

Near Death

on Franklin's face that my comments were hitting home. As Billy had taught me, so I taught Franklin. Then Franklin smiled and pursued other lines of personal investigation. When our discussion ended we arrived at the Billy Graham School of Evangelism. I wrote Franklin's message and organized the upcoming crusades in the west.

In 1990 it had been seventy years since Franklin's grandfather Dr. L. Nelson Bell went to China. The Bells are natives of Virginia. March 1990 saw two twin Virginian crusades. The first was in the Bells' hometown of Lexington, Virginia. This town was steeped in American historical tradition. It was here that Ruth (Bunny) Graham first gave her testimony. From 1990 to 1996 she gave her testimony many times, especially in Canada.

The television crew traveled from Boone to Lexington to tape this crusade. Franklin was appearing monthly on the John Wesley White program. My program generated a mailing list of 17,000 names. These names were added to the names already associated with Samaritan's Purse. We would hold approximately ten John Wesley White crusades across Canada annually. Franklin had a friend named Bill who was a professional television producer and taped the Franklin Graham-John Wesley White crusades regularly over the four years 1990 to 1994.

In Lexington, a burly and curly haired man named Tommy with a big deep voice, came up to me and said, "I've got to get right with God." His dad had died, and now he needed a heavenly Father. Franklin preached fervently at this crusade. He was rapidly growing as a preacher.

In the 1990s Franklin and I held a dozen crusades per year under the banner of Franklin Graham-John Wesley White Crusades. Franklin's father talked to him about the '90s and added people to assist us with our crusades. Two of these personalities on the platform were Tom Bledsoe and Ted Cornell. These men brought twenty years of experience each through three decades, the '70s, the '80s and the '90s. They joined our platform with Dennis Agajanian's band over a quarter of a century ago. In the '90s Tommy Coomes and the Praise Band were the featured performers.

In September 1990 we held a crusade in Dayton, Ohio, in an area that held 10,000. It was only half full. Franklin, now a member of his father's board, had access to the BGEA crusade crew. This would enable our crusades to increase in both quantity and quality.

Suddenly Silenced

The year 1991 arrived, and the Franklin Graham-John Wesley White crusades were in full swing. Grover Maughon became the chief coordinator of our crusades. He had eight assistant coordinators helping him. They were Hank Beukema, Lewis Blanchard, John McGregor, Sherman Barnett, Wendel Rovenstine, Danny Little, Herb McCarthy, and Bill Marti.

At the height of our success, tragedy struck. John Wesley White Junior was killed when his twin-prop plane crashed shortly after takeoff in Northern Quebec.

Wes was en route to the Arctic, where he worked with the Inuit people. For ten years Wes had been flying the big jets with Worldways of Toronto. He flew across the Atlantic and the Pacific. He also flew his private Comanche. He'd fly into the north and buy the soapstone carving of the Inuits. This was a great economic boon for a community that often knew poverty and hard times. Wes became a hero to these people. His last presentation had been to actor Paul Newman, whose Indy car had won a world-class race at the Molson Judy in Toronto that summer. Wes left his work to his wife, Sandra. Peter Durrant later relayed the message to us that in Quebec, diesel gas had filled Wes' regular internal combustion plane engine. This undoubtedly caused the crash.

Kathleen and I had met Wes at Shopsy's deli one day. Shopsy's was across from Toronto's O'Keefe Center, Canada's number one festival hall. Broadcasters, newspaper columnists, lawyers with their clients, and entertainment types would lunch over a reuben sandwich and a bowl of pickles. Wes offered the prayer, and we discussed our trip that upcoming weekend to New York. We asked him if he would fly us there. At Shopsy's Wes' eyes lit up, sparkling sky-blue like his mother's when she's excited. He said he would try, but he just might have to go instead to Cape Dorset in the upper Northwest Territories to buy a fresh supply of Inuit carvings for his Eskimo art gallery down on Queen's Quay. It was acknowledged by many to be the finest store of its kind in Canada. Currently his inventory was in short supply, so he just might have to take a rain check on the New York trip. There was, he said, the possibility that his brother Randy, also a pilot, could fly us down, provided Randy brought the plane home in time for Wes to go on up north.

Near Death

And then came that last proposal: "Dad, some of the Inuits up there are Christians, but most are not. They know you from television. How about coming up with me when you've finished those autumn crusades? You and I will just climb into the Comanche and go back up to Cape Dorset, and we'll have a crusade with the Inuits. How about it?" I agreed instantly.

Wesley would have liked to take us down in his twin Comanche and be with us in what was doubtless the largest evangelistic gathering ever to assemble in the Western world. Over one-quarter million people attended. It was also my honor to offer the invocational prayer. I was seated on the front row of the platform between the world's two foremost gospel singers, George Beverly Shea and Sandi Patti. Behind me sat Kathie Lee Gifford, who testified, and across the narrow aisle was Johnny Cash, Wes' favorite singer. He was the one who sang that infamous song titled "A Boy Named Sue." Franklin appreciated Johnny Cash too. He was particularly comforted by that Cash classic "The Orange Blossom Special," which railroaded its way all the way up to the Alaskan jukebox upon which Franklin happened to be leaning in 1970. I remember clearly that when Johnny sang I especially wished Wes had been there to see it.

Outside Shopsy's, Wes clamped on his helmet, mounted, started the motor, and turned his big Honda motorcycle around sharply. We watched him lay into a westward curve from Front Street into Yonge. He couldn't resist the temptation. He liked to lay even just a little rubber. It was his way of displaying his wheelie artistry. This would be the last time that Wes' mother and father would see him on this earth. Our last memory of Wes is technicolor sharp and blue.

During the very first moments after the news was received the White family was stunned, in shock. Time stopped; the earth stood still. I recall that spot on the driveway where we pulled in. To our right we noticed Kathleen's three sisters driving by and then backing up. The taillights seemed to be flashing blood red. Mary got out of the driver's seat and Ruth from the passenger side; at first, Jean remained in the car. None of them smiled. Their heads were bowed down. Mary came to Kathleen and Ruth to me. It was odd for Kathleen to go into the house first. They went inside, with Jean now trailing close behind.

Suddenly Silenced

Ruth, known to the family as the truth-teller, is the youngest of Kathleen's five Irish sisters. Petite and pretty, this time she looked pale and frightened, and her voice ratcheted up in pitch as she blurted, "I've got terrible news!" The anguish on her face was unspeakable.

I was totally unprepared for what was to come. "Wes was killed yesterday in his plane in Quebec!"

My head went into a dizzy whirl. I couldn't breathe. The world, as I had known it, had come to an end. I gazed at the faded pink unilock bricks in the driveway. They flamed as if coming red-hot out of the kiln, rising like fiery cannon balls, scorching me. The noonday sun seemed to descend like a star drawing too near, yet dampening darkness wrapped me in a dank shroud. My knees went rubbery; my heart leapt into my mouth. My head continued to spin as if bolted to a paint shop mixer. Was I slipping over the edge to insanity? Shafts of pain coursed through me. For a moment I thought the hammering of my heart was a massive, fatal heart attack. If so, I want to go quickly; how about right now? If Wes was gone I want to go too.

As Ruth burst into tears, I heard Kathleen inside the house shriek to her soft-spoken sister Mary, "Where is he? What hospital is he in?"

I wandered around like a zombie. Wes was everywhere. There were those moments when the mind would find its way back to certain vivid remembrances and time would disappear into recollection. Wes had ridden, driven, or walked through that corner of our driveway perhaps ten thousand times. And it was the spot from which as a teenager he perfected his hockey slap shot, which terrorized goalies from Toronto to Boston to Chicago to St. Petersburg, Florida.

This was the moment that I crossed from middle age into old age. Former prime minister Pierre Elliott Trudeau spoke of losing his son Michel, who was swallowed up in an avalanche in British Columbia on November 13, 2000. Trudeau exclaimed that at the time of his son's death he was a young seventy-nine. But he became an old eighty! September 28 is a date that will stick with me for as long as I live. It is a date of twin tragedies. Our beloved son John Wesley White Jr. perished at exactly 3:10 p.m. when his twin-prop plane crashed in northern Quebec on September 28, 1991. Our family mourns. Pierre Elliott Trudeau perished at exactly 3:10 p.m. when he succumbed to death on September 28, 2000, in Montreal, Quebec. Our country mourns.

Then came October 3, 1991, and with it Wes' funeral. Franklin Graham presided over the solemn occasion, and he chose Psalm 23. Sandra, Mr. and Mrs. Frank Duff, Kathleen and I had made the arrangements. He has been a close friend of our family for thirty years. So when we called, he said he would come any time, day or night, and even if he had another engagement, he would cancel it and come.

And with Franklin would come Dennis Agajanian, all the way from San Diego at his own expense. He'd sing Wes' favorite song, "Nothing but the Blood":

What can wash away my sin?
Nothing but the blood of Jesus.
What can make me whole again?
Nothing but the blood of Jesus.
(Robert Lowry, 1876)

In all our crusades since Wes' funeral, Dennis has sung that song and dedicated it to Wes' memory. And if it moves the crowds as much as it has moved me for years, then I feel the Lord may have Dennis sing that one before the hosts of heaven in eternity. Maybe I'll request it!

Then came the crowds of people, well-wishers of every description. Family, friends and the Billy Graham family descended upon us like doves. Wes' funeral was held at The Peoples Church, traditionally known as Canada's largest Protestant congregation.

Franklin and Dennis spent most of their time with Kathleen. "Why, Franklin, do you—and why did Wes—have this seemingly irrepressible urge to fly?" she asked.

"Because" replied Franklin with the utmost of empathy, "it's in your blood. You're like a human bird. When you take off and ascend into the sky, that's where you really feel free! A real pilot is someone who just has to fly."

Every time since when Kathleen has seen Franklin, she asks him the same question. And he gives her the same answer. It's a cyclic conversation that will perhaps go on for years to come. And it's as regular as clockwork. But it's therapeutic. Each time she and Franklin have that verbal exchange, she tells each of her sisters on the telephone.

In a letter to Kathleen and I dated October 4, 1991, John Wesley White Jr. was remembered "In deepest sympathy and with my prayers":

Suddenly Silenced

Several weeks ago I watched a [CTV network] documentary report on Wesley's work with the people of Canada's north. The phrase "They trusted him" impressed me. I didn't realize at the time Wes was your son, but I know I admired the wonderful relationship he had with those dear people. You certainly gave Wesley a tremendous legacy, which enabled him to be trusted by the natives, who have often seen betrayal as a way of life. May the knowledge that in his short life he touched the lives of many with God's love, by giving them a purpose in life, give you strength and peace during your time of sorrow.
God bless and keep you.
Most sincerely,
Bonnie Booth
Toronto, Ontario

After the funeral I was due to start a large, area-wide crusade in Tucson, Arizona. On the Saturday two days after the funeral, we had a family discussion. Paul had to return the next week to Baylor University in Texas, Bill the next month to Thailand, and Randy was off to fly in the north. Should I leave the family home too? Should I go to Tucson?

We decided I should. That's what Wes would have wished. He believed totally in what I was doing. I felt about as much like going as Jonah felt initially about going to Nineveh. But Kathleen had her sisters and two of the boys. I delayed one day, but that sad, sad Sunday the planes on which I flew seemed to be going the speed of an early nineteenth century wagon train.

Alone I would brood. Kathleen would cry. All the while she would kiss the various pictures of Wes, and I would hear her saying over and over again, "My son, Wesley! My son, Wesley!" Since Wes' death this haunting reprise has been the theme of Kathleen's evening prayers.

Kathleen's best comforts were the Lord and her three Irish sisters. They feathered our nest every day for weeks.

We had eight days of crusading at the arena in Tucson. I took the first half, and Franklin took the second half. I was seated forlorn and alone in a row of seats before I was to preach. Earlier that dreadful Sunday I called Billy's pastor, Calvin Thielman, for some moral sup-

Near Death

port. I could hear the shock in Calvin's voice, and he exclaimed, "My three boys live. Your boy Wes is in heaven." Through his sobs Calvin compassionately suggested that the text in my message that night should be John 3:16. He summed it all up. "We know what you're going through, but nobody knows like God the Father. He gave His only begotten Son, so He knows."

"For God so loved the world, that he gave his only begotten Son, that whosoever believeth in him should not perish, but have everlasting life" (John 3:16). I felt the Lord assuring me that this was the right message for that night. It would be John 3:16! What did God the Father give when He sent His only begotten Son? For the first time in the fifty years I had been delivering this text, I really understood the pain that the Father (God) had for His crucified Son (Jesus). I was Wes' father, and he was his father's son.

There were hundreds of decisions made for Christ in the 9,000-seat arena that week, but one stands out in my mind. It was that of the sheriff of Tucson, who had 1,100 officers under him. He came up to me later that week and said, "Your sermon on John 3:16—I have been able to think of nothing else all week. It has had an enormous impact on me personally. Your ministry to the people during this time of bereavement has profoundly touched me."

Franklin took his message from the prophet Daniel, who had dreamed the dream the Lord had given him: "Then was the part of the hand sent from him; and this writing was written...*This is the interpretation of the thing...God hath numbered thy kingdom, and finished it...Thou art weighed in the balances, and art found wanting"* (Daniel 5:24-27). Franklin's message was a message of judgment concerning death and procrastination. He said, "Come to the Lord before it's too late."

The second memorable decision of the week was that of a rich and powerful Jewish man name Bernard Rubin. He was a real estate tycoon from New York City who had been traveling around the United States. He reminded the wary listeners of the story of Belshazzar, who waited too long to make his decision for the Lord and in the night perished among his earthly delights. And a historic kingdom crumbled! Bernard Rubin was killed a week later as he was crossing the street in Tucson. A speeding car struck him down. But he had made his decision for Christ.

Suddenly Silenced

Kathleen and I continued on to Yuma, Arizona, for another crusade that ran into early November. From there we traveled to the Imperial Valley in Southern California. In late November, we crossed the continent again to a crusade in Wilkes Barre, Pennsylvania

Then, on December 27, Kathleen and I flew into the USSR. At the stroke of midnight on December 31, the U.S.S.R officially became Russia. Anatoly Sobchak, a professor at the University of St. Petersburg and the mayor of the city of St. Petersburg, was in attendance at the historic pre-revolution Opera House as I preached. Sobchak was a mentor to his protégé Vladimir Putin. In March 2000, Vladimir Putin was elected president of the largest country in the world, Russia.

It was 1991. Even with Wes' death so fresh in my mind, I couldn't help but be amazed at the inarguable fact that I was now preaching in the historic Opera House in downtown St. Petersburg. Until very recently this was the seedbed of Communism in the world. I was anointed and delivered a sermon for the ages. I again assailed John 3:16. I preached to fresh ears and unreborn souls. *"They gave to me...the right hands of fellowship"* (Galatians 2:9). They came for two or three hours to shake hands as I sobbed through the enormous blessing of the Lord.

Kathleen and I returned to Toronto from St. Petersburg, Russia. We spent two months grieving the death of our son Wesley. Then we moved on. We departed Toronto for a Bible conference in Florida. Following the conference I preached a funeral in Atlanta for Martha Mahon, Grover's first wife. Then Kathleen and I returned home to Toronto.

I was about to appear on Peoples Church TV and was quickly descending the stairs of my home when suddenly it felt like an elephant was standing on my chest. I dropped to the floor in the library. Kathleen shrieked. Our sons Paul and Randy called in our next-door neighbor Lloyd Nesbitt, who was a podiatrist. He had nothing to do with cardiology, so he phoned for an ambulance. Only scant months after Wes died I was rushed in a screaming ambulance to North York General Hospital near my home.

Electric paddles were clamped onto my chest, and volts of electricity surged through my heart. TPA clot dissolver was injected, and I was snatched from the jaws of death. Through the blaring din of noise and strange separating mist, I considered the sermon I had prepared. It was on heaven and was crafted from my vivid recollections of Wes' death. I found comfort in thinking about that now, as I lay supine and totally powerless. I felt close to God, the true caregiver, as they worked on me. Doctor Richard James later informed me that my heart had stopped. I was five minutes from being brain dead, something some people think actually happened!

I wondered what my good friend and colleague Franklin Graham would do if I were out of commission for any time at all. God was taking care of that too. Grover had called Franklin, asking him to take over our crusade in Eugene, Oregon.

Franklin was with Dennis Agajanian in India at the time and later recounted that he wondered how on earth he would fulfill his duties for Samaritan's Purse and take over for me at the crusade too. Franklin did the right thing; he took his problem to the Lord, and he got his message from heaven. As Franklin wrote in *Rebel with a Cause:*

> I was feeling broken inside. "Lord, You blessed me with the leadership of Samaritan's Purse. I've tried to be faithful to You all these years. If I have sinned, forgive me. You have given me life. You can do with me as You see fit, I am Yours…I will not quit preaching the gospel. Give me the strength to deliver Your Word for the spiritual battle that will rage in the arena tonight. And Lord be with John. If it be Your will, give him a complete and full recovery."

Franklin flew to Eugene, Oregon, to stand in for me at the Franklin Graham-John Wesley White crusades, and I am ever grateful to him for that. Franklin received further blessing from the Lord as people streamed down the aisles giving their lives to Jesus. As stated in *Rebel with a Cause,* he heard the Lord say, "Be faithful to Me, I will take care of the rest and will give you strength for the task." He thought of Isaiah 59:19: *"When the enemy shall come in like a flood, the Spirit of the LORD shall lift up a standard against him."*

It was only six weeks later when I rejoined the Franklin Graham-John Wesley White crusades. I was still weak, but raring to go. We held five crusades from March to July.

During the period from July 12 to 19, 1992, three crucial events took place. On July 14, Franklin Graham turned forty; that night we packed the stadium at Arvada, Colorado. Wendel Rovenstine, the coordinator of the crusade, introduced Bill McCartney, the founder of Promise Keepers' rallies, to Franklin and me. In addition to this great responsibility, Bill is also the head coach of the University of Colorado's football team. Three years later, on June 30, 1995, at a Promise Keepers' rally in Indianapolis, Indiana, Franklin Graham preached before 71,000 men. Thus began Franklin's Promise Keeper's rallies, which have been attended by hundreds of thousands over the past years. As it happened, I spoke at the Minneapolis Metrodome before 61,000 men that July.

That Thursday Ricky Skaggs was scheduled to perform. But his bus had an accident in the mountains en route from California to Denver. His guitar was on that bus. Wendell Rovenstine introduced me to Ricky. I cajoled Ricky into giving a thirty-five-minute personal testimony, which grabbed the crowds right where it counted—in the heart.

Then Melvin Graham ascended the platform to give a short testimony. Since the 1980s, Billy Graham's nephew Mel Graham Jr. has remained a close friend of mine. He is an enormously successful real estate businessman and has a heart that equals his wealth in size. Mel once called our youngest son Randy a "rock star."

Additionally, Catherine McElroy's husband sat with us. Catherine McElroy is Billy Graham's sister. That Thursday night I was especially anointed. It was a great blessing to have Ricky Skaggs connected to Franklin Graham.

In September 1992 in Fredericton, New Brunswick, we held a Franklin Graham-John Wesley White crusade. There were hundreds of decisions made for Christ here. One of those rises out of the sands of memory above all the others. It was the story of a beautiful and talented young girl in high school. She made her decision for faith on a Wednesday evening. Katie Dawn White became the head of the high school Christian Fellowship. She held morning prayer meetings with her fellow students and always led an exemplary life. She was unquestionably popular and sweet. She came from a prosperous farm five miles from town. Perhaps the greatest of Katie's testaments in life was the winning of many of her high school friends to Jesus Christ.

Then tragically, one Saturday morning twenty months later, Katie was killed in a freak farm accident. She slipped and toppled down

Near Death

about thirty feet in a haystack to the cement floor of the barn. They rushed her, unconscious, to the hospital. She lay in a coma for four hours before she was pronounced dead of a brain aneurysm. It was a tragedy in rural Canada.

Katie's family belonged to a small Baptist church, which was packed to the rafters the day of her funeral. They formed lines inside and outside and upstairs and downstairs. Seven hundred people came to mourn the intelligent and pretty girl that they so admired. Many students were so moved that they rededicated their lives to Jesus Christ right at the service. Katie Dawn White made the headlines of the four Maritime province's leading newspapers, and a feature film was made about her life. It was simply titled *Katie Dawn White*. I made special mention of this somber event on our television program. In August 1994 I was featured on the *Hour of Decision* radio program and told the world about Katie Dawn White.

April 24 to May 1, 1994, we held a Franklin Graham-John Wesley White crusade in Charleston, West Virginia. I preached the first half from Saturday to Wednesday, and Franklin preached the second, half from Thursday to Sunday. Franklin's father joined us at our crusade. He was just returning from delivering the funeral address for Richard Milhous Nixon. Four former presidents attended this funeral: Gerald Ford, Jimmy Carter, Ronald Reagan and George Bush. The then president, Bill Clinton, likewise attended.

At the meeting I had the privilege of sitting between father and son—Billy and Franklin Graham. The stadium that held 12,000 had standing room only. Franklin became very nervous, because he had always been afraid of being compared to his father, and here he was about to preach right in front of him. It's hard enough being an evangelist without having to be an evangelist in front of your own family!

One particular night in Charleston before the meeting, in a room to the side of the stadium, I recall that Billy, Franklin and I were inundated with reporters from various newspapers and local radio and television stations. They had been following Nixon's funeral and wanted to probe the event further. In addition to this, the reporters wanted to know about Billy's health and his ability to carry on as CEO of the BGEA.

In January 2006, a tragic mining accident in Charleston, West Virginia, made world headlines. Thirteen men were trapped under-

Suddenly Silenced

ground as one of the Seco mines collapsed. Twelve men lost their lives, and one single man named McCloy survived. Any number of those thirteen men perhaps attended our crusade.

In 1995 we held eleven crusades in all. Franklin's first five years as an evangelist were spent gaining experience with the Franklin Graham-John Wesley White crusades. Franklin gained much experience also through his ongoing preaching assignments at the Promise Keepers' rallies.

Returning to Toronto that June, Billy Graham delivered his crusade at the SkyDome. At noon on Tuesday before he was scheduled to preach he fainted on the platform. All of us on the platform went into shock. We called for an ambulance, and Billy was rushed to hospital. It was discovered that Billy was bleeding from the colon.

I telephoned Ruth Graham, who made Franklin very anxious to learn of Billy's hospitalization. I then contacted Franklin immediately to let him know that Billy was in the hospital. He and his sister Anne flew to Toronto. But the committee decision was to replace Billy with Franklin, not another much qualified associate evangelist, Dr. Ralph Bell.

In 1995 Franklin and his father had much business of a practical nature to consider. Billy was getting older and was getting considerably weaker every year. But Franklin had a profound understanding of his father's desire to deliver the gospel for as long as he could. Franklin wanted to be a support for his father, and he felt that it was perhaps time to face his own deepest fear. Franklin began preparing himself to share the pulpit with his father.

The crusade committee in Saskatoon invited Franklin and his father to crusade there. On a Sunday in October 1995, Franklin and Billy set an all-time record for the number of people turning out to a single crusade. The crusade was held at the indoor stadium at Saskatchewan Place, and 20,000 people packed the house. They were wall to wall and overflowed into the outdoor seating area.

On November 7, 1995, Franklin Graham was by unanimous decision voted in as the leader of the BGEA when his father, after a long lifetime of service, decided to step aside. This was Franklin's great honor, and his father was well pleased. Franklin was the first vice-chair of the BGEA. Billy said, "Franklin was selected by the board of direc-

Near Death

tors to be the first vice chairman; and as a father, I am both proud of his capacity for leadership and humbled in gratitude for the Lord's blessing on him" (*Decision*, February 1996). As of November 2000, Franklin is the chief executive officer.

Franklin and Billy joined the other 400 members of the BGEA team in Fort Lauderdale, Florida. Here Billy made the formal announcement of Franklin's appointment as first vice-chair of the BGEA. With great joy in our hearts Franklin and I gave a detailed account of the previous five years and sixty meetings of the Franklin Graham-John Wesley White crusades. In the Church of Antioch the evangelists Paul and Barnabas were anointed in the Holy Spirit and went out into Asia and Europe, as written in Acts 13. Franklin and I were at the team meeting when it was decided that Franklin would take over his father's itinerary, which included a trip to Australia in the new year, 1996. Then we retraced the footsteps of Paul and Barnabas. We went to the church of Jerusalem.

When Franklin was elected first vice-chair of the Billy Graham Evangelistic Association, he was in the midst of many projects through the work of Samaritan's Purse and World Medical Mission. He was also busy preaching at crusades, like the one he was about to preach at in Australia the next month. Franklin invited me to assist him in writing the illustrations for the festival.

A Franklin Graham-John Wesley White crusade had been planned in West Toronto in March 1996. However, Billy Graham had been confined to his home for the previous six months due to debilitating health problems. Franklin was called to stand in for his father for four festivals in Australia. This was a terrific opportunity to expand his worldwide evangelism. He would preach in Sydney, Cairns, Townsville and Brisbane.

Dr. Ralph Bell was called in as a substitute for Franklin. Now it was the John Wesley White-Ralph Bell crusade in West Toronto. This crusade lasted nine days. During this crusade I was suddenly called away to be with Franklin. I packed in a hurry and flew to Australia.

We returned to Brisbane to the Royal Agriculture and Industrial Association, Australia's largest showgrounds, where in 1967 I had preached five days and Billy preached three days. I had a funny feeling. This part of the world looked exactly the same to me as it did years

Suddenly Silenced

ago, but it was somehow different this time. For one thing, crusades were now referred to as festivals, and there was a greater appeal to the young people than there used to be. This set the stage. Christians were schooled in "Christian Life and Witness" classes. Four hundred homes were visited, gathering food for the needy. Two thousand volunteers and 700 churches worked in unison preparing for Festival '96.

Rob Adsett, the executive chairman of the evangelistic festival, spoke to the unity of the churches. He declared, "I've never been involved in anything with such trust and unity. The Australian media are rough on evangelists, but when Franklin Graham held a press conference, every television channel and newspaper was here. They liked him. I think that's because of the unity."

Thursday night was a dedication meeting, and I preached. The chairman of the festival, Dr. Peter Hollingworth, presided. Seven thousand dedicated themselves to Jesus that night as I spoke. I was greatly anointed. I could feel the Holy Spirit descend upon me and lift me up and bring God's Holy Word.

I spoke about Matthew 9:35–38. My first point was a "Complete Communication." What is it we are trying to do and say? We read, *"And Jesus went about all the cities and villages, teaching in their synagogues, and preaching the gospel of the kingdom, and healing every sickness and every disease among the people"* (Matthew 9:35).

The second point in this message was a" Commiserate Company." *"When [Jesus] saw the multitudes, he was moved with compassion on them, because they fainted, and were scattered abroad, as sheep having no shepherd"* (Matthew 9:36). As with "Complete Communication" He looked at this "Commiserate Company" of wayward wandering people, we read, He was moved with "Compelling Compassion" on them. The word *compassion* comes from the Latin and means "to feel pity," from *com*, "together," and *pati*, "to suffer." So compassion means "to suffer with"; to love someone so much that you crave to absorb his or her suffering in yourself.

Point four was "Commanded Communion." Jesus gave His disciples this point from which to begin: *"Pray ye therefore"* (Matthew 9:38). It was not a possible option but a positive opportunity. Indeed, it was more. It was a commanded communion.

Point five was the "Committed Commission" that Jesus advanced.

Near Death

"The harvest truly is plenteous, but the labourers are few; Pray ye therefore the Lord of the harvest, that he will send forth labourers into his harvest" (Matthew 9:37–38).

Seven thousand Christian counselors, choir members and stewards were anointed, instructed, and enabled to assist with those who would make inquiries at the invitation. Archbishop Peter Hollingworth turned to me during the benediction and declared, "Dr. White, your message tonight was good Anglican biblical theology." This first night had been dynamic and had successfully set the stage for Franklin's Friday night extravaganza.

Friday night the showgrounds filled with 25,000 young people. The people of this city also beheld an enormous spectacle of fireworks. Their ears were flooded with popular Christian music. They were inundated with relevant and heart-filled testimonies. And a spellbinding message by Franklin Graham led them to the Lord. Over 1,000 people responded to the invitation.

Franklin exhorted, "God has forgiven me. I don't deserve it, because I have broken God's laws. Tonight I'm talking about coming to Jesus Christ, God's Son, by faith. You need to say to Almighty God, 'I have sinned, and I want to know that I'm forgiven, that I'll go to heaven for eternity.' God is offering a pardon to all of us if we are willing to believe that Jesus Christ died for our sins." Even young girls fell under the spell of the Holy Spirit. A seventeen-year-old girl wailed, "I've had an abortion; will I get my baby back when I get to heaven?"

In the mornings, as a part of Franklin's team, before many of his Australian friends I preached a series of seven messages from the text of 1 Timothy 2:1: *"Supplications, prayers, intercessions, and giving of thanks."* Worship, adoration, grace, glorification, and benediction provided other substance for my morning messages.

Brisbane and the entire Australian Festival 96 was an enormous blessing. The message was carried, spoken and received. God was present in Brisbane and in Australia, and He chose to move his great hand upon the masses.

Upon returning to Toronto in March, I was quoted from my book *Where Is Wes?* "One of the greatest joys of this servant of Jesus is to share in the crusades with Franklin Graham—the most recent series being in Australia. This year alone, God willing, Franklin will be

Suddenly Silenced

addressing, face-to-face, one half million people scattered throughout two hemispheres."

That April I resumed taping my television program. The substance of my series on the *John Wesley White Television Program* was taken from the format that I had used in my messages at the Australian festival. There were nine programs in all. They were broadcast three times each Sunday, afternoon, evening and midnight, beginning May 5 and running into July. My program had been broadcast for a quarter of a century.

The last of this series, which ran 4,000 miles across Canada, was viewed by over one million people each week. The sad irony was that I was confined to a bed and viewed this series from the Queen Elizabeth Hospital. In the hospital, I was propped up on plump pillows. I could speak only one word—Jesus. I watched myself on TV delivering the message under the power of the Holy Spirit and could feel the cinders of a past lifetime still smoldering. But I was reduced to the silence of the stroke and the cold foreboding hospital room. I cried!

April 28, 1996, was the day the preaching stopped. Fifty-two years of evangelizing ended. I was suddenly stricken with a devastating stroke.

For fifty-two years of my life I had given the invitation while the choir sang "Just As I Am." But late in the dark night before, I was suddenly overwhelmed—struck with a dumbfounding thought. "I shall ask the choir to sing "I Surrender All" at the invitation tomorrow evening." The next evening, the last evening, the choir cast their haunting voices upon the crowd. They sang "I Surrender All" just as I had envisaged:

> All to Jesus I surrender;
> All to Him I freely give;
> I will ever love and trust Him,
> In His presence daily live.
> I surrender all, I surrender all,
> All to Thee, my blessed Savior,
> I surrender all.
> (Judson W. Van DeVenter, 1896)

Today, I get chills running up and down my spine as I think of that moment. This song has been my theme song since that fateful day, April 28, 1996, the day the preaching stopped!

Near Death

Scores of people came streaming out of the bleachers and onto the gym floor. The first man who came forward said that he had been convicted of a sin. "I want to ask God to forgive me and to take the sin out of my life," he said. He prayed to receive Christ (*Decision*, July 1996). This man was a surgeon, Dr. Mark Patterson from Greeneville Memorial Hospital. His son, also a skillful surgeon, was on the crusade committee. This man had counseled me not to preach that night due to my health.

Dr. Patterson Sr. was an alcoholic who had been snared by the beckoning gleam of the social elite. But now he was dizzy and disillusioned and was the first person to come to the front to Christ. Kathleen informed me later that his son had been in tears when his father came forward. The younger Patterson at that moment was torn in two. He was overcome with the joy of knowing that his father was one day going to join him in heaven but was despairing about that fact that I had suddenly fallen to a severe stroke.

Kathleen found me in our hotel room staring into the dark void. I could no longer respond to the external world. I was entombed in my body. My face was askew and my arm and leg dangled limp. My brain had given way to a paralyzing stroke. The left side of my brain burned out.

At 11:34 p.m., the sobbing Kathleen made that phone call. "Send an ambulance quickly," she screamed. "I think my husband is dead." Yet, I lived! Death had been staved off. The doctors must have met us at the emergency entrance. I must have been rolled into the operating room. They must have hooked me up to the various machines. An oxygen mask must have been placed on my face. I must not have been conscious for any of this.

In hospital I began the sojourn up the long, thin tunnel toward consciousness. I fought to return to the world I had been jolted out of. Darkness gradually gave way to an opaque light, and the deafening silence of a mute world began permitting a smattering of indiscernible auditory fragments into what was left of my frazzled brain.

The first biblical passage of my new life made it through the previously impenetrable vault of my mind. It was Psalm 39:10: *"Remove thy stroke away from me: I am consumed by the blow of thine hand."*

In May 1996, John Pollock, a Cambridge scholar and the premier evangelical biographer of Billy Graham's, wrote me a letter. In it he spelled out his thoughts and feelings concerning my stroke. John Pollock spoke of God's providence. Franklin Graham must now carry on God's good work in bringing the gospel to the world. A little Bible verse crossed my mind as I reclined in my quiet world. "*Promotion cometh neither from the east, nor from the west, nor from the south. But God is the judge: he putteth down one, and setteth up another*" (Psalm 75:6,7).

I envisaged being replaced by the brilliant and charismatic associate evangelist, Ross Rhoads. Following my stroke a decade ago, Ross indeed began partnering with Franklin Graham.

There were three giants who hailed from Ross Rhoads' hometown, Philadelphia, the "City of Brotherly Love." The first was Donald Grey Barnhouse, a preacher to the world. The second was Percy Crawford, the world-renowned evangelist. And, the third was Ross Rhoads, a father and a lawyer. The first two distinguished evangelicals were a mighty influence on Ross.

Ross was a Wheaton College freshman in 1952, the year of my graduation. While at Wheaton, Ross became one of four prominent students at the school. In the summer of 1954, he traveled to Belfast for an Ian Paisley crusade. Kathleen met up with him there and became fast friends. Paisley was famous and infamous for his dogmatic, fundamental views. He was both a preacher and a politician.

Ross went on to Fuller Seminary, where he graduated, and then he traveled for fifteen years as an evangelist. In the 1960s, he became an independent evangelist. Tens of thousands of young people have come to the Lord as a result of hearing Ross. Michael W. Smith, a now legendary Christian rock musician, was converted at a Ross Rhoads crusade. Michael W. Smith has been a regularly featured performer at both Billy and Franklin Graham crusades and festivals for two decades.

Billy Graham's autobiography *Just As I Am* identifies the two prominent radio programs of the day: "Dr. Maier and Charles Fuller were virtually the only preachers on national radio at the time." After Charles Fuller died in the 1960s, Ross Rhoads succeeded him.

In the 1970s, Ross was the pastor of the Calvary Presbyterian Church in Charlotte, North Carolina, which had a 700-member roster. In the 1980s that number exploded to 3,000. This church was connected to a seminary of which Ross was both the founder and the president. Ross became the official chairperson of Samaritan's Purse a quarter of a century ago. Each year Ross is involved in Ruth Graham's brain child, the missionary program Operation Christmas Child. Seven million shoeboxes filled with toys and gifts were sent to needy children around the globe in 2005.

Over the ten years following my stroke, Ross has shed tears for my condition and has been compassionate with me always. He has been with the Franklin Graham festivals for a decade and has given the morning dedication regularly with a deep commitment. Ross, Carol, Kathleen and I remain close friends.

CHAPTER XVI

Phoenix: Rising Up from the Ashes

The phoenix—the bird of fire—rose up from the ashes to spread its wings across the great sky once more. Franklin preached alone that Monday following my stroke. I remained at the Laughlin Memorial Hospital in Greeneville until Wednesday morning, when Billy Graham graciously provided the jet that carried Kathleen and me to our destiny. To this day I recall the quizzical looks on the faces of the team gathered around me as I left Greeneville. Those well-wishers, people I had known for many years, squeezed out grins, supposed-to-be smiles, reflecting the pain of watching me lie supine and speechless. We were driven to the Greeneville airport. On a gray Wednesday morning just after the sun had risen behind a bank of clouds, I was flown by an air ambulance, a Learjet, to Mayo Clinic in Rochester, Minnesota.

Aboard I could sense the constant motion of the jet. This bird flew high—as high as I had ever flown. In all the commercial airliners I had taken in my travels around the globe, we flew at a height of just over 30,000 feet. This time I was winging 45,000 feet in the air. I was closer to heaven than I had ever been in all my sixty-seven years of life. We raced northwest through the still air of 1,000 miles to Mayo and to help.

The screaming jets were but a faint buzz in my ears as I lay helpless on that stretcher on that plane. I was almost smothered by the oxygen mask, which was connected to a five-foot cylinder and a tube that I wore tightly, like a young boy wears his toque on a cold winter day before a hockey scrimmage. My eyes were shut most of the time, but

Suddenly Silenced

when I managed to pry them open all I saw were Kathleen's sky-blue azure eyes. Kathleen's were the only words I could hear distinctly. She attempted to compact her small frame beside me. I recall that she spoke words of love and hope softly into my ear as we made the journey across country from Greeneville, Tennessee, to Rochester, Minnesota. This trip was my long journey as my heart pounded like a tribal drum in my chest.

As we approached the runway I was told that slowly melting drifts of snow still lined the tarmac. It is cold in Minnesota sometimes into May. I was rushed from the airport by ambulance to Mayo, again smothered beneath a mask. Every movement seemed perilous. I was afraid to move, and I felt like I was in suspended animation—in a deep freeze, locked into a time vacuum.

The vehicle made its way into the midday traffic. Sunlight beamed through the window as I squinted my eyes, to see only the penetrating lights of the low ceiling. How often had I pulled over to get out of the way of some approaching siren? Now I was a prisoner in this vehicle causing others to stop and make way.

When we came up to the emergency dock at Mayo we were greeted by the quizzically smiling yet kindly Fred Durston, a fellow Canadian and team member from the Minneapolis office whom I had known for two decades. Fred had come the distance. The BGEA office was a 120 miles from Mayo. Fred and Kathleen checked me in to the hospital ward. The looks on their faces told me that they were still gravely concerned about my condition.

As I entered the dizzying corridors at Mayo, I was a man caught in a crazy maze. The dim light was barely enough for the hospital emergency staff to run my four-wheeled gurney, narrowly missing the walls, to my dank, dark room. I could recall having to put my life so completely into the hands of other human beings only during my heart attack episode. But I had known that Jesus was the copilot on the plane that day, and He was with me at Mayo.

When I could finally sit up a little I felt my back give. Muscles have a strange way of tightening up when they have been held in one position for too long. I arched my aching back enough to lean over just slightly to peek out of my hospital window. My view was a portrait of a lonely city bar at night on a narrow street. The blue and red neon lights pierced the night. They flashed intermittently into my room. On the blazing face of the saloon I could read "Hamm's Beer."

Through the meandering days and nights at Mayo I caught glimpses of shadowy Irish and Scandinavian drunks stumbling out after a binge, perhaps for an old stogie that looked like it had a puff or two left. Alarmingly, my surgeon would make his daily rounds rolling up to my bedside in his own wheelchair. I had to believe that this man knew his stuff.

I would lie there sleepless and in terrible pain. At four a.m. each day the pain would climax. My head felt like it was an overfilled hot air balloon about to pop. My chest strained with every beat of my heart, and my whole body ached with the lack of use. During the night I was experiencing acute attacks of excruciating pain on the lower right side of my abdomen. Acute and searing pain would flare up. I was in agony, yet I couldn't let anybody know about it. Later that year the reason for the pain was revealed when my gallbladder exploded! But at Mayo in my lonely ward, my mind was flooded with images past. I remembered T.W. Wilson, Billy Graham's right-hand man, having told me about his gall-bladder attack in the recent past.

I beheld through that misty atmosphere the outline of two friends: Franklin Graham and his best friend, Dennis Agajanian, stood by. They offered prayers of healing and tears of sorrow. I began to understand that the stroke was not the paramount event that took place. The love and camaraderie of companions over so many years is of greater significance to a stroke victim. Love overcomes loss.

When Billy Graham called me about my stroke, I struggled for the tens of thousands of punch lines to as many jokes that I had told over the decades. But they had evaporated into a questionable pause. I had been eloquent and loud, but now all I could do was manage a nervous laugh. Billy then read me a Bible passage that I will never forget. It comes from the first epistle of Peter, 1 Peter 1:3–9. This simple message bound me and kept me safe. I knew that Billy was proud of me. He then honored me further by acknowledging that once I had the use of three languages, and now I had but one word: Jesus. I knew that somehow Billy understood what I was going through. But I hurt so.

I learned to dream while awake. It is possible, you know, to force vivid recollections forward to screen out reality. Alone, so alone—but

Suddenly Silenced

Jesus was there, and with Him sometimes came the blessed gift of a moment's real sleep.

Immediately following the news that I had had a devastating stroke our sons made their ways to my side. Bill traveled from Toronto to Minnesota to be with me for two weeks. He was deeply interested in my treatment at Mayo, and he wondered whether there was anything he could do for me, particularly in the area of preventing further damage to my brain.

Paul, who had been teaching day and night, also hurried to be with me. Paul is sensitive, and our relationship through the years has been markedly intellectual and compassionate. He was still shocked and concerned at my condition. He insisted that I take as much time as I needed to get well and not hurry my recovery to get back to work. Equal to the devastation I felt as a result of my stroke was the stabbing mental pain I experienced as I watched my sons standing over my bed, unable to hide the fear and anxiety they felt from seeing me in this terrible condition.

My speech therapist was a pretty divorced woman who had an eleven-year-old son. She found Paul interesting! She would be forming mouth gestures in attempts to show me how to speak words when she would suddenly become distracted and turn her head from my view to gaze at Paul. She batted her eyelashes at him. Secretly I found this more inspiring to my recovery than any therapy could be.

Randy was in South Africa when I suffered my stroke. It was impossible for him to reach me right away. He piloted a Dash 7 jet to Israel, where he was delayed for three days due to the prime ministerial elections in that country. When he did get to me, like his mother he tended to me. He made sure that I was given everything that I needed.

My brother Hugh and his wife Aileen, along with my sister Betty and Kathleen's sister Mary, drove together over a 2,000-mile return trip to be with me. I finally attempted to communicate my feelings to someone. Somehow I got the message across to the four ladies—Kathleen, Mary, Betty and Aileen—that I was in severe pain at night and couldn't sleep at all. I was desperate to get sleep. I felt like a left-handed, one-armed bandit, grasping for my little plastic bottle of comatose. I wanted my sleeping pills. For five years following Wes' death I had been addicted to those little pills. The women were deeply sympathetic about my condition, but

Phoenix: Rising Up from the Ashes

the doctor had told them that he wasn't sure that the sleeping pills were a good idea, as they tended to slow my heart rate, and that could be deleterious to my condition. So, Kathleen, Mary, Betty and Aileen made the tough decision not to let me have the pills. However uncomfortable I was in the short term, I am ever grateful for their decision.

When Hugh, my seismologist brother, tiptoed into my room, he was concerned about not causing a tremor, as he could see that I was indulging in a precious moment of sleep. He wiggled the big toe of my right foot. I did not wake up. Hugh discovered abruptly that I did not have any feeling on the right side of my body! My prairie brother, Lewis, left the family farm to come to my side. I found great sustenance in Lewis' recollections of days gone by and the recent events of the places of my youth.

Roy Gustafson, an associate evangelist for forty years, was a tour guide with the BGEA. Roy had led 153 tours over a generation. Roy would phone me each day at noon for a one-sided fifteen-minute witty and biblical conversation. He somehow knew how much it meant to me to have his contact each day. Roy would share his adventures in a personal way that I could only respond to with laughter. Somehow Roy understood me. But that was the way with Roy. He always saw deeply into the human condition, and he had the gift of connecting with people as they were.

There was another who made his way down the long hallway to my room. I hoisted myself up in bed a little, just after sundown. I heard a distinct clinking and clanging approaching my room. It was the sound of boot spurs on the hard hospital tile floor. Then the figure of a man standing in the frame of the door presented itself. The darkly dressed man in the doorway had a bushy handlebar mustache that seemed to overshoot the frame. The man wore a black ten-gallon cowboy hat and was clad from the neck down in denim. I knew instantly who it was. It was Brent Smith, the most classic southwestern cowboy I had ever known. He had come to take up residence beside me.

I recall that a nurse scurried into the room behind Brent, announcing that the hospital had strict regulations and that he would have to go. I was located in the Roman Catholic quarters, and the nurse was an authoritarian nun. Brent, in his deep southwestern and gravelly drawl, politely roared back at the nurse, saying, "Excuse me, ma' am. I've

Suddenly Silenced

known this old sidewinder for many a day. In fact, we have shared a platform in your Minneapolis Metrodome. Just nine months ago Dr. John here and I spoke before over 61,000 of your finest men, and I've come to pray and talk to my friend."

The apprehensive nurse swallowed in fright and squeaked, "I guess it will be all right if you stay for a while then, but no rough stuff; he needs all the rest he can get."

Brent retorted, "Oh no, ma'am, I'm here for the night. I stay right here."

"What?" the nurse stormed. "You are not! You'll leave at a decent Christian hour so that Dr. White here can get the rest he needs!"

Then Brent barked, "No, ma'am, I'm truly sorry, but as I've said I've known Dr. John for a long while, and what he needs is prayer and fellowship—I stay!" Then Brent laid down beside my bed and took up residence—on the floor!

Harold Salem, the comedian team member from the days of the moon shots, came to see me at Mayo too. Harold came all the way from his Baptist church in Aberdeen, South Dakota. Once again Harold began firing his volley of jokes. I appreciated his visit more than I can express. The old saying "It only hurts when I laugh" was not true in my case. It hurt all the time. But I loved Harold's stand-up visits. I remember as though it was yesterday that Harold Salem, a man of both humor and deep human compassion, was the chairman of our John Wesley White Crusade in Aberdeen in July 1969.

My son Bill came to see me at Mayo. He divulged that once he came down the hallway toward my room and saw funny Harold Salem gripping the wall outside my room. Harold was sobbing profusely, Bill recounted. Bill stayed back a distance until Harold recovered.

Scores of Billy Graham people marched in and out of my room over the next few weeks. I was of course happy to see them all, but there is a certain stress when those so desperately ill receive visitors. Receiving comfort has never been one of my strong suits. I have sought to comfort rather than to be comforted. But agonizingly, the tables had turned; the world had been turned upside down for me. Prayers and blessings were poured over me continuously, as was the indomitable spirit of love, and the need of forgiveness came upon me. It helped to salve the wound and stop the bleeding of the silence.

Phoenix: Rising Up from the Ashes

Even in the darkest moments there can be flashes of light and humor. For me one of those moments came when my physical therapist, a hockey fanatic, had me stumbling around on one leg. He would make jokes about how I would never be drafted by the Colorado Avalanche if I didn't learn to skate on my bad leg too. He had the most uplifting and spirit-filled communion with me.

In 1982, we had held a week of crusade meetings at the John F. Kennedy Coliseum in Manchester, New Hampshire. There were 1,000 decisions for Christ made that week. On a crucial night, Stephen Merrill was one of 232 who repented and came to the Lord.

In 1992 Stephen was elected the governor of New Hampshire. To this day, Stephen and I correspond by letter and telephone regularly. Four years ago he was appointed to the board of directors of the Billy Graham Evangelistic Association. As it happened, I was scheduled to preach a Franklin Graham-John Wesley White crusade on the east coast of New Hampshire. Franklin would have to go it alone. I had been suddenly silenced.

While Franklin was in New Hampshire he contacted Governor Stephen Merrill. Stephen was a wonderfully spiritual man and was made the honorary chairman of the Franklin Graham-John Wesley White crusades. I once again had the pleasure of speaking with Governor Stephen Merrill at the BGEA headquarters in Charlotte in 2004.

Yes, I guess I knew that I'd had a stroke, but I thought it was only a hiccup. I was terribly homesick. I wanted to go home. I realized that when one is hurting badly there really is "no place like home." I wanted things to be back to normal again, but I was beginning to see that this prospect was not favorable.

The acceptance of the stroke was starting to set in. When I first arrived at Mayo I denied anything had really happened. As I lay night after painful night in my lonely bed in my dark room I cried out to God to "please heal me." I would do anything to be well again. Where once I had been flying around the world in a state of almost total physical freedom, I was currently restrained in the human dog kennel referred to as my bed. I was angry, frustrated, despairing and hopeless about what had happened. Why me? Why now? Was it something I had done? No! I knew God to be my loving Savior and Billy had selected the right chapter and verse for me.

Suddenly Silenced

There were times too when I felt low, depressed some people called it. Looking back I guess that is natural for an evangelist who had lost his greatest tool—his voice—and the use of his right hand, the writing hand for twenty-three books. I recall spending four hours handwriting each sermon prior to the crusades.

The silence was permeating. There was nothing in me that wanted to accept being in this condition where I was. One day as Kathleen made arrangements for me, I was alone in my room. I made a desperate attempt to escape. I twisted my aching body around in a convoluted way in order to slide myself down out of bed. I toppled to the floor. I strained to get myself up so that I could hobble to the doorway. I collapsed again. I reached the doorway and glanced down the hall. The way was clear, so I began crawling down the hall, which was flooded with artificial light. Through the stench of antiseptic I crawled until I hit a dead end. I was stopped abruptly by a matronly nurse.

My love of Jesus remained strong, and I had the faith that He still had a purpose for my life as an evangelist, but I discovered the battle of the two natures—human and spiritual. Every nerve in my body wanted out of that hospital. Or else, "Jesus, take me now!"

Kathleen and Bill both knew how desperate I was to get out of that hospital. They also knew that I was still in delicate health. So they faced another difficult decision—what to do with me! It was clear that I could not stay in Mayo much longer. They talked it over and decided that my psychological health was inextricably linked to my physical health. They put two and two together and, knowing that I was homesick, made arrangements to have me moved to Toronto General Hospital in downtown Toronto.

I found myself aboard another ambulance jet, this time from Minnesota to Toronto. The five intervening weeks between my arrival at Mayo and my coming home gave me enough of a chance at gaining strength that the jet ride was tolerable. In the air, I became exhilarated about the prospects of going home to the "White house." Bill, Paul and Randy had done so much talking about our house that I had mistakenly thought that I was being taken straight home.

After landing at Lester B. Pearson International Airport we hit the highway and sped to my disillusionment. In the ambulance I lay looking out the window, day-dreaming about being in my own bed.

Phoenix: Rising Up from the Ashes

Suddenly I recognized a highway sign that told me we had turned south from Highway 401 and onto Highway 427. I knew that this spaghetti configuration of concrete led downtown. I got the picture. In one fleeting moment my elation was dashed into depression. I felt my blood pressure surge with rage as we turned again onto the Gardiner Expressway, the last leg en route to Toronto General Hospital. Had I the strength I would have been furious. The ambulance did not stop. I knew nothing of how long I would be there. But I knew that any amount of time was too long.

The Toronto General Hospital was being operated by the zealous and very talented David Allan. Initially, Linda Davis, my niece, the daughter of my sister Betty, had recommended to Bill that we connect with David Allan. Linda suggested that Mr. Allan was a capable and reliable authority on the subject of strokes. As it turned out, he was more than capable.

On the recommendation of David, after a week of examination I was moved to the Queen Elizabeth Hospital for further treatment. Of some incidental interest to me was that David had been the goalie for Richmond College's rival team twenty-five years before. He was a member of the Christian Brethren believers and each Sunday for twenty-two years had seen my television programs.

Half of my nurses were Caribbean Christians. It appeared to me to be almost filmic as they tried to cheer me up by flashing their movie-star pearly white teeth while singing familiar Christian songs. Such dedication to recovery I had never realized existed! These nurses had seen my programs regularly on Sunday afternoons and evenings for twenty-five years. I was not known at the Mayo Clinic, but here in Toronto I was treated like a celebrity.

The head of the department of neurology was Dr. Hajik, a mature Hungarian Jewish woman of remarkable compassion. She was the foremost authority in stroke research in Toronto. Dr. Hajik was very bright and was always encouraging to me. She would always smile when she dropped in for a visit. This was a great relief to me, as I had spent so much time at Mayo, where I had been confronted by the cold countenance of the hospital staff.

Dr. Hajik astutely developed a series of exercises that involved raising and lowering my arms above my head. Although secular, Dr. Hajik had heard of me through a variety of sources. She took the time to read the entire *Of Wheels and Wings*. Following this she allowed me to personally hand out three whole boxes of my book to other suffering stroke victims in the hospital. I had a deep desire to minister to these stroke victims, for I knew exactly what they were going through. Although I couldn't speak, I could smile and laugh with them. The rest I had to leave up to Jesus Christ; my book would do the testifying. I confess that my little hospital ministry helped me to recover as much as it helped the other stroke victims.

Along with the enormous physical discomfort that I had, I was experiencing violent mood swings. I would ride the crest of elation, joyous at being alive at all, and then drearily I'd fall, crashing into despair at the ongoing plight of having to rebuild my life from the very grass roots. Adding to my difficulty was the relentless mental confusion caused by the medication that I was taking. This, combined with the confusion that I'd suffered due to the damage done to the left side of my brain, was causing me almost unimaginable distress.

My son Bill was not at all pleased with the interpretation of my condition. He is not a specialist regarding aphasic strokes, but he would pursue whatever avenues it took to discover the truth or falseness of the speech therapist's findings. The speech therapist's findings were as follows: "He'll never speak again." At these words I shut down. Stroke victims ought to prepare themselves to hear almost everything during the course of their recovery. Above all, they must remember that Jesus is Lord.

I had the luxury of having a private room, so the therapists could work with me on an individual basis, without distraction. Dr. Hajik appointed the three top stroke therapists to my case. Two of my therapists, the physiotherapist and the vocational therapist, were absolutely superb.

The physiotherapist was abundantly kind as she guided me through my efforts at rehabilitation. It was a matter of adding just one baby-step each day. My first step was taken in July. Only those who have traveled the path of recovery really comprehend the joy of continuous improvement from such debilitation. I am most grateful for my physiotherapist's inexhaustible patience with me. It came as a shock that I had lost an astounding fifty pounds. That meant that when I finally made it to the hallway, one of our boys could easily take me in one arm and brace me while I got my balance. They kept me from falling—again.

My other therapists were not only experts in their fields but also remarkable human beings. In fact, they took the time to read *Of Wings and Wheels*. I appreciated the type of personal attention that I was receiving at the Queen Elizabeth Hospital. Again, I could see God's Hand at work in my life. As a bonus, this therapist had familiar sky-blue azure eyes. I was daunted at the great physical challenge of getting dressed.

The patient blue-eyed therapist took me through a regimen of bending down to tie my shoelaces. Then away up I came to fasten the buttons on my shirt. Then, standing tall, I would fumble with my tie with my left hand. For fifty years straight I had tied my own tie and had gone to work. The tying of the ties stopped! Day after day I would practice the simple everyday things. I can tell you that I gained a sense of deep and abiding compassion for those who are crippled. The vocational therapist's father had been a rugby player at Oxford in the 1950s. I may have known this man back then.

The speech therapist was discouraging me with a wooden exercise regimen meted out in a strict manner. She determined that I would never again be able to string coherent syllables together; thank the Lord that she was ultimately proven wrong. As I have alluded to earlier, this proclamation blasted me into a frozen purgatory. This single interpretation of my condition more than any other possible event threatened my recovery. I am an evangelist. My life has been my preaching. After the stroke, I faced another battlefield—the psychological battlefield waged in the mind. It was doubt and fear against faith and hope.

However grateful I was for the careful and loving attention I was getting, a month later I was still peering through thick double-pane hospital windows from a room that could be found in any dismal corner of any inner city anywhere in the world. I wanted to go home. At the Queen Elizabeth Hospital at least the boys and the rest of my family and friends could have easy access to me. I could get the sense that I was one step closer to my home.

At times visitors would form a human chain down the hall to get in to see me. There are no words to adequately express how much their

Suddenly Silenced

good thoughts, love and prayers meant to me. *"And now abide faith, hope, love, these three; but the greatest of these is love"* (1 Corinthians 13:13).

Collectively, all these blessings provided a platform, and the stage was set from which I could begin my ascension—rising up from the ashes like the immortal phoenix!

Russell Wells, my close friend, came to see me no less than twenty-three times over the seven weeks that I was in the Queen Elizabeth Hospital. It was no doubt difficult for Russell, who tried to initiate the kind of two-way dialogue that we had enjoyed for so many years. He found out in short order that I could speak only one word—*Jesus*. Still, Russell would sit with me and fill me in on details of things I would find relevant and interesting. What a precious friend he is to me to this day. I also came to know the Peoples Church pastor of the day, John Hull. John kindly visited me in the hospital. He honored me with a portrait of Jesus. This was a special gift to me. I had been connected with the Peoples Church for thirty-five years as a member, preacher and elder.

Sam Hamilton was another close friend who visited me during this time. Sam and his wife, Doreen, were marvelous Christians. Sam had been converted one day while viewing *Agape*. While I preached, George Beverly Shea sang. Sam began singing at Peoples Church, and I liked him so much that I offered him a job singing at my crusades and on my television programs. Sam was with me for twenty years.

My friend and fellow evangelist Bill Newman came all the way from Australia to see me. The last time I had seen Bill was half a year earlier in March; I had been his dinner guest at the Hotel Marriott in Brisbane. We'd shared conversation and laughs at the Franklin Graham festival, which more than 30,000 people had attended. Bill was saddened and shocked to see me lying on my hospital bed. He had always praised my oratory eloquence, but he was now faced with my silence. We moved to the lunchroom in the Queen Elizabeth Hospital, and suddenly he was surrounded by a roomful of stroke patients frozen in a suspended stillness. Fifty people—not one word spoken. Bill made every attempt to cheer me up, but still I could not speak!

I had a TV in my room so that I could watch my program, the news, and the Blue Jays. I had been the assistant chaplain to the

Phoenix: Rising Up from the Ashes

Toronto Blue Jays for the previous fifteen years. Over the years, scores of players had made their decisions and dedications to Christ in my presence. I guess that they wanted to pay me back. To the nurses' amazement my room filled up with ball players and others. Jerry Howarth, the "Voice of the Blue Jays," came to visit me. In fact, Jerry has been kindly toward my entire family and to my facilitator, Stephen Trelford. Jerry Howarth took us out to the ballgame. Jerry and David Fisher, the full-time Blue Jay chaplain, led the players in. John Olerud, the former Blue Jay and American League batting champion, is a humble Christian, who had to duck to get in the room. He stood an enormous six feet seven inches tall. He was more than happy to sign autographs for the children of the nurses. I was a Blue Jay fan, and the players knew it.

All the way from Hollywood in south Florida came the tall Perry Ellis. When I was taken to the hospital's gymnasium for my therapy, Perry would join us. The nurses and the therapists alike couldn't get over his awesome six foot nine inch size, his giant personality—the size of his native state of Texas—or his voice, at least a couple of octaves below Lorne Greene's. Perry provided the highlight during the week that he visited me.

Sterling Huston and his son came to visit me from Rochester, New York. In the 1970s Sterling's wife, Esther, prayed for their little son, who then came to faith while I preached in Nampa, Idaho. Sterling was a brilliant and superb organizer.

David Mainse found the time to come to visit me at the Queen Elizabeth Hospital. Although he was busy in the extreme, he stayed with me for forty minutes, praying and passing his best regards to me. Then he pressed on. I had hobbled down the hall to see David out when without warning my right leg gave way. I fell flat on my face on the grass. I am thankful that this is the only place that David has seen me fall flat on my face—physically!

Preston Parrish, now the vice president of BGEA, and his two teenage boys flew from North Carolina to see me. They encouraged me with the passage from 1 Peter that Billy had sent me soon after the stroke. Preston ministered to me about the loss of my speech. He spoke of the trials and tribulations that face men and how through Jesus Christ we might overcome them.

Suddenly Silenced

Elwood McLean, my boyhood friend and spiritual comrade, traveled over 2,000 miles to be with me in the hospital. Elwood was ample in size and had the personality of a prince. He would actually lumber up onto my bed and lie beside me. He shared Bible verses and prayed dramatic prayers for me. He was gracious and extended great hope to Kathleen and our sons. In 1998 Elwood was diagnosed with rectal cancer. I guess Elwood has firsthand experience with hardships and hospitals.

James Wetheral and his wife, Evelyn, also visited me at the Queen Elizabeth Hospital. Evelyn is a direct descendant of Napoleon Bonaparte. She lives in stark contrast to her ancestral forefather. Napoleon had been a dictatorial warrior, whereas Evelyn possesses the charm of a princess—ever gracious. That summer their son Gordon had toured Switzerland, so they had a great deal to talk about.

Never more accurately was my condition reflected than when Kathleen's brother-in-law Albert came from Ireland, where open displays of emotion are more readily accepted. The whole tribes of Whites and Calderwoods showed up at my room. But it was old Albert who broke down wailing in prayer over my condition. He cried prayers of healing and prayers of hope and, in a staunch Irish brogue, pronounced his blessing before the assembled. I was blessed by this Old World outpouring, but the New Wonders were quite simply embarrassed, especially Ken and Roy Sommerville, who were all too aware of the nurses' reactions in the hallway.

Gordon Freeland updated me for about half an hour. It was then that I took my left hand and with great consternation gripped it. I persevered to get the pen to a tiny scrap of paper, where I managed to scribble one word—*Jesus*!

It was August 17, 1996, and for all the world it felt like the first day of my life. Although I had been enormously blessed by having so many wonderful people express their love for me over the past three and a half months, I still had a deep longing to go home.

As I was helped into our white Buick Skylark I noticed that the left tire in the driver's side was as thin as canvas. I was, however, too excited to get home to motion my interest in pulling into a service station to get the tire changed. I managed to glance back at the Queen Elizabeth Hospital. I looked, but I did not stare. I looked ahead instead;

my way home was filled with vivid colors of buildings and trees. Even the graffiti etched on the walls of Yonge Street appeared like the renderings of famous artists.

A sense of newness welled up within me. The sun shone its summer light high in the sky—no shadows were cast. The wheels spun, and the car made its way through the familiar streets of the inner city and on to the green-green grass of the suburbs. My senses drank in every bit of the trip. My heart pounded, this time in the excited anticipation of coming home, sweet home.

As we turned off Bayview Avenue and wound our pleasant way onto Argonne Crescent, I instantly noticed that the tall bare trees that I had last seen in April had exploded into full green leaf. My skin began to tingle with little goose bumps—my dream was coming true. I had survived to see our home again.

We turned into the driveway, avoiding the six-foot load of rich black earth that had been scattered by the wind and the passage of time since it had arrived there back in the early spring. I had intended to give our sweet little Lhasa Apso dog, Chang, a proper burial. As it happened I had almost given myself one.

The wheels stopped revolving, and I waited as Kathleen got out and came around to my side of the car to open my door. The door did open, and I was flooded with the immediately recognizable aroma of the "White house." I glanced up to see our steps that lead to our double front doors. For half a lifetime I had climbed these steps—home.

This time I wondered how I would negotiate them. Kathleen took me by the arm and slowly walked me, one foot in front of the other, to the steps. I kind of leaned on the wall while being propped up by Kathleen as I ascended my mountain. My right leg was limp and weak, so it had to be dragged behind me as I made my way.

The boys greeted me as I entered our house. A welcome could not have been warmer for a prince or a king. Even when I had delivered a particularly moving sermon that I knew God had anointed me to preach, I had never felt the joy of being appreciated as I was at this time. I was in rapture. The boys had expressions on their faces that were exquisitely cherubic. Angels were all I could see, each one stepping in front of the other to help their poor old dad through our vestibule and up the long stairs to his bedroom.

Suddenly Silenced

My family helped me grip the winding banister as I deliberately placed one foot, then the other, on the long procession of curving stairs. Up I stumbled. The family was hushed in profound consternation until I reached the summit.

The stairs had been conquered for the first time since I had bounded down them what seemed like eons ago. Our whole family has a way of bounding up and down stairs. This time we all took them at a snail's pace.

Then before my eyes it lay. My very own bed, in my own room. I think I let go a tear of joy before I collapsed into the sheets and into a world of blissful dreams. I was home again—at last!

When I awakened I was told that five Jewish neighbors had dropped by to welcome me home. This kindness was monumental to me. Three of the gentlemen were doctors and two were lawyers. I guess I hadn't really known what a friendly street I'd lived on until that moment. When I returned to a moment of quiet concern, that very moment outside our house in the front yard our next door neighbor, Dr. Lloyd Nesbitt, suggested to our sons that now they must go to work to teach me to speak again.

Then I was assisted through the dining room and out onto the balcony veranda. From this precipice I could cast my glance over our backyard. A virtual garden of Eden spread out before me. It was summertime, and my whole world was in bloom. The branches of the trees became loving arms that in not quite reaching me to give me hugs softly waved their hellos. The fragrance of delicately blooming roses wafted indescribable essences upward, and my nostrils flared with delight. I could feel the warm summer sun bathe my cheek, and an indescribable sense of well-being swept over me.

Squirrels darted through the trees, their tails waving a welcome. I thought that I saw their eyes blinking approval at me. The sounds of varieties of singing birds were entirely jubilant to my ears. Even the dog's gleeful barks from across the street somehow lifted my spirit with hope of the new days to come. Woodchucks had become bold since our dogs, the quick Wimp and the ever-vigilant Chang, were no longer standing sentry for us. Now the snapping of delicate twigs could be heard from the distant reaches.

I was treated to the sweet sound of a passing bumblebee making its

Phoenix: Rising Up from the Ashes

way to a sprig of clover and its honey reward in the garden below. Monarch butterflies hovered in the corner of the yard just above Wes' beloved and buried Wimp. Cicada bugs harmonized in a splendid song of greeting high in the weeping willows that accentuated the stunning blue dome just a little below heaven.

A jumbo jet silently crossed my path. It appeared to be hovering or perhaps gliding in its descent en route to Lester B. Pearson International Airport. It seemed so close to me that I thought that I could reach out and shake the hands of the pilots whose faces I imagined were smiling at me.

Like my father I find McIntosh apples especially delicious. So in the '60s the boys had planted a small stand of apple trees in the northwest quadrant of the back forty perpendicular to my position aloft on the veranda. This day, these majestic trees appeared absolutely robust.

We were at this time of the year in deep privacy. The farthest boundary to the north gave way to infinity. No sign of human life could be seen beyond our property line. There was just the great expanse of blue and the treetops. I lifted my eyes to the sky to give thanks, and I could see soft cottony clouds changing form. This kind of cloud has always seemed to me to take the form of God's creatures—animals of every sort. The sky was a kind of Noah's ark in motion on the great ocean of the sky. Then I cast my eyes downward to catch a look at our boys frolicking and laughing in the warm, sparkling water of our swimming pool. The whole world seemed resplendent, ineffably beautiful as I stood in silent gratitude.

Even while I was in my quiet world, unable to utter a word, my family knew what I was feeling, and that was connection. *Oh! Thank You, Jesus, You have blessed me beyond words.* I now, again, felt like a modern-day Job. Like the phoenix, I had risen from the ashes!

I must have looked an incredible sight as I attempted to swim in our pool. I flailed around in the water, paddling frantically with my left arm and leg. My right side acted like an anchor dragging me down. I was clasped into a life preserver, like I had been when I was a child. It kept me afloat then, and it kept me afloat in our blue pool this splendid day!

Randy, like his mother, was a bit overcautious about my aquatic efforts. Paul, on the other hand, was motivating. He encouraged me to try to extend my swimming capabilities—within reason.

Suddenly Silenced

It was great to be back at a Blue Jay game. Jerry Howarth had been kind enough to offer me a couple of tickets. I have always enjoyed having tickets to a baseball game. When I looked them over to see where Jerry had me seated, I noticed that the tickets read "handicapped." We invalids have special privileges, you know. I was placed right behind home plate. Paul and I went to the game. I rolled up to my special spot in the park in a brand new deluxe wheelchair! The Baltimore Orioles were in town, and they were leading the American League's Eastern Division. It was a good game, as the Blue Jays were contenders.

This day, only a short time after coming home, I had my little battery transistor radio pressed up to my ear in the ninth when all of a sudden I heard Jerry bellow, "There she goes!" Ed Sprague blasted a tremendous shot over the wall to win the game. Paul rolled me out of the park elated.

One day when Kathleen and I had been out shopping we turned on the radio to listen to the Blue Jay game. This too meant a great deal to me.

The first Sunday morning that I was out of the hospital, Kathleen, the boys and I went to People's Church. When we entered the building we were engulfed in well-wishers and good Christian fellowship. I ambled along, shaking people's hands with my left hand. This must have been uncomfortable for people, but they came to me anyway.

John Hull's service was being broadcast on TV across Canada. He announced my being seated in the service. He spoke for a minute about my stroke and miraculous recovery. It was both humbling and comforting to be recognized this way. I was overjoyed to be home. Kathleen and I then resumed worship at my nephew Roy's Baptist church.

Another friend came from afar to extend to me his best wishes. It was Arthur Sheppard, my boyhood friend from the prairies. Art was now living in Vancouver. I couldn't take my eyes off Art. He stood before me like a time machine to my past. My mind flooded with sweet memories of my boyhood and the youthful adventures Art and I had engaged in. His compassion for my condition brought out feelings of deep connection to my roots. What a blessing it is that, even in the worst travail, the mind mostly recalls the pleasant memories and discards so much of the painful ones!

On two of the last days in hot July 1977, I was preaching in a wind-blown field to 10,000 "Jesus People." They were strewn among the grass on the borderland of Brantford, Ontario. These followers of Christ were camping, squatting and laying about, many with only their Bibles in hand.

One evening, Pastor Benny Hinn and I spent two hours together at the Brantford "Jesus People" festival. We found ourselves walking up and down the lonely winding roadsides of the country much the same way they did in the wake of the resurrection. I recalled the biblical parallel:

"Why do you seek the living among the dead? He is not here, but is risen! Remember how He spoke to you when He was still in Galilee, saying, 'The Son of Man must be delivered into the hands of sinful men, and be crucified, and the third day rise again.'" And they remembered His words. Then they returned from the tomb and told all these things to the eleven and to all the rest…Now behold, two of them [disciples] were traveling that same day to a village called Emmaus, which was seven miles from Jerusalem. And they talked together of all these things which had happened. So it was, while they conversed and reasoned, that Jesus Himself drew near and went with them. But their eyes were restrained, so that they did not know Him. And He said to them, "What kind of conversation is this that you have with one another as you walk and are sad?…O foolish ones, and slow of heart to believe in all that the prophets have spoken! Ought not the Christ to have suffered these things and to enter into His glory?"…And they said to one another, "Did not our heart burn within us while He talked with us on the road, and while He opened the Scriptures to us?" (Luke 24:6–32).

In July 1968 Benny Hinn had emigrated from Israel to Don Mills, a suburb of Toronto. Just prior to this I was with the Billy Graham team visiting Richard Nixon in his hotel room in Portland, Oregon. Billy, being already overbooked, had no time to keep his appointment with Bobby Kennedy. So, as previously mentioned, he asked me to stand in for him. When I met with Bobby, and he and I walked and talked together outside the hotel room for a distance of three blocks. Twelve days later Bobby Kennedy was brutally assassinated in the Ambassador Hotel in Los Angeles.

Suddenly Silenced

Then in September Billy introduced Kathleen and me to Richard Nixon. That week in the First Presbyterian Church in Pittsburgh, at the Billy Graham School of Evangelism, I spoke the words of the devoted apostle Paul to the Corinthians:

For if I preach the gospel, I have nothing to boast of, for necessity is laid upon me; yes, woe is me if I do not preach the gospel! For if I do this willingly, I have a reward; but if against my will, I have been entrusted with a stewardship. What is my reward then? That when I preach the gospel, I may present the gospel of Christ without charge, that I may not abuse my authority in the gospel (1 Corinthians 9:16–18).

Yes, that day it had been Benny Hinn, the rookie, who handed me, the veteran, the outline for my preaching in Pittsburgh:

1. The Woe (1 Corinthians 9:16–18; Isaiah 6:3–7).
2. The Worship (Luke 4:18,19; Revelation 4:11).
3. The Way (John 14:6; Acts 16:17).
4. The Word (Jeremiah 20:9; Luke 24:32).
5. The World (Mark 16:15–18; Matthew 28:19).
6. The Winning (Proverbs 11:30; 1 Corinthians 19:23).
7. The Watch (Mark 13:37; Matthew 16:3; Revelation 4:1).

In 1972, Benny Hinn was saved in Don Mills, and in 1974 he received a second blessing at that First Presbyterian Church. I had spoken to 1,200 ministers and their wives at the Billy Graham School of Evangelism. As a rough count, 30,000 ministers and their wives had by 1977 the benefit of hearing Benny's outlined message over twelve years at the Billy Graham School of Evangelism.

Yes, that First Presbyterian Church in Pittsburg had been significant both for Benny Hinn and for myself.

In July 1977 Benny and I talked and prayed and found each other in the Spirit in Brantford under the sun and the Sonship that day. It was precious fellowship that bound us as spiritual brothers. Many times in airports on my way to crusades I would cross paths with Benny, and we would take the opportunity to fellowship and give praise to our Lord and Savior Jesus Christ for His generosity of Spirit. Benny and I spent the next twenty years busy with evangelism.

Phoenix: Rising Up from the Ashes

In January 1992, Kathleen and I had just returned from Russia. While performing our privileges with Franklin's Samaritan's Purse board down in West Palm Beach, we visited Benny's Church in Orlando, Florida. We were packed in like sardines in our pews. It was George Parson who brought Benny and me together again.

There were over 3,000 people in Benny's church at that time. This blessed event was tinged, however, with grief, because the White family was mourning in the wake our son Wes' sudden death. I had traveled extensively with Wes, and he had companioned with us on our crusades. The pain was indescribable. His whole life flashed before our eyes. Now the bright light was extinguished. He was dead.

During the 1990s George Parson was one of the coordinators of Benny's crusades worldwide. In the late '60s and through the '70s George was the head of Grason's Publishers at the BGEA in Minneapolis. Grason's was one of the world's largest publishers. They have published in excess of 100 million evangelical books to date. George has remained my agent through the publishing of my twenty-three books.

Indeed, Benny Hinn presided that day in Orlando, but it was George Parson who greeted us in our pew and walked us up that long meandering aisle to the platform, where Benny asked for the prayers for us from his congregation in the muggy twilight following Wes death. Kathleen stood there, almost frozen, with her sky-blue azure eyes beginning to stream as we prayed with Benny. We were overcome with emotion. Our son had gone to heaven while we remained on earth. George Parson was a dear friend to us in our time of grieving.

Benny's meeting lasted for four hours. Four hours seemed like scant minutes as the Holy Spirit descended on the congregation and took time away. It was Shekinah!

Then, on April 28, 1996, the preaching stopped. I was suddenly silenced. Fourteen months earlier I had preached to 61,000 men in the Minneapolis Metrodome. Randy Phillips, the president of Promise Keepers, informed me that a record 9,000 people had made decisions for Jesus Christ that Friday night.

Then I completed my seven years of twinning with Franklin Graham at our festival in Australia. The climax of this festival was at Brisbane, where 30,000 people attended on one night.

Suddenly Silenced

In September 1996 following my tour of North America's hospitals, I limped to Kitchener, Ontario, where Franklin was holding his festival. Ten thousand people had come to listen as an anointed Franklin preached the Word of God. I was on the platform beside Franklin, and as the song came up Tom Bledsoe turned to me and remarked, "John, you're singing. John, just listen to you sing in tenor!"

I was ignorant. The words emanating from the left side of my brain had been entirely obliterated by the aphasia. But the right side of my brain remained intact, so I could sing the words of the songs, and all I could see through my tears was the crowd.

In October 1996, Benny Hinn held a packed rally in Toronto's Maple Leaf Gardens. Indeed, 20,000 people had come to witness the man in the white suit wave his hand and palm people in healing. George, Kathleen and I sat in the front seats on the platform. The substance of Benny's message that night was the apostle Paul's: "*God worked unusual miracles by the hands of Paul, so that even handkerchiefs or aprons were brought from his body to the sick, and the diseases left them and the evil spirits went out of them*" (Acts 19:11,12).

Benny, standing in white there in Maple Leaf Gardens and commanding me to stand, announced John Wesley White to the crowd. I could say nothing. He asked me to step down from the platform onto the floor at the front. I was slightly embarrassed; I'd suffered my stroke only months before. But Benny commanded the Spirit of Jesus upon me in a very gentle way, and I came under the blessing of God. Benny had me repeat a prayer, alternating one word at a time. First Benny, then me. Then Benny, then me. When I came to the Gardens I could speak not one word. But standing there in the beam of that light I could—yes, I could—repeat the prayer. The crowd exploded. Another four hours telescoped into what seemed like only minutes as Christ's eternity loomed. I was singing, and yes, I had spoken. Yes, I had spoken.

The *National Post* declared Benny Hinn as powerful as ever. Benny Hinn "does not give the impression of a miracle healer on the wane," wrote the *Post*. On the Canadian Broadcasting Corporation during prime time television, there appeared back-to-back programs on "Miracles" via Benny Hinn. Whether you believe that Benny works as God's divinely ordained and direct agent or not, a hundred million plus have tuned in to see his miracles performed on stage on his television

Phoenix: Rising Up from the Ashes

program *This Is Your Day,* which airs daily in our region on the Crossroads Television Network. I have tuned in to this program regularly for the past ten years.

Thousands still pour into Benny's meetings as he trumpets down the power of the Almighty. They come to the front in wheelchairs, in iron lungs and on crutches. Benny takes one affliction at a time to Jesus, as the evangelist snaps out his palm and the ailing fall to the platform. One by one the lame walk, the weak are made strong and the breathless breathe again. Miracles are plentiful and are strung together in chains of glory to the Lord. Benny and his team have a friend in Jesus. Over the years Benny has visited countless stadiums, arenas and parks in nations around the world.

In the 1990s Evander Holyfield went to the Mayo Clinic. It has been reported that he was diagnosed as having a hole in his heart. The boxing commission barred him from boxing because of his medical condition. Then Evander Holyfield attended a Benny Hinn rally and came to the platform for healing. Benny called on the Holy Spirit of Jesus, palmed Evander in the forehead, and laid him out on the floor. When Evander finally got up—he was healed! In the '90s the doctors back in Mayo were dumbfounded. They pronounced him healed, and for five years and into the new millennium, Evander Holyfield was been the reigning heavy weight boxing champion of the world. Then, in July 2007 the world was again told of Evander Holyfield. The media trumpeted that the boxing titan outworked and outclassed Lou Savarese, winning a ten-round unanimous decision to remain undefeated in his comeback. Holyfield, 44, started and ended the fight with a hard left to the head of Savarese.

In Atlanta, Georgia, in 1994, at another Billy Graham crusade, before 65,000, former president Jimmy Carter was seated on the platform with Evander Holyfield. Billy Graham introduced these two great American Christian "heroes."

For sixty years I have held to the doctrinal statement put forth by Dr. R.A. Torrey. But William Cowper said it best:

God moves in a mysterious way
His wonders to perform;
He plants His footsteps in the sea

And rides upon the storm.
(William Cowper, 1774)

In August I had begun a program of rehabilitation at St. John's Convalescent Hospital, a mile from my home. At first Kathleen drove me to the hospital; then I began stubbornly sneaking out to limp up there by myself. I guess that I needed to prove to myself that I could do something for myself. I visited St. John's as an outpatient three times weekly for speech, physical and vocational therapy. They were really starting to work on my arm and my leg in earnest.

Two of my three therapists were evangelical Christians. My vocational therapist, Donna Barker, looked after my arm. Donna was extremely kind to me. She dealt with my condition for seventeen months, always making sure that I got the maximum allowable time for rehabilitation under the prevailing government regulations. Her father was the head of the mathematics department at the University of Toronto and the longtime chairman of Pastor Alf Rees' Banfield Memorial Church.

My second physical therapist, Pauline, was from India. She stood only four feet ten inches tall, but she had a heart the size of a house! She was an expert in her area, and she was greatly dedicated to me. Her father, while in India, had seen Alf Rees preach and was born again. He and his family immigrated to Toronto in the 1970s. I am thankful that he did. His daughter Pauline is a brilliant therapist who graduated from the University of Western Ontario. Her father became a Methodist minister.

Pauline would pray for me aloud. She knew that I could only speak one word. She read *Of Wheels and Wings*. This way she had something definite that she could talk to me about. Although I was already tired of people's monologues, I appreciated that they tried hard to converse with me.

The third therapist was my speech therapist, who was rough with me. In fact, she appeared to me to be prejudiced against evangelical Christians. In the beginning she worked strict forty-five-minute sessions. By October she had reduced my therapy time down to paltry fifteen-minute sessions. That was just about enough time for her to socialize in the hallway.

Phoenix: Rising Up from the Ashes

When I got the news about my stroke, I was crushed. The only other time that I felt this depressed was when Kathleen and I lost our son Wes. A long six months I was praying, "Lord, if You have finished with me preaching the gospel, then please take me home to heaven." I know that this was selfish of me, but this is really how I felt during my time of despair. The day I was told that I would never speak again I lost control and sobbed uncontrollably. I experienced some of the loneliest hours of my life. I wandered up and down my street for three hours in a foggy haze. Bill found me in despair and made me the solemn promise that I would one day preach again.

In October I faced another threat to my life. Ever since Mayo I had been awakened at night with searing pain on my right side. It felt like a dragon was blowing flames on my abdomen. The pain was so excruciating that many times I believed I would just pass out from it, never to wake up. The trouble was that I was effectively mute—I couldn't tell anyone.

All of a sudden, while at the Airport Holiday Inn, I was taken by enormous pain. I groaned and doubled over in my chair. Those assembled gasped and leapt up to see what was wrong. Apparently I had turned green, then white, as I began drifting into oblivion. I imagined that I was experiencing the degree of agony that mothers experience when giving birth. I was rushed home to bed, where I spent the night alternately rolling around, then lying as still as I possibly could, according to the ebb and flow of the stabbing pain in my side.

This was the longest night that I could ever remember. In the morning Bill saw me and rushed me to the emergency ward of North York General Hospital. When the doctors got a look at my gallbladder, it was so inflamed with toxins that they deemed it too risky to operate. They had to wait until the inflammation subsided, so that the incision wouldn't flood my system with a lethal dose of poison.

For ten days I waited in hospital. Finally, the surgeons felt the odds were good enough to take a chance on surgery. The head surgeon approached Kathleen solemnly. He told her that he gave me only about a fifty-fifty chance of surviving the operation. I had said a prayer with Kathleen and told her that there was as much a chance that I would be seeing Wes again as there was the chance that I would see her again. I squinted to see her sky-blue azure eyes. This time they were filled with tears.

Suddenly Silenced

When I came out of the operating room the surgeon told Kathleen that in all his thirty years of performing such operations he had never seen a gallbladder as bad as mine. I had flirted with death once more! Upon entering the recovery room I immediately became aware of one of my four roommates. He was wailing in pain. I found this circumstance less than encouraging. After the anesthetic wore off completely I had five more hours of pain. John Hull came to see me. We prayed.

I had a ten-inch incision on the lower right side of my abdomen. I had been cleaned like a fish. I had had time to reflect on the surgeon's words about having a fifty-fifty chance of survival and prayed vehemently about my continuance of life on earth. I had experienced another close shave.

This time, I spent an entire month in North York General Hospital. Nothing could be further than what I desired. Kathleen visited me daily. Paul came up from Purdue again to see his dad. I felt like I was having an instant replay of my Queen Elizabeth Hospital experience. Kathleen's sisters and my sister Betty and brother Hugh came to visit daily. So did Russell Wells. He was still attempting to spark up a dialogue with me. Still I could not speak.

When I was released from hospital in December, Bill put a program of recovery together that included videotapes, audiotapes and flash cards. Bill was convinced that the only thing that could stop me from preaching again was negative thinking. I have come to believe that I was being tested by Jesus Christ. I believe also that it was only faith and hard work, which began immediately after my stroke, that got me better again. I worked fourteen hours a day for three months. That resulted in my being able to utter a few intelligible words.

There were three things that got me better: one: work; two: more work; and three: even more work! Bill had been thinking about my recovery. He had been reading about strokes. He had put together several computer-based programs for me. Each morning at 6:30 we would sit at the basement computer while Bill took me through the rudiments of "see and say" computerized word games.

For an hour each morning at 9:00 a.m., members of the team would phone me with updates concerning the crusades. They prayed about my condition. This custom began before my surgery and continued until well after I had recovered. Then the team went on to Farmington, New

Phoenix: Rising Up from the Ashes

Mexico. They never failed to telephone me at 11:00 a.m. sharp, Toronto time. Each member would take a turn on the phone praying for divine intercession for me. Oh! How I missed the Franklin Graham-John Wesley White team!

It was a brutal winter. In December, I came home. Then Christmas was upon us. I remember that during that Christmas season it just kept snowing. It was frightfully cold outside. But it was warm in our house. Paul had come home from Purdue, and Bill was around that year. Randy was flying up north, but he came home for Christmas.

Christmas Eve was, however, punctuated with calamity. I had been upstairs sleeping when Kathleen took her tumble—right down the long, winding stairs. Apparently she shrieked in pain, and that brought Paul running.

Kathleen was lying at the bottom of the stairs, gripping her ankle. I managed to sleep through this, as I was exhausted. My day had begun at 6:00 a.m., and my family did not want to disturb me. I was still quite fragile.

An ambulance was called and arrived just as Randy was coming in the house. He exclaimed, "Is it Dad?"

Paul blurted out, "It's okay. It's only Mom!"

Randy was really confused. Paul explained, "What I mean to say is that now both Mom and Dad have only one good leg." Paul continued, "Mom tumbled down the stairs, and I think that she broke her ankle."

Randy retorted, "What else can possibly happen to us?"

When they could gather their senses, Paul and Randy woke Bill up. They all accompanied Kathleen to the hospital.

In the dark of the night, I awoke. I wandered out of my room to find myself at home alone. I thought that perhaps Jesus had forgotten me in the Rapture at the second coming of Jesus Christ. Anyway, I was terrified! Where were Kathleen and our sons? The minutes that passed until the boys phoned seemed like an eternity. It was Christmas morning by now. But where was the celebration?

When the phone rang, I managed to hobble over to pick it up. Bill was on the other end. At least I felt a little better knowing that my family was still alive! The boys came home to pick me up to go to the hospital. I cried when I looked into Kathleen's sky-blue azure eyes. Yet I

Suddenly Silenced

couldn't tell her what I felt. I could only kiss her on the cheek. She managed a little smile.

We ate our Christmas turkey in the hospital cafeteria. Kathleen was in rather severe pain; she had shattered her ankle. It had swollen up to become as large as a football. She couldn't walk for the first thirty-six hours after the cast had been put on. Her ankle remained swollen. She was released from the hospital ten days after she had fallen.

When again, finally, the family assembled together, we all looked at each other, wondering what else could happen to us. It was clear that we had to build a new life for ourselves and be ever vigilant to pray for God's mercy in our lives.

But life goes on, and Paul had to go back to Purdue, Randy was scheduled to fly back up north, and Bill went to Cuba. There were two of us in the house. We were marooned, as neither of us could drive the car.

I still could not speak at all, but Kathleen would whisper a little phrase thousands of times in my ear: "Jesus is Lord! Jesus is Lord! Jesus is Lord!" This was the first phrase that I learned to speak.

This was the crucial month for me. I was determined to speak. I just couldn't imagine life without speaking and preaching again. Jean, Mary and Ruth, Kathleen's sisters, would come over in the afternoons and make a delicious dinner for us. They would also clean up our house.

A turning point for us came when Kathleen and I visited our favorite Jewish deli, which we have frequented for the past twenty-five years. During dinner a huge sweeping feeling came over me. In a flash I was taken and I stood up, declaring in a dramatic, almost theatrical voice, "Jesus is Lord."

Kathleen burst into a smile and exclaimed, "John, you're preaching again!" This was my first sentence. The roomful of sated diners applauded their approval with exuberance. I was back in the pulpit. Thankfully, I was well known in this place by both the waiters and the clientele. They had seen my television programs and were greatly surprised at my first post-stroke sermon.

It had been nine months since I had spoken any word but *Jesus*. I could not help but think about Mrs. Ike Jacques' class in Black Oak Sunday School when I was just a shy boy of six years old. I had stood up with my knees shaking. I trembled before my classmates as I recited, *"Jesus wept"* (John 11:35). I sat down abruptly. I felt like the whole

Phoenix: Rising Up from the Ashes

world was watching, and my face was as red as a beet. Certainly my declaration that "Jesus Is Lord" overshot this mark measurably. Therefore, I was back speaking again. For two-thirds of a century I had thought about my little statement *"Jesus wept,"* the shortest verse in the Bible. How I wept—with joy!

Throughout my life I have memorized thousands of verses and have recited them around the world. Then, on April 28, 1996, my mouth stopped! I came to parallel another very special person, Ruth Graham, who was likewise unable to speak the thousands of verses that she had memorized when she fell from her grandchildren's tree house in Milwaukee a quarter of a century ago. She plummeted fifteen feet, banging her head on the ground, plunging into a deep coma. When she came to she could remember—not one verse! Throughout my recovery I have considered Ruth's story countless times. In the '70s Ruth's memory was restored. For the past ten and one half years I have studied the Scriptures diligently from Genesis to Revelation.

In January 1997 Franklin Graham telephoned Kathleen and me. He likened the account of my stroke to that of Zacharias in the book of Luke. Franklin instructed Bill to hire for me the three best therapists in Toronto. Bill hired Ron, a speech therapist who used traditional means of therapy directed towards the gradual reinstatement of my speech. Kathleen and Ron and I would form a triangle and practice my responses in the usual conversational modes.

It was clear after about six months that I would have to move outside the traditional lines of therapy if I were to progress at an accelerated rate. So I stopped seeing Ron.

A kind speech therapist named Elise from Washington, D.C., came over to our house twice a week beginning in February 1997. She worked with flash cards, attempting to get my mouth reconnected with my mind. To some degree this worked.

However, after eighteen months I was impatient and began working exclusively with Stephen Trelford, who has been with me since that crucial month, January 1997. Stephen is an evangelical. Bill has known Steve since they were teenagers. In the early '70s, Bill and Steve traveled throughout North America together. Steve is now a professor of communications. He specializes in English, grammar and public speaking. He is a graduate of Bishop's University, located east of Montreal. He was training to be an Anglican clergyman but went into teaching. In 2003, Steve was conferred with a doctor of literature degree.

Steve was originally hired to take me through exercises that would assist me in recognizing simple sentence structure. Although these exercises were tedious, we discovered that we worked wonderfully well together. Therefore I felt that we could begin working on preliminary sermons. I was interested in returning to the pulpit as soon as the Lord made it possible.

Steve has worked with students of every description, from everywhere. He possesses the practical combination of an innately compassionate nature and a highly developed ability to take semblances of words and utterances and then to construct them into meaningful sentences. Using an anthropological metaphor, Russell Wells commented that, "Stephen has the ability to take a single buried bone and then to reconstruct the original animal from it." For so long I could utter only fragments of words. Steve had to listen intently and decipher what I meant to say. Remarkably, he is able to key into the text complex meanings that he has taken from the fragments of words and then create stylistic, poetic prose, rich in vivid description. In addition, Steve continuously demonstrates his unique style of hearing the intended meaning of my words and uniting that meaning with a strong background in grammar. Said another way, the result is a theatrical writing that has the reader living the narrative. I believe that God has anointed Steve to undertake our work. Steve modestly echoes my sentiments. We both felt that he was the ideal candidate for reconstructing my preaching life.

When Steve arrives each day to work on sermons, TV programs and my autobiography, I meet him at the door with a smile. We are both delighted to work together. I enjoyed working with Ron and Elise, but Steve and I have become close friends. We make working together fun. Steve says that for the ten and a half years that we've worked together, he has never felt that what we do is work. It's more like a spiritual and intellectual holiday, he declares! We spend hours together working and laughing—and that might be the very best form of therapy of all. Maybe having a stroke has had its benefits!

In March 1997 Kathleen, Paul and I went to the city that gave birth to the rock and roll legend Elvis Presley—Tupelo, Mississippi. Before

Phoenix: Rising Up from the Ashes

Franklin's festival our eighteen-member team got on our knees in a circle for two hours of prayer. Among the prayers offered to God were those said for me. When it came time for Kathleen and I to speak, we boldly exclaimed, "Jesus Is Lord! Amen!" The team burst into laughter and tears. Some of them thought that a miracle had just occurred, while others felt a deep sadness for us.

After the crusade we visited Graceland in Memphis, Tennessee. Paul was excited to see the place where Elvis had lived. We spent a full three hours there. From Tennessee we flew to Boone, North Carolina, for the Samaritan's Purse Board meeting. There are many doctors on the board, and they recognized my condition as similar to others they had dealt with. They suggested that the board pray for me. I was filled with the joy of the Holy Spirit and the love of my colleagues.

Upon returning home, I badgered Kathleen to call Norma Jean Mainse, David's wife. I was desperate to get back on the air. David was very supportive of my returning to television. Kathleen and I were invited to appear on *100 Huntley Street*. I was elated but realized that I had a lot of work to do in preparation for the program and the big moment of my return to television.

When the program opened, David announced to the country that I would be returning to television for the first time since my devastating stroke. Kathleen and I were interviewed. While Kathleen did the talking, I just sat on the couch and smiled. I occasionally exclaimed, "Jesus is Lord."

Then it came time for my segment. It was Easter. I spoke in stumbling utterances for a few minutes on the seven sayings of the Lord. I managed to shatter the English language in every way possible.

Though David was gracious, my return to television was premature. Family and friends telephoned me after the program. They tried to disguise the disappointment they felt at seeing me humiliate myself the way I did.

In retrospect, I am not entirely sure that this television appearance, which was viewed around the continent, did much for my calling. What it did do for me was provide me with an opportunity to build my courage and self-confidence. I had the nagging feeling that if I waited too long for my return to television I may never be able to face a camera again.

Suddenly Silenced

During spring training Jerry Howarth caught this program while in the airport in Florida en route to a Grapefruit League game. He called me that night and expressed his belief that because I was speaking again, a miracle had indeed occurred. He encouraged me for even having the gall to get back on television. The theme of those very early television and preaching events was "Miracles."

Immediately following my stroke I could no longer handle our family's financial affairs. I inadvertently missed mailing my annual income tax return. As it happened I owed income tax which amounted to $1,900. Kathleen appealed to Revenue Canada for special consideration, due to the circumstances surrounding my stroke. Further, we sought the best counsel for advice in this matter.

We telephoned John Brooks. He went to work. When he phoned us back, he informed us that he had seen me on *100 Huntley Street* and he had been greatly moved by my situation. In fact, he told us that he had wept when he saw me stuttering hopeful utterances. He joyfully announced that we needn't worry about the taxes owed. He then passed on his apologies from Revenue Canada for any trouble that they might have caused us.

In the spring of 1998, my second post-stroke appearance was in Boone before Franklin's team. In my usual post-stroke fashion, I had rehearsed my message 300 times. This extensive rehearsal practice became a habit for five years. The substance of my message was designed to parallel Franklin and Billy with Joshua and Moses respectively. I had learned to deliver my message with slow precision. My delivery was clear this time, and I used the eraser end of a pencil to guide me word by word through the text. I was so anxious to communicate the central words of the message that I had the tendency to overlook conjunctions, articles, pronouns and prepositions. The use of the pencil ensured that I spoke every word. Though I spoke in a staccato voice, I was clearly understandable. This helped to generate an optimistic attitude toward the possibility of recovering my ability to preach again. Everyone was surprised and relieved.

Franklin was greatly moved by my performance. He walked to the pulpit with a visible determination and gently put his arm around me. Then he asked the thirty-eight members of the team to kneel and pray for me—that I might preach again. Each and every person in the room

Phoenix: Rising Up from the Ashes

took their turn praying over me. I felt the great Hand of God move once more, and a great blessing came upon me.

After the prayer meeting, Reverend John McGregor of the Billy Graham team and pastor of the Alliance church in Saskatoon, Saskatchewan, took me aside and personally invited Kathleen and me to his church. He announced that he was coordinating a crusade in November. He invited me to preach four meetings there.

In 1978, John McGregor had emigrated from Ulster to Vermilion. He had become involved with a terrorist organization in Northern Ireland. At age nineteen, John was born again in a fiery baptism of the Holy Spirit. Then, ironically, he was called to preach the simple Word of God. When John first arrived in Canada, he began a career as an accountant and lived with his wife and four children in a small house.

Then, in November 1980, I conducted a ten-day area-wide crusade Vermilion, Alberta, where I met John, who had volunteered to work with the crusade committee and coordinated the crusade. He spoke to me of nothing but his love for his work with the Lord. For fifteen years John coordinated the Billy Graham associate evangelist crusades, including those seven years when I twinned with Franklin Graham. Notably, John coordinated the Billy and Franklin Graham crusade in Saskatoon, Saskatchewan. Then at this crusade John was called to preach the Word of God. He went on to pastor an Alliance church in Saskatoon, where he settled. At the turn of the millennium, he began taking his brilliant and biblical crusades across Canada.

By June 1997, I was preaching an average of four times a month in churches around Metropolitan Toronto. I was steadily improving my delivery. That July, I was given an opportunity to deliver the message at the Billy Graham School of Evangelism before 800 ministers. Tom Bledsoe is now the head of the Billy Graham Schools of Evangelism. I rehearsed this message 300 times. Our son Paul recommended a funny illustration about Mike Tyson, the boxer, for the meeting: "It's rumored that Mike studied Shakespeare in prison. It seems to me that while Mike was fighting, he was inspired by those great words of Shakespeare: 'Friends, Romans and *Holyfield*, lend me your ears.' Ministers, please lend me *your* ears for a few minutes." Mike Tyson had bitten off part of Evander Holyfield's ear during a 1997 rematch.

Suddenly Silenced

The ministers roared at this joke and enjoyed my speaking. They applauded loudly as they understood that I had suffered a stroke, yet I had delivered my message with some appreciable "unction and utterance."

In August, Sam Hamilton arranged for me to speak at Bramalea Baptist Church. This church had a seating capacity of 1,200. I again expounded an eight-minute message. Each time I got up into the pulpit I improved.

Russell Wells is a friend of the born-again Michael Coren. They both were aired on CFRB 1010 in Toronto, Canada's most-listened-to radio station. Michael and his family showed up at the church in Bramalea and shook my hand after I spoke. Michael, though born Jewish, now had a strong faith in Jesus Christ. He had the number-one rated talk show in Canada, and he sincerely congratulated me. I was really on my way!

In September 1997 Kathleen and I were invited to travel to Kingston, Ontario, for three days of meetings at a Free Methodist church. A neighbor of ours had moved to the Kingston area to pastor this church. When we arrived we located our good-looking Spirit-filled friend Pastor Gary Shearer. Gary was well known for his success in working with young people. He had a flourishing church.

I preached on the Sunday morning of that weekend on "Nero, the emperor." An idea for the sermon originated during a trip from Charlotte to Boone, North Carolina. Will, Franklin's son, announced that the Old Testament figure of Jacob was the second strongest man who ever lived. Nero was the third strongest man. He had forty wrestlers wrestling for him. They would cry, "We the wrestlers, wrestling for thee, O Emperor, to win for thee the victory and from thee the victor's crown." The great royal Roman emperor commanded his men into the arena and lions' den. The sermon was a classic illustration of power hungry madness, which took listeners through twisting emotional turns. It was a story of Nero's men turning away from the egocentric tyrant and toward Jesus Christ. When Nero found out, he sent a message: "If there be any among your soldiers who cling to the faith of the Christian, they must die!"

The wrestlers were ordered to strip in the Alps of Switzerland by their general, Vespasian, and thirty-nine of these men ultimately

Phoenix: Rising Up from the Ashes

declared that they would rather freeze to death than come back to their former emperor. Only one coward renounced Christ and returned to Nero. The persuasive and bold decision of the thirty-nine brave souls was so profound that the world-renowned general threw off his clothes, article by article, and joined his men in declaring, "Forty wrestlers, wrestling for thee, O Christ, to win for thee the victory and from thee the victor's crown."

The invitation after this sermon was spirited: *"Whoever confesses Me before men, him I will also confess before My Father who is in heaven. But whoever denies Me before men, him I will also deny before My Father who is in heaven"* (Matthew 10:32,33). The altar, filled with people making their decisions, kneeling before their God. I was greatly anointed to preach the Word of God. It had been eighteen months since Greeneville.

In October, on Thanksgiving Sunday, I preached before a congregation in St. Catharines, Ontario. After I finished preaching I shook hands. I had a flashback memory of four years earlier when David Boyes, a member of Canada's world champion rowing team and a gold medalist, was converted as I preached.

It was November and time to leave for Saskatoon. I spoke at those four meetings at the crusade and for the first time had a slight feeling of being my old self again.

On the plane back to Toronto from Saskatoon I had a brainstorm. I began developing the idea for a Christmas program for Huntley Street. It would be called "The Five Old People in the Christmas Story."

Immediately upon arriving home Steve and I got to work on the script. Our work was especially inspired at this time. We had managed to create methods of writing that suited my specific needs. My stroke had meant that we had to change our ways of working to accommodate my ever-improving abilities. Sometimes these changes had to be developed over again. Our five old people were Zacharias, Elizabeth, Herod, Anna and Simeon.

The use of the teleprompter meant that I could adjust the speed at which the text scrolled up. This suited my developing reading abilities very well. I could read at my own speed. Again, this was crucial. In contrast, this Christmas program went off without a hitch. I had practiced scrolling the script in preparation for taping. I worked with the use of the teleprompter. The script was written into the computer, and Steve then converted the document to text and displayed it on the screen. He would coach me in the proper pronunciation of the words.

Of my early post-stroke sermons, "Old People" was heralded as my best. David Mainse was exuberant about my comeback. Calvin Thielman spoke positively about this program with Billy and Ruth Graham and Patricia Claremount, the world famous author, at "Little Piney Cove."

In March 1998 we came back with another sermon for television on *100 Huntley Street*. I delivered this message after being interviewed by the capable and compassionate Moira Brown. I had made another quantum leap forward. This time we went for a topic that has been near and dear to me for the majority of my preaching life: prophecy. We developed seven main points that revealed the circumstances in the world that represented the signs of the times and Christ's Second Coming. The seven points were

1. Nuclear Weapons
2. The World's Changing Climate—El Nino
3. Thinking the Unthinkable—Armageddon
4. Cloning: Immortality
5. Moral Crisis in the World
6. Great Earthquakes
7. Religious Revival

When it came time to tape the program, I had been rushed. Normally Steve and I would rehearse each script 300 times before it went to air. But this time I went to air having rehearsed the script only a few times. I stuttered and paused. Moira was sympathetic, but I was embarrassed. It was a calamity.

Billy Graham brought the gospel to the world as his single commitment. But Franklin was dually charged with evangelism and Samaritan's Purse. In April, I gave a fourteen-minute dissertation on my stroke. It was my commissioning of Franklin to carry on God's good work without me, since I had fallen with a stroke. I was nervous because I felt my message was crucially important. When I got up to speak I found that God had greatly anointed me. The following excerpt

Phoenix: Rising Up from the Ashes

contains some of the words that more or less flowed from me (Luke 4:18):

To Franklin:
Your father is a preacher. You, Franklin, are a preacher and a healer. Franklin, you parallel Jesus in Doctor Luke's gospel: You, Franklin, have been anointed to preach the gospel to the poor. You, Franklin, have been sent to heal the brokenhearted. You, Franklin, will preach deliverance to the captives. You, Franklin, will bring recovery of sight to the blind. You, Franklin, will set at liberty them that are bruised, and you, Franklin, will preach the acceptable year of the Lord.

At the end of the message, Franklin instructed Chairman Ross Rhoads to pray. Ross was in tears. After ten seconds Franklin instructed another team member to pray. I was enormously grateful when following my speech Dr. Richard Furman, a surgeon and one of the founders of the World Medical Mission, walked up to me. I could see that he was in tears. He wrote something on my script. When I looked down to see what he had written, I read, "John, this is one of the most moving addresses that I have ever heard." I was stunned and greatly blessed.

After leaving the meeting place Kathleen and I traveled eighty miles to Calvin Thielman's manse in Montreat. Calvin had about fifteen guests for dinner that evening. Everyone seated at the dinner table was a close friend of ours. The guests included Chaplain Al Christensen and his wife, Marion, who had come from the "Cove," John and Paula Wallace, who were visiting from Tennessee, and Ruth Graham.

After a gracious and delicious meal Dr. Dick Furman asked me to pass my address to Ruth. Ruth read the address and then turned to Kathleen and me and declared, "John, you are the one man responsible for our son's preaching at crusades." I was honored and greatly humbled by Ruth's kind comments.

In June I was asked to go to Ottawa, where Billy Graham was holding his crusade at the Corel Centre later that week. George Beverly Shea, Canada's national treasure, was born in a suburb of the nation's capital city.

It was arranged that I introduce three people on Huntley Street on concurrent days. These programs were being televised from the lawn of the Parliament buildings and shown across North America. My introductions of George Beverly Shea and surgeon Melvin Cheatham went superbly, as did my introduction of David Mainse. However, when it came to introducing Franklin Graham, my performance was a catastrophe.

We were seated outside, and it began to rain. I protected my script for as long as I could, but the ink ran and blotted when I removed it from my raincoat. I had to read it. Exacerbating my difficulties was the awkward fact that my glasses were steaming up and I was a victim of Kathleen's well- intentioned support. Every time I stumbled through a line, Kathleen would reach into the sightline of the cameras and try to help me with my lines. She was both visible and audible to the television audience.

Billy was watching this spectacle from his room. I can only imagine what he was thinking. Billy was proud of his son and must have felt that Franklin deserved better than to have his introduction bungled and battered so badly. That was the day David introduced Franklin and the brother-in-law of former prime minister John Turner. I felt badly about my fiasco. Again, I was a fool! David Mainse is a long-standing friend of mine. Instead of reprimanding my awful performance that day he asked me if he could use a foreword that I had written years earlier for his republished autobiography, which would run tens of thousands of copies around the world.

In July I spoke back-to-back with Pastor John Hull before another 800 ministers at the Billy Graham School of Evangelism in Toronto. This time my topic was "Strokes." I hoped to shed light on this very misunderstood and under-researched medical condition. John Hull was impressed with my newfound abilities. He asked me to preach to his Peoples Church congregation on Thanksgiving evening. This invitation delighted me no end. Peoples Church had been my home church for over three decades.

Interestingly, Kathleen introduced me that night. She spoke about my stroke and how the Lord had blessed our lives with my recovery. She presented a heartfelt and articulate speech that night. My twenty-seven-minute sermon was the longest I had spoken since my stroke. I used humor extensively in this sermon. It began,

Phoenix: Rising Up from the Ashes

It's Thanksgiving, and recently Kathleen and I went to Koo Koo Roos on Yonge Street in Toronto. It's one of those restaurants where you take a number and wait your turn. I was pondering my message at our table. A woman stared at me. "Are you ninety-five?" Perplexed I said, "I am old, I had a stroke, but I am no ninety-five!"

That broke the ice, and the congregation howled with laughter. I was off to the races. Only moments later I followed with:

The world has a new virus called country-and-western-itis: You may recognize these lines: "She got the goldmine—I got the shaft." And "I'm so miserable without you—it's almost like having you here." And "Walk out backwards—I'll think you're comin' in."

They say the 1999 Chrysler's been "born again." But, it's Christ through whom in 1999 "you must be 'born again!" It's Christ, not the 1999 Honda, who can make you "feel like a brand new person!" It's Christ, not the 1999 Mazda, who "just feels right!" In 1999, it's Christ, not the 1999 Toyota, "Oh what a feeling." It's Jesus Christ, not the 1999 Jaguar, who is the "Sovereign one!"

After my sermon, Jerry Howarth joined me on the platform. He was still chuckling. The night was a terrific blessing for us.

CHAPTER XVII

Y2K and 9/11

On September 11, 2001, the world changed. The World Trade Center had been dissolved to rubble by terrorists. North America had long ignored warnings of impending terrorist attacks. No one knew the extent of devastation the Israeli-Palestinian conflict would bring. And, of course, there were those notorious foes: Saddam Hussein, holed up in his squalid little spider hole, and Osama Bin Laden, darting mysteriously in the shadows. On December 30, 2006, Saddam Hussein was hanged by the neck until dead. But the world still plays hide-and-seek with Bin Laden. It spins its circuitous route toward chaos. It is Armageddon sooner or later.

At the emergence of the new era, perhaps the era that history will record as the era of terrorism, the world had been knocked off kilter. My life had similarly been permanently altered. For the first half decade after being suddenly silenced, I struggled to get myself afoot. Then, after a very conscious and deliberate process of therapy, although I had not regained control of my speech, I was crystal clear in thought, and my connection with Jesus had never been more fulfilling.

I had recovered much of my health and was motivated to resume my *John Wesley White Program* on television. It would mean a great deal to me to get back on the air. So Stephen Trelford and I went to work preparing scripts for a thirteen-program season. For me, it was a whole new ballgame. Where once I had been able to speak intelligibly, I was now relegated to the basement of our home to assist Stephen in writing specifically arranged short sentences that featured boldface words that would enable me to emphasize meanings in the text.

The lines of text were double-spaced in a large font for easy reading. Once written, Stephen would convert the copy to a text format so that it could be transcribed to the teleprompter. This way I could comfortably scroll the text on the screen. This is what most television celebrities and politicians do. However difficult our task was, our job was further exacerbated by the rather uncomfortable fact that we were working to deadline. Scripts in various stages of development had to be mastered weekly for airing nationally on Vision TV.

When reading, I still missed articles, prepositions, conjunctions and other small words when I spoke. This frustrating idiosyncrasy made my message difficult for the audience to understand. Stephen would assist me with the recitation of the material until our voices gave out. Then, alone, I would rehearse it 300 more times prior to airing.

Taping the programs posed other difficulties. Lloyd Knight, with whom I had a close association during the '80s and '90s, and his son trucked their film equipment to our home. We would use our living room as the set. We dressed the room in a warm and homey manner so that the viewing audience got a feeling of being with us in our home. Stephen assembled the computer right beside a camera and placed the teleprompter within a natural sight line of the lens. Everything was spatially specific.

In my hand I clutched the remote control for the text. Happily, I could control the speed of my reading. I would sit in my easy chair, and Lloyd and Kathleen would straighten my suit jacket so that my paralyzed arm, which had the unfortunate tendency to raise itself up almost like it was levitating into the view of the camera, would stay put and mostly out of sight. Stephen was perched on the arm of the sofa, so close to me with his copy of the script that his arm once crossed the sight line of the camera and somehow appeared in the final edit. Steve would mouth words that I would miss. He functioned as an earphone would.

Frequently, when I missed something badly enough that it would obscure the message for the audience, Steve would signal "cut" and the taping would cease. I would have to be tended to again. My tie would have to be adjusted. The knot of a tie is never quite right when someone else ties it. My jacket cuff would be pulled down with some difficulty, as my arm was still trying to levitate. And my body was re-situated in the deep chair.

To get up to speed for television, I would practice the first words of the next sentence before the cameras started rolling again. This way I could dovetail the words with the rolling of the videotape. It took a considerable amount of effort and time to complete the half-hour programs, with introductions and conclusions delivered by Kathleen, who managed the project. My nephew Roy Sommerville made regular appearances. Prior to my speaking, he would painstakingly explain to the audience that I had suffered an aphasic stroke and that the left side of my brain had to be reconnected. Yes, it took a while to get the programs in the can.

The whole project, which spanned two years, although difficult made me feel like I was getting back to normal. All in all the programs went off well enough, though admittedly not up to the standard of my pre-stroke programs. We featured two celebrities on our new *John Wesley White Programs*. Jerry Howarth, the voice of the Blue Jays, gave his testimony on one program, and ex-Toronto Maple Leaf hockey player Mark Osborne, who had been converted at one of my meetings in Toronto in the '70s, gave his testimony. The experience was exhilarating and fun. Vision TV contacted us, relaying the encouraging news that the Neilson ratings had us as the second most widely viewed program on air across Canada in the year 2000.

Then I received a letter from Franklin after sending him tapes of some of my programs. Franklin recognized both the effort and the quality of the new series; however, he felt that I might do damage to my image if I continued with my stuttering attempts to return to television. The last thing that people see is the first thing that they remember. Franklin suggested that I discontinue all public appearances.

I was devastated. In the dark of my lonely nights I cried out to the Lord to guide my next moves.

However discouraged I felt in the short run, Franklin had been correct. Indeed, I might do irreparable damage to my ministry if I persisted in attempting to resurrect my media persona. However, I was reaching some people for Christ.

Once again, I lay wide-eyed in bed, praying for direction. Then a thunderous bolt of lightning crashed in on me during a dark and very stormy night. The penetrating and inspiring thought overcame me that I would begin rerunning my programs from the early '90s. Excitedly, I began airing the reruns of the *John Wesley White Program* on the CTS Broadcasting Network and on the Miracle Channel.

Pastor Charles Wesley Price and Hilary Price are a team of ministers. They gathered up their children, Hannah, Laura and Matthew, and emigrated from England to Canada in 2001. Immediately upon entering the New World, Charles was thrust into the driver's seat as our senior pastor at the Peoples Church. He worked tirelessly and with great enthusiasm. He championed the Lord Jesus Christ.

Charles has made a name for himself, and in my opinion, at the doorway of the third millennium of the Christian era, Charles Price is the best preacher in Canada, both from the pulpit and across the nation on television. The theological and spiritual messages of Charles Price travel the world via the Peoples Church television broadcast. As a motivated man of God he crisscrosses the globe carrying God's Word to lost souls. Yes, by way of introduction to a new job, a new congregation and a new continent, Charles Price came out of the gate like a racehorse. Charles has endeared himself not only to those assembled in Peoples Church, but also to a nation thirsty for a brilliant, witty and straight-shooting preacher.

Charles Price hails from the countryside abutting the city of Hereford, England, in Ross-on-Wye River Village, approximately a dozen miles south of Hereford. A magnificent cathedral is situated in Hereford, for which the picturesque city is well-known. Charles is the second of five sons and one daughter. Curiously, my family was one of five sons and one daughter. Another Wesley, his older brother, was John Wesley Price.

Charles' great-grandfather was converted at an historic revival in Wales at which tens of thousands of souls were saved. Charles' Jewish father made a living as a sheep and cattle farmer. When he became a believer in Jesus Christ, Charles' family regularly attended the Brethren Hall. Yes, Christianity has long been the guiding light of the Price family.

In his own words Charles declared of himself, "I was not Christian, but I became a Christian on a Saturday night when I was twelve years of age after seeing Billy Graham's film *Shadow of the Boomerang*." As a strict Brethren Hall member, Charles hadn't seen a "worldly" film

Y2K and 9/11

until he was twelve years old. He became bored. He was a curious boy with an active mind.

One Saturday night, a fervent Christian man in his city invited Charles to come to the town hall, where there was a meeting of interdenominational churches connected with a Youth For Christ rally. It was that evening Charles Price saw the Billy Graham film.

With the world still dizzy in the wake of 9/11, in October 2001 Charles hit the pulpit hard, delivering a captivating personal testimony. It was televised across Canada. Charles revealed:

> After seeing the film that night I knew that I wasn't a Christian. I said, "Lord, please take over my life." I didn't know if anything happened at all. But the next day I went to the church that I had been to all of my life. And that Sunday morning for the first time, the service was interesting. I went back on Sunday night, and again for the first time in a long while, the preacher's sermon made sense. I thought to myself "this is incredible, these people have changed overnight." I soon realized actually what had changed was that something had happened to me. Before it was dull and boring. Now it was interesting and alive and God proved to my heart what he puts into all of our hearts—a hunger and a thirst for righteousness. I had a bad track record in righteousness…So, I rededicated myself to Christ.

At sixteen years of age Charles was dedicated to Christ by his dynamic mentor Major Thomas, the founder of Capernwray Bible College. Some time later, Jill Briscoe of Cambridge University met Charles in person. He had come up to her home while going door-to-door for Christ. It was at this time that Charles became recognized as a street-corner soul winner. Seeing his burgeoning potential, Jill invited Charles back to her husband, Stuart, who had succeeded Major Thomas at Capernwray.

As a sixteen-year old rookie, he proclaimed the words of the prophet Jeremiah, "*I will not make mention of him, nor speak any more in his name. But his word was in mine heart as a burning fire shut up in my bones, and I was weary with forbearing, and I could not stay*" (Jeremiah 20:9).

Suddenly Silenced

Charles graduated from Glasgow Bible School; then he obtained his BA, then was conferred an honorary doctor of divinity degree from Tyndale University in 2005. Charles immersed himself with great enthusiasm for three years prior to his esteemed appointment as principal at Capernwray.

His wife, Hilary, has picked up a mantel of her own. She is the chairperson for the Anne Graham Lotz Angel Ministries in Toronto. Charles was carved out of a Mount Rushmore clay, as was Billy Graham; so Hilary was smithed from a mighty metal in the likeness of the "Iron Lady" Margaret Thatcher.

Annually, on Mother's Day, Hilary Price commands the audience at the Peoples Church with forthrightness, wisdom and wit. On Mother's Day 2007 Hilary addressed the crowd with her usual grace and charm. She proudly announced that her eldest child, Hannah, was leading a tour from the University of Calcutta. Hannah was taking students on missionary excursions. Then Hilary happily announced that her next daughter, Laura, was nursing in Guatemala.

Of her son, Hilary revealed that Matthew is a normal sixteen-year-old. She shared that when she comes to pick Matthew up at school she follows his instructions to the letter. He asks that she wait away from the school, near the park, in the car. She is to wear sunglasses, keep the window up and remain incognito so that no one will recognize her. Then Matthew tarries no more. He slinks away from his friends and has his rendezvous with his mother. Matthew always says of his mother, "She has eyes in the back of her head."

But all of his dedication to his work took its toll on Charles. In the late '90s Charles, like me, suffered a life-threatening heart attack. His ministry was endangered. Dr. Bentley-Taylor, also my brother Hugh's surgeon, cared for Charles. Charles recalled the most relevant biblical promise and struggled to hold it in his mind: "*I shall not die, but live, And declare the works of the LORD*" (Psalm 118:17). He, just into his fifties, was given only a fifty-fifty chance of survival, just as I was in my time. Yes, like me, Charles lives, having received the promise of the Lord!

In our home we receive Charles' services on Sundays at 9 a.m. on the Crossroads Television Network, then at 10:30 a.m. on CTV Television, then at 1 p.m. on the Vision Channel, then on the Miracle Channel via satellite at 5:00 p.m. Kathleen and I watch the reruns of

Y2K and 9/11

Charles' services to catch a sharper image of his countenance and his message, which wings its way around the world. Then Kathleen and I go to the Peoples Church. We sit in the back pews. These services are like multi-media flashbacks of the years that I spent with Billy Graham.

Notably, with wit and humor Pastor Charles wields the cutting voice of a master orator. Charles speaks with a pitch that cuts into the ear. The edge of this pitch I have been privileged to hear in sharp relief, up close and personal for forty years with Billy Graham. There are the dramatic gestures too. The abrupt swivel of Charles' head instantaneously commands the attention of an entire congregation. And perhaps most notably, he has the same penetrating steel blue eyes, protruding jaw and chiseled Mount Rushmore features. Charles whisks his light auburn hair back much in the same fashion. Charles commands the Word of God boldly. These anointed men of God possess the charisma of the prophet Elijah of the Old Testament and of John the Baptist of the New Testament.

The other divine message that I received was that Steve and I were to work on my autobiography towards airing it as a thirty-eight-program radio series. With introductions and conclusions read by our son Bill and substance read by Steve, the successful radio program has aired on the WDCX 99.5 FM radio network from Buffalo, throughout New York state, the Ohio Valley and into Southern Ontario. Then CJYE (Joy) Radio picked up the series for airing.

After my stroke I discovered that there were thousands of my twenty-three books packed around my house and garage. I made arrangements to deliver the boxes and boxes of books to Peoples Church, 100 Huntley Street, Canada Christian College and Tyndale University for distribution to the public. The remainder of the books I mail to people around North America. And I carry with me some of the books on my evangelistic excursions up and down Argonne Street. I make gifts of these books to my neighbors. Each night, post-stroke, I go walking up our street in silence. Along with handing out books, I limp along praying and attempting to memorizing Scripture. After the stroke I could speak not one word. In 2010, I have memorized hundreds of verses and phrases of Scripture.

Each month Steve and I produce a dozen or so pages for Franklin Graham on the biblical perspective as related to current events. This work is our monthly "Letter to Franklin Graham." This alone makes Steve and I rather prolific, considering the challenge of overcoming my stroke to make sense of it all. If that weren't enough, we prepare our "Dear Friends" letter each month, updating people of the activity of my Join The Family Christian Ministries.

Some time ago, I was very much focused on memorizing Scripture when an interesting thought occurred to me. I recalled that fifty-five years ago, D.L. Moody was personally responsible for bringing 75,000 people face to face with the Lord. David the Psalmist joyfully explained, *"He who continually goes forth weeping, Bearing seed for sowing, Shall doubtless come again with rejoicing, Bringing his sheaves with him"* (Psalm 126:6). Then, the king's son Solomon appropriately stated, *"The fruit of the righteous is a tree of life, And he who wins souls is wise"* (Proverbs 11:30).

With this as my theme, as I passed by a three-garage mansion I noticed a man outside. I approached him with a will and a witness for the Lord. I reached out, handing him a copy of the book that I had written following the death of our son, *Where Is Wes?* The man gently smiled and took the book.

A week later, en route up the hill, I glanced at the sizable home that I was again passing, and just then the man hauled open his door and came right out to the street to meet me. This time his smile was wide and warm. He looked me in the eye and said, "Your book, it is interesting." I humbly confess to have passed out hundreds of *Where Is Wes?* books to Jews, Chinese, Indians, Pakistanis, Iranians, Russians, and Czechoslovakians in my diverse and trendy upper-middle-class suburb and to the multicultural mosaic that is Toronto.

Recently, as is my habit, I hobbled up Argonne, where I came upon two Czechoslovakian brothers. I discovered that one devout Roman Catholic brother was visiting the other. In my fractured English I started a conversation with them. I handed the one who lived on my street one of my *Where Is Wes?* books. In turn, this man handed the book to his visiting brother, who, glancing at the cover, excitedly piped up, "Billy Graham! To us Billy Graham is the pope." Apparently this man had been to a Billy Graham crusade in Prague, Czechoslovakia. The man was obviously overcome with adulation. In an enthusiastic staccato utterance I blurted that I had been a Billy Graham associate

Y2K and 9/11

evangelist for forty year. The visiting brother managed to reply, "I will try to read this." It then struck me that these men would be interested in an account that happened in the ordinarily still air of August 2002.

That same month on a Monday afternoon I stepped into my backyard and was abruptly jolted, caught completely off balance, by a roar of swirling winds. I squinted skyward and to my amazement saw multiple low-hovering helicopters, the beams of which brightly scanned the ground. I noticed that these helicopters held a militaristic formation in the sky. These were the post-9/11 days, so the dust cyclone created by these hawks in the sky sent ominous chills through me. Was it a terrorist attack in my own backyard? I shuddered.

I again forced my eyes to squint into the cloudless blue and saw that these whirling Apaches were swarming a particular pattern in the air. They were mighty close to me.

Beyond curiosity, I trundled up Argonne to see what was really going on. By the time I crested the top of the hill, I glanced down Bayview Avenue, and then I realized what all this meant. The pope was in town. Incredibly, he was staying within a stone's throw of our house.

I moved down the street and from the sidewalk into a grassy knoll. I leaned into a wire fence that encompassed the periphery of the Jesuit seminary of St. Joseph's Morrow Park. I clung onto the fence, and all at once there he was, the pope, meandering by in his popemobile. He was a mere six feet from my awe-stricken face. Without expectation the pope turned and craned his neck. We were at once eye-to-eye. I reeled back a bit, as it struck me that the eyes of the pope were the same blue eagle eyes that I had come to know over the decades in the evangelist Billy Graham. I trembled at the thought of what incarnation really means. Without a word, I think, the pope knew me. Then I relaxed my grip from the fence and the pope rolled away into the cloistered grounds. In my turning, I doffed my cap and hobbled out of sight and down the hill.

A little while later I was hobbling again, this time up the street like any crippled old man, when I stumbled upon two beautiful teenage girls. As I approached them I noticed that one was on her cellphone, perhaps to her boyfriend. To the other I handed another copy of *Where Is Wes?* The girl quizzically glanced up from the curb and at my offering exclaimed, "Cool!" I felt my step quicken and my hobble a little more

Suddenly Silenced

sprightly. "*Now king David was old and stricken in years*" (1 Kings 1:1.)

A little farther on I stumbled to the sidewalk again, in front of our house, to find our Iranian neighbor across the street on the sidewalk in front of his house. This man had crutches nestled underneath his arms. I inquired as to what had happened. First, the soft-spoken man admitted to being alone, as his Persian wife and daughter had flown to Iran. The man glanced up at me with a particularly quizzical expression. Then in a firm voice he exclaimed that the other day he had been chopping wood for his fireplace and had made an unfortunate slip. Off had come his big toe. He was rushed by ambulance to North York General Hospital, where almost miraculously they stitched his big toe back where it had been chopped off. This day, the man was singing praises to modern medicine: "They sewed it back on! They sewed it back on!" So I took this man under wing and prayed with him—and gave him my book *Where Is Wes?*

Whereas I had lived in suits, twenty of them, in 100 countries around the world, I now live in blue jeans. A lifetime of memories was conjured up when I recently viewed those suits on a rack. I have now brought them out of the closet and delivered them to appreciative preachers and to the Salvation Army.

In 1996 I was in painful disillusionment, but today I am happy. In 2003 Kathleen underwent cancer surgery and received chemotherapy treatments. She was scheduled for surgery two months after the date that her cancer was diagnosed. We all felt that this was too long to wait for surgery, given the aggressive nature of the cancer. So I put a call in to Billy Graham, who then called the surgeon who had treated him so well during his visit in 1995. Kathleen had surgery five days later. She has recovered well and is also quite happy.

For the first six and a half decades of my life I was caught in the maelstrom of perpetual motion. After the stroke I work steadily along, and I frequently find myself reclining in reverie. Where I had been on thousands of platforms before countless television cameras and a multitude of microphones, I now spend time in solitude and attend The Peoples Church in the back pews. As John the Baptist so accurately expressed, "*[Jesus] must increase, but I must decrease*" (John 3:30). Now I know that "*Godliness with contentment is great gain*" (1 Timothy 6:6).

Y2K and 9/11

Regularly in the morning and in the evening, on my knees I chant, "Jesus Christ is Lord, Jesus Christ is Lord, Jesus Christ is Lord," one hundred times. Fifty times I chant, "Praise the Lord" and another fifty times I chant, "I lift my hands to the Lord." Then I repeat the Lord's prayer two times. I repeat this sequence three consecutive times each day, to this day. The entire process takes me approximately seven minutes each time.

It is now 2010, and I reflect on my motto of sixty years. I have signed thousands of autographs using it. It has been the foundation of my Christianity throughout my life. And it was said best by the apostle Paul 2,000 years ago: *"That I may know him, and the power of his resurrection, and the fellowship of his sufferings, being made conformable unto his death"* (Philippians 3:10).

Finally, I cite the Hebrews benediction:

Now may the God of peace who brought up our Lord Jesus from the dead, that great Shepherd of the sheep, through the blood of the everlasting covenant, make you complete in every good work to do His will, working in you what is well pleasing in His sight, through Jesus Christ, to whom be glory forever and ever. Amen (Hebrews 13:20,21).

CHAPTER XVIII

Lessons from a Stroke

For sixty-seven years of my life I knew nothing about strokes. Previously, I had believed that strokes were for grandmothers. Grandmother White fell to a stroke, but she was eighty-one years old, and I was too young to understand what it meant to suffer a stroke.

It was an undeniable fact that my heart stopped for two minutes. My mother and father had suffered fatal heart attacks. Kathleen's parents had died of heart attacks, and my brother Hugh had undergone quadruple bypass surgery following a heart attack, so I knew something about heart attacks. However, I remained abysmally ignorant concerning strokes.

Lesson One: For the first eight months following my stroke, I was despairing. Our son Bill had tried to bolster my confidence about my future while at St. John's Convalescent Hospital. Yet my female speech therapist had made that ominous proclamation: "He'll never speak again." As a result of that short sentence, I hit the kind of bottom that I'd hit when our second son, Wesley, perished when his twin prop plane crashed in 1991. Then Bill started me working with simple language-oriented software computer programs. One of these programs rated the language centers of my mind. It tested my IQ. This test was a highlight, because it indicated that even following my stroke my mind remained clear. When attempting to convey my condition to others, I use the analogy of a four-cylinder car: three cylinders were fully operational; one cylinder was dead. *"God has not* *given us a spirit of fear, but of power and of love and of a sound mind"* (2 Timothy 1:7).

Lesson Two: For nine long months following April 28, 1996, I was without speech, even though Kathleen had made a consistent effort to get me to speak again. Professor and surgeon Melvin Cheatham, a distinguished close friend and member of Samaritan's Purse International, had traveled around the world to over 100 countries during his lifetime, bringing the Word of God to people of all races. He made a rather frightening observation. He explained that there was only one other person he had known who had suffered the same fate as I had. Likewise, in Dr. Luke's gospel, Zacharias, after his stroke, *"asked for a writing tablet, and wrote, saying, 'His name is John.' So they all marveled. Immediately his mouth was opened and his tongue loosed, and he spoke, praising God"* (Luke 1:63,64).

Lesson Three: On April 29, 1996, a dozen Billy Graham team members surrounded my bed in the Greeneville Hospital. It so happened that, in the very early '70s, I went as bald as a bowling ball. Ted Dienert, in charge of videotaping *Agape*, demanded that I go out immediately and purchase the most expensive hairpiece that I could find. So, I did. In the hospital following my stroke, I lay there in a diaper, covered by only a thin sheet. My bald head protruded from beneath the sheet, and those gathered around managed to snicker through their tears. They were thinking, "John, you're bald." *"Go up, you baldhead! Go up, you baldhead!"* (2 Kings 2:23).

Lesson Four: I would give times and dates. I often wanted to get things done "yesterday," and I reflected on something that I'd done "tomorrow." I had my *yesterdays* and *tomorrows* backwards. Thank God, *"Jesus Christ is the same yesterday, today, and forever"* (Hebrews 13:8).

Lesson Five: A person having fallen prey to a stroke often suffers many startling and confusing affects. As far as I was concerned, one of the first examples of this was that when I was asked a direct question I responded with a rather disconcerting "Yes—No—Yes"! I knew very clearly which way I wanted to answer. However, the simple words *Yes* and *No* somehow got reversed. *"With me there should be Yes, Yes, and*

No, No? But as God is faithful, our word to you was not Yes and No" (2 Corinthians 1:17,18).

Lesson Six: Equally embarrassing was my unfortunate tendency to confuse gender in my fractured speech. I would refer to *he* when I wanted to say *she*, and I said *his* when I wanted to say *hers*, and so on. "[*The Lord*] *made into a woman, and He brought her to the man*" (Genesis 2: 22).

Lesson Seven: There are three Greek words to express the different forms of love: *agape, filios* and *eros*. Prior to marriage I was a virgin, and I have been faithfully married to my wife for fifty-seven years. Billy Graham used to warn of three perilous pitfalls: pride, money and sex. Prior to my stroke I was always careful to avoid these pitfalls. So in scores of countries I only shook hands with people. In September 1996, following the Franklin Graham festival in Kitchener, Ontario, and my stroke, I was enjoying fellowship. Suddenly, I grabbed a beautiful woman on the elevator and boldly gave her a hug and a holy kiss on the cheek. I suddenly became aware of a man—the woman's husband. He was fuming. The woman in the elevator was a complete stranger to Kathleen and me. So, the rumor began that John Wesley White, formerly a street corner preacher, had now become a street corner Casanova! Since my stroke I have observed the exhortation to "*Greet all the brethren [sisters] with a holy kiss*" (1 Thessalonians 5:26).

Lesson Eight: The left side of my brain had been seriously affected by the stroke. In September 1996 I couldn't speak a single word except *Jesus*. I attended a Franklin Graham festival of 10,000 people that night in Kitchener, Ontario. It was here that the country singer icon Ricky Skaggs dedicated a song to me. I sat between Tom Bledsoe, our song leader, and Franklin. Tom heard me singing "Blessed Assurance" on the platform, as I had for the past twenty-five years. Tom whispered in my ear, "John, just listen to you sing in tenor." For us that night it was *"psalms and hymns and spiritual songs, singing with grace in [our] hearts to the Lord"* (Colossians 3:16).

Lesson Nine: In the early '70s, concerning our nationally televised program *Agape,* I employed a rather unusual technique that was a gift from the Holy Spirit. I could play a recorded message into my earphone from a tape player in my pocket. This enhanced the delivery of my more articulate messages, because I could relay, verbatim, information that I had previously compiled. The one caveat concerning this technique was that there was a millisecond delay between the time I heard the message and the time it took my brain to synchronize it. It is written of our Lord that "*'When He ascended on high, He led captivity captive, And gave gifts to men'...some to be...evangelists*" (Ephesians 4:8–11).

Lesson Ten: My stroke paralleled the stroke of William Manchester, the Winston Churchill biographer. We were both writers, and we both suffered a stroke. Manchester spoke intently about the difficulties faced by an author who previously "couldn't write fast enough to keep up with his thoughts." But now, due to the aphasia that accompanied our strokes, we faced enormous frustration when sitting down to compose sentences on paper, and we found that our everyday tasks became dreadfully slow. Manchester could manage to write only one letter a day. Frustratingly, for five hours one day I struggled to write a single page to Billy Graham's brother Mel, but I made so many errors that I had to quit. My facilitator, Stephen Trelford, had to write the letter. "*One thing I do*" (Philippians 3:13).

Lesson Eleven: There were times when I became so frustrated with my inability to speak that I would lose my temper and shout, causing Kathleen, our family and friends to be embarrassed. For example, I would bellow with my loud evangelistic voice, "I don't know, I don't know, I don't know." "*'Be angry, and do not sin': do not let the sun go down on your wrath*" (Ephesians 4:26).

Lesson Twelve: Bill Frist, the Republican senate majority leader, traveled to Billy Graham's "Cove" in October 2003. So did I. I had the opportunity to meet with the potential presidential candidate. Interestingly, Senator Frist, one of America's leading surgeons, came from East Tennessee, close to where I'd suffered my stroke. I was self-conscious about not being able to speak. When we met face-to-face there was a discernibly uncomfortable pause. I stood in front of him in mute silence, blushing. I am grateful that Russell Busby, Billy Graham's personal photographer, politely explained to Senator Frist that I was an

Lessons from a Stroke

Oxford graduate and had been an associate evangelist with Billy Graham for forty years. Russell also told how I had for seven years prior to my stroke twinned with Franklin Graham. While Russell was talking, my heart was palpitating. The diplomatic senator, having understood the situation clearly, dropped into a compassionately conversational tone and attempted to dialogue with me for a few minutes. *"Aspire to lead a quiet life, to mind your own business"* (1 Thessalonians 4:11).

Lesson Thirteen: Since my stroke in 1996, my close friend Russell Wells faithfully has come to our home for two hours on Saturday mornings. This is "the highlight of the week" for me. After I greet him with a friendly "Good morning," he reads five or six chapters of the Bible. We discuss politics and current events. We have added something new to our Saturday morning meetings. I volunteer this prayer regularly: "Jesus Christ, bless the Wells family: Russell, Lois, John, Mark, Grant, Margaret, Jennifer and Joel." One week I took a ten second pause as Russell was leaving our home, and then I said a friendly "Good morning!" Russell just laughed. He knew what I had intended to say. *"My voice You shall hear in the morning, O LORD"* (Psalm 5:3).

Lesson Fourteen: In high school I got a perfect 100 percent in algebra. Following my stroke, I got scattered by merely trying to count to ten. Dialing the telephone was a near impossibility for me. I would stare at the dial pad, at all those numbers, and would try to press one number, then the next, then the next, and so on. I would frequently misdial and then have to repeat the confusing constellation of numbers. Even today, I attempt to dial a phone number an average of seven times before I get through to the party that I wish to speak with. I would frequently attempt to phone my close friend Calvin Thielman, the pastor to two generations of Grahams. He was both brilliant and compassionate. Calvin had suffered a stroke himself. I had contacted Calvin hundreds of times, but following my stroke sometimes I would not get through. *"The number of them was ten thousand times ten thousand, and thousands of thousands"* (Revelation 5:11).

Lesson Fifteen: I believed that work—lots of work—would help to reconnect my brain. Much to my disillusionment, when I began to work with Kathleen, my family and Steve, I found that the small words in a sentence—the articles, conjunctions and prepositions—would somehow disappear from my view. Curiously, I believed that if I got the more complicated words correct, the audience would clearly understand my meanings. This caused much difficulty. With direction, I'd rehearse my simple scripts 300 times to ensure that I would catch the small words on the paper. Where I had been an Oxford University graduate, now I was like the apostle John. *"John...[was] uneducated and untrained"* (Acts 4:13). That was me!

Lesson Sixteen: For seventeen months after the stroke, I took physical therapy as an outpatient at St. John's Convalescent Hospital. I worked with Donna, my therapist, who had recognized that I would now have to begin writing with my left hand. I'd kept telling her that my hand would skate around on the desk like the surface was made of ice. So, three years after I had begun therapy, she gave me a sticky placemat that remained fixed to the desk. As I put pen to paper, my pages didn't shift around, making it easier for me to work. Her ingenious pad has enabled me to write the names of 700 people each month. I have printed the return address on the envelopes, but each and every name and contact address has to be painstakingly copied onto the center of the envelopes from cards that I have written out. At first the addresses on the envelopes appeared in childlike penmanship. Additionally, characters and numbers were missing on my envelopes, and many envelopes had to be trashed and new ones begun. I would spend many hours per day writing names and addresses. I prayed over each name as I write it. But remember that Ehud, a judge in the Bible, *"[was] a left-handed man"* (Judges 3:15).

Lesson Seventeen: What troubled me most was that the people closest to me, the people on whom I most heavily relied, made an incorrect assumption. They believed that I had regressed into an infantile state and that they were dealing with a child. Our son Paul's wife, Paula, is a professor of French at Purdue University in Indiana. Paul announced on the telephone that our six-year-old grandson William and our four-year-old grandson Izzy were like their grandfather. They were "talking machines" in English and in French. Our son phones us regularly, and our grandsons speak incessantly into the mouthpiece. Once a man of three languages, now I would just listen, then stutter a few words into the phone. *"When I was a child, I spoke as a child, I understood as a child, I thought as a child"* (1 Corinthians 13: 11).

Lesson Eighteen: That first Christmas following my stroke, while I slept, Kathleen fell down the stairs in our house and broke her ankle. The boys alone rushed her to the hospital. Kathleen was awaiting the surgeon and was in a great deal of pain. When I arrived at the hospital I waited with my sons. As we waited, I got my exercise by pacing up and down the hallways. All at once, I came across a noisy man. He must have been crazy. He had broken free of his nurses. He lunged out of bed and scrambled into a chair in the hallway near to Kathleen's room. The nurses may have been trying to summon the hospital security. The man stared at me with an alarmingly angry expression. Then he began shouting nonsense at the top of his lungs. Suddenly, this man paused and then stood up. He came within eighteen inches of my face. I was almost overcome with halitosis. Yet I managed to come, smiling, boldly eye-to-eye and toe-to-toe with this man, and all I could do was laugh. Then this man began laughing and laughing and laughing some more. He continued to laugh with me as I paced the hallway. I had found a laughing friend at the hospital. Wise Solomon chided that there is *"a time to laugh"* (Ecclesiastes 3:4).

Lesson Nineteen: A soulmate of mine concerning strokes, Alfred Rees, the ex-senior pastor of Banfield Memorial Church, had a heart attack at the same time that I had mine in 1992. He also suffered a stroke in India just prior to my stroke. Alf was left with a limp like Jacob had after wrestling with the angel. I too would limp, up and down on our street. Al's first wife died years back, and our son informed me that Alf had remarried. One day in 1996 I hobbled, enthusiastically, a mile and a half to Banfield to see Alf, and I discovered that his new wife, Bernadette, was a beautiful brunette from Michigan. I could see how spiritual she was and how she was supportive of Alf's condition. However, my stroke had left me oversensitive. I realized that Bernadette meant well, but following our introduction, Bernadette exclaimed, "Dr. White, you were a TV star, but now you have been humbled by the Lord." I managed to smile at her. But I skulked home like a dog with its tail between its legs. Alf and Bernadette made their way over to our house frequently to coach me concerning the regaining of my speech shortly after I fell to the stroke. *"God resists the proud, but gives grace to the humble"* (James 4:6).

Lesson Twenty: One evening during prime time in July 2004, Kathleen happened to be channel surfing through the TV when she suddenly stopped on Much Music, the secular rock music channel that airs across Canada. The host of the program probed the studio audience, inquiring, "Who is the Messiah?"

Then a youth from the audience piped up, "It's John Wesley White."

The audience broke up into laughter. Kathleen's chest swelled with pride. When I heard this I was proud, so proud, in fact that when I stepped outside I tripped and fell on the brick driveway. My right side is paralyzed, so I had to struggle for a full three minutes to get back on my feet. As the Psalmist David so appropriately stated, *"Though he fall, he shall not be utterly cast down; For the LORD upholds him with His hand"* (Psalm 37:24).

But some of the greatest lessons that I have learned and needed for my own recovery are the importance of prayer, persistence in seeking physical health, and meditation on verses from the Bible about healing, in both the Old and New Testaments. After all, God is the Great Healer.

Acknowledgments

The apostle Paul declared,

Lest I should be exalted above measure by the abundance of the revelations, a thorn in the flesh was given to me, a messenger of Satan to buffet me, lest I be exalted above measure. Concerning this thing I pleaded with the Lord three times that it might depart from me. And He said to me, "My grace is sufficient for you, for My strength is made perfect in weakness" (2 Corinthians 12:7–9).

I turned eighty-one on September 15, 2009. But on April 28, 1996, I was suddenly silenced. I fell to a devastating stroke and spoke not one word. For nine months I sat at the bottom of my life. Just like John the Baptist in prison, I was questioning everything. But John the Baptist was beheaded. I was left with my head! So I had to ask myself what I was to do.

I would like to dedicate my autobiography, *Suddenly Silenced,* to Kathleen, my wife of fifty-seven years, who, throughout her enduring agony of being married to a man who has suffered aphasia and is an unquestionable workaholic, once again has supported me behind the scenes, permitting the long writing of this book. The feat of writing this book in itself seems incredible, since during that brutally cold winter of 1996-1997 I had but one three-word sentence: "Jesus is Lord." Kathleen had whispered this simple sentence into my ears so often it cannot be counted. Subsequently, I defeated a therapist's gloomy prediction that I would never speak again when in one unforgettable moment I seized an opportunity. I stood boldly and declared in a booming voice, "Jesus is Lord."

I am in debt to Franklin Graham, the evangelist, CEO of the BGEA and president of Samaritan's Purse. I had the privilege of twinning with Franklin for seven years. In September 1995 Billy and Franklin Graham twinned for the first time in my home province of Saskatchewan. At the Canadian BGEA headquarters in Calgary in April 2006, Franklin made the announcement that The My Hope India Festival was the costliest evangelistic effort in history. Perhaps it would be the last time that Billy and Franklin Graham twinned. The seeds were sown. The harvest was reaped. Yes, the largest ever evangelistic project, The My Hope India Festival in December 2006, involved 61,000 churches throughout India. There were 1.3 million people trained as counselors for this effort. The festival was publicized through TV spots, billboards and newspaper ads. The enormous event was translated into fourteen languages and aired on five different television programs on more than fifty television networks. As of June 2007, 8 million people had made decisions for Jesus Christ. They are the harvest of the festival.

A jovial David Mainse of *100 Huntley Street* took joy in thoroughly reading the manuscript. He inspired me with his friendly chuckles at the humorous forays contained within. Many thanks go to David for writing a thoughtful and compassionate introduction to this book. He found time in his busy schedule to come to me in our basement. That was January 1997. That same brutal winter following my stroke, I worked with a traditional female speech therapist. After a few weeks she moved on, as I could still speak only one word: *Jesus*. Since January 1997, I have been working exclusively with Stephen Trelford.

In March of that year David held my hand through one of the most embarrassing moments in my life. He afforded me the opportunity to get back into televangelism. He knew that, for me, to sit idle was to perish. So, in a sacrifice of Herculean proportions, he agreed to slot me in for a segment on *100 Huntley Street*—to get me back on my feet. Yet my dismal performance proved that it was too early to attempt such an undertaking. When I appeared on live television I was enthusiastic, but I simply stuttered and stammered. Awful. Realizing the extent of my stroke, David burst into tears, but he never let me down.

For David, my stroke was only strike one. The awful performance

Acknowledgments

was strike two. So he sent me back to the plate for another at bat. By that Christmas I had recovered sufficiently to step up to the plate again. This time I would belt a home run. *Five Characters in the Christmas Story,* a program for which I had rehearsed 300 times, was a smash hit. By that time my brain was successfully reconnecting. The program went to air.

David's encouragement has flowed through the years following my stroke, and in the winter of 2007 he made another house call. He brought with him much encouragement when he visited Kathleen, Stephen and me. David has remained my dear friend for forty years. I thank you, David.

Kathleen and I watch Charles Price's People's Church broadcasts of his Sunday morning services after we have attended them. Over the past five years I have considered the dashing Charles the best preacher in Canada from the pulpit or on television. Not only has he captivated the congregation of one of Canada's largest churches, but he also subtly weaves into the tapestry of his messages colorful illustrations that attract those in the pews and in the living rooms of the nation. Personal testimonials like his daring leap of faith, his bungee jumping from a bridge high above a raging river in New Zealand, make him truly a people's preacher. He bravely soldiers on in the fight to Christianize the world as he circumnavigates the globe, bringing the gospel to people in the trenches and everywhere. It is frontline combat for Charles Price, who is devoted to the Holy Word of God.

In his home district of Hereford, England, Charles was converted to Christ at the age of twelve after seeing *Boomerang*, the Billy Graham film. At sixteen years of age he was appointed the foreman in a crew that traveled to Rhodesia, Africa, for a year. Yes, at a tender age Charles toiled in the hot sun, getting his hands dirty in the soil of farm life. Then, upon returning to England, he found a dynamic mentor in Major Thomas, his principal at Capernwray College, where Charles himself later ascended to the principalship.

When Kathleen was diagnosed with cancer in 2005, Charles made a compassionate visit to our home. Both Kathleen and I were greatly encouraged by his visit. Charles, we thank you, too.

In 1999 in Ottawa, we met with Bob Paulson, the editor of *Decision,* who had sent me the entire forty-seven-year run of that magazine. He suggested that my autobiography should contain an expansion of the substance of the October 2003 article published in *Decision*, aptly titled "Suddenly Silenced."

I would like to express as best I can my deep and abiding gratitude to the many who offered suggestions for this book. After much prayer and rumination I would set a *fresh* course. I would pour my life onto the burning pages of my autobiography. I found new vigor. At just the right moment our son Bill called on his close friend Stephen Trelford to facilitate my voice. Yes, Stephen took the chair at the computer in January 1997. In an anthropological metaphor, Russell Wells once declared of Stephen, "He is uniquely capable of taking a single bone and reconstructing the original animal from it." This has been true, and this book is the evidence of such a skill. Stephen and I have worked together an average of ten or twelve hours per week to this day. Of all the contributions to the writing of this book, Stephen's is the most significant. Without his patient listening ear, his insightful interpretive power and his creative vocabulary, all transferred into text, this book simply would not exist.

To date approximately fifty people have read various editions of my autobiography. I am incapable of adequately expressing how greatly I appreciate the various enlightened comments that have emerged from those readings. Suffice it to say then that I am most grateful for their faithful service to me in the difficult memory work of cross-referencing pertinent dates, times and places identified in the book.

In the earliest days following my stroke our eldest son, Bill, and his wife, Nok, who traveled from her mother's home in Thailand, made the sacrifice and read the original sketches. Our son Randy and his wife, Lorraine, thoroughly read various editions of the book and made valuable comment as to the direction the text ought to take. They did not hesitate to make specific references to corrections wherever they found them necessary. Professors Paul and Paula kept in contact with us regarding the development of this work.

My brother Hugh and his wife, Aileen, visited our home to read sections of the book aloud. Their daughter, Sheryl Chrighton, read it too. My brother Lewis and his wife, Clara, perused the first edition. Their cousin, my mentor, the scholar Earle Cairns, gave me fresh eyes and ears for the printed word. My sister Betty, her son Charles, his

Acknowledgments

wife, Jennifer McVety, and Linda Davis all took time to look over the pages. Our nephew Roy Sommerville read the entire volume of *Suddenly Silenced*. The comments that these family members at home offered did not fall on fallow ground.

In England, John Pollock, Billy Graham's award-winning biographer, took rare time to comb the manuscript. His masterful notes regarding relevant additions and deletions crossed the Atlantic Ocean by mail. Maurice Rowlandson, the head of the BGEA in Britain in the 1980s, was a willing recipient of the rough manuscript.

Russell Wells, the friend who has been stationed at my side throughout the development of this book, regularly shared his vision of this work with me. George Beverly Shea and his wife, Karlene, read the book and offered their direction. Billy Graham's brother Mel found the time to read the entire manuscript. He offered many words of encouragement. Mel then passed the book on to his son, Mel Jr., who read it. Calvin Thielman accepted the mailing of the manuscript. His advice and encouragement I found eminently valuable. Calvin suffered a stroke of his own a quarter of a century ago. I am grateful, too, to Ross Rhoads, who took over my post as associate evangelist with the BGEA, and his wife, Carol, who were most concerned that I record the events of the crusades with the dignity and the accuracy they deserve. They went through the manuscript two times.

Old friends are not forgotten. My friend from Wheaton College, Professor Frank Nelsen, joined with his wife, Lois, to go through the book. Joe Yukich took out his blue pencil, marking up the margins where he deemed necessary. I am indebted to my former secretary Beatrice Ann Jackson, who put a seasoned editor's eye to the work. Marilou Wilson, to whom I am also indebted, diligently devoured the complete manuscript, weeding out inconsistencies and highlighting the necessary grammatical changes.

Huntley Street's Moira Brown swept over the work, ensuring accuracy of detail. I am thankful to Brian Kempster, who has been the Join the Family lawyer since the 1970s, for looking over the text and for giving critical comment. I wish to thank Sandy Trelford for patiently keying out the early editions of the book. Finally, George and Wendy Parson, my agents for forty years, added their usual spot-on direction with prophetic illumination.

Suddenly Silenced

The apostle who wrote the Gospel of John mentioned, *"There are also many other things that Jesus did, which if they were written one by one, I suppose that even the world itself could not contain the books that would be written. Amen"* (John 21:25). *Suddenly Silenced* is dedicated to those souls living and those gone to heaven.

Definition of a Stroke

April 28, 1996: the night the preaching stopped. Strokes are the fourth leading cause of death in North America, where in 2006 over half a million people were afflicted with strokes. In twenty years, the number of strokes will have increased by 50 percent annually. Today, when far more is known about strokes and people are more outspoken about them, we know that they can happen to anyone at any age.

Apoplexy is a condition of unconsciousness and paralysis caused by a disturbance in the blood circulation in the brain. The word *apoplexy* means "stroke," and this name is often used for the disease. The most frequent cause of stroke is a break in the wall of a blood vessel in the brain. This type of stroke is known as a cerebral hemorrhage.

Stroke caused by hemorrhage in the brain occurs in older people who have hardening of the arteries or other diseases of the blood vessels. A blood vessel may break because of sudden increased blood pressure, extreme physical exercise, or emotional strain. Another cause of stroke is the formation of a clot, or thrombus, in one of the blood streams to the brain from some other part of the body. It is often part of a larger clot that has formed on the lining of the heart. A clot that is carried in the blood stream is called an embolus.

Often when an attack occurs the patient collapses and paralysis develops, although the trouble may occur in a part of the brain that does not lead to paralysis. One side of the body, one leg and arm, and one side of the face and tongue become paralyzed. The side affected is usually opposite to the part of the brain that is injured, depending on the exact level at which the injury occurs. The person may be unable to speak and may remain unconscious. The pupils of the eyes are sometimes unequal in size, and the pulse may be slow or rapid. Fever sometimes develops.

A person who has just had an attack should be kept quiet until a physician arrives to give the proper care. Recovery from an attack is slow. The patient regains use of the leg first, then of the face, tongue, and arm.

During convalescence, the paralyzed muscles should be massaged. Later they should be exercised carefully to restore their action. In exercising and massaging, increase in blood pressure must be prevented. The patient should avoid emotional strain.

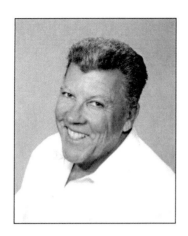

Stephen Edward Trelford Bio

Stephen Edward Trelford was born in a northern suburb of Toronto, Ontario, Canada. Raised in an upper-middle-class family, he was from an early age surrounded by actors, writers and creative people. At the age of nineteen Stephen found the Lord and dedicated his life to educating himself and to serving the Lord through writing and teaching.

He achieved an honors B.A. in religion from Bishops University, a private institution outside Montreal. He furthered his education at Bishops within the graduate school of education. In 2003, Canada Christian College conferred a doctor of literature degree on Stephen and three Canadian icons: The Honorable James Flaherty, the minister of finance of Canada; the Honorable David Onley, the lieutenant governor of Ontario; and the hockey sensation Paul Henderson.

Stephen teaches a variety of communications courses at Seneca College in Toronto. He developed and provided the voice for the thirty-eight-program radio series *Suddenly Silenced,* which has aired throughout the eastern United States and Canada. He has worked on the *John Wesley White Program* for television and is involved in numerous writ-

Suddenly Silenced

ing projects. For the past fourteen years Stephen has committed himself to service as the facilitator for John Wesley White.

Index of Names

By Chapter in Order of Appearance

Chapter 1
Shakespeare, William
Hawking, Stephen
Churchill, Winston
Blair, Tony
Clinton, Bill
White, Kathleen
Cornell, Ted
Ellis, Perry
Thielman, Calvin
Dillon, John
Bledsoe, Tom
White, Paul
Graham, Franklin
Graham, Billy
Phillips, Randy
Smith, Brent
White, John Wesley Jr.

Chapter 2
White, John Wesley
White, Charles Earle
White, Martha Jean
Wesley, John
Kirk, John
Kirk, Gordon
McClung, Nellie
Strand, Dr.
Sheppard, Harry
Hollands, Fred
Hollands, Harold
Clews, Mrs. Charles
Peden, Sister
Andrew, Sister
Hollands, Aunt Emma
White, Frank
Wagner, Linda
White, Lorraine
Calderwood, Billy
Cox, Harvey
White, Roy
White, Elmore
Steinbeck, John
White, Hugh
White, Aileen
White, Lewis
White, Clara
Cairns, Earle
White, Betty
McVety, Elmer
McVety, Charles
Apps, Syl
Drillon, Gordon
Metz, Nick

Hewitt, Foster
Hitler, Adolf
King George
Elizabeth, Queen Mother
Graham, Glenna

Chapter 3
Cantalon, Howard
Lowry, Oscar
Torrey, R.A.
Smith O.J.
Moody, Dl.
Crawford, Percy
Graham, Ruth
Landry, Tom
McGee, J. Vernon
McVety, Hugh
MacLean, Glen
Pritchard, Lorne
Sheppard, Arthur
Pattison, Jimmy
Carpenter, Jerry
Dynna, Gilbert
Dynna, Lillian
Dynna, Harold
Dynna, Dole
Shea, George Beverly

Suddenly Silenced

Chapter 4
Barrows, Cliff
Graham, Morrow
Radar, Paul
Jones, Bob
Twist, Arlo
Janecek, Ed
Janecek, Janine
Ayers, Lou
Janecek, Phil
Harrison, Dr.
Cook, Bob
Hustad, Don
Kendall, Ron
DeBoer, Lester
Nunn, Arthur
Benjamin, Dwayne
Whitefeather, Chief
Templeton, Charles
Smith, Paul
Wilson, T.W.
Wilson, Grady
Shuler, Jack
Roswell, Merv
Johnson, Torrey
Pierce, Bob
Christensen, Al
Ford, Leighton
Mosienko, Bill
Nelson, Frank
Musial, Stan
Williams, Ted
Holiday, Don
McClintock, Mrs. Bill

Chapter 5
Carter, Clarence
Criswell, W.A.
Lee, Robert
Rogers, Adrian

Paisley, Ian
Lynas, Lynda
Harris, Trevor
Baird, Sam
Baird, Trevor
Baird, Clifford
Baird, Neville
Baird, Stephen
Freeland, Gordon
Stiller, Brian
McRae, William
Sherrard, Sam
Humbard, Rex
Calderwood, Billy
Wetheral, Jim
Wetheral, Evelyn
Abraham, John
Paskett, Louis
Paskett, Shirley
Manning, Ernest
White, Aunt Beryl

Chapter 6
Sargent, Jean
Calderwood, William Sr.
Monaghan, Rinty
Calderwood, Mina Wilson
Wilson, Woodrow
Sommerville, Dorothy
Sommerville, Albert
Sommerville, Kenneth
Bullock, Bruce
Bullock, Jean
Matier, Billy
Briggs, James
Briggs, Mary
Calderwood, Ruth
Robb, John
Hendry, Gordon
Stuart, Jimmie

King Olaf
King George VI
Queen Elizabeth
White, Bill Charlton
James, Homer
Duff, John
Graham, Mel
Graham, William
   Franklin Sr.
Pilate, Pontius
McDougall, Douglas
Pickering, John
Pickering, Olive
Findlay, John
Gray, James
Upritchard, Harry

Chapter 7
Allan, Tom
Blinco, Joe
Ford, Leighton
Einstein, Albert
Mann, Allan
MacArthur, Douglas
Finney, Charles
Chapman, Wilbur
Sweeting, George
Presley, Elvis
Alderdice, David
Scriven Joseph
Dobbie, Orde
Debbie, Florence
Dobbie, William
Walker, Hugh
Taylor, Mick
Stephens, Arthur
Innis, John
Iverson, Hubert
Williams, Garnett

Index of Names—By Chapter in Order of Appearance

Winstone, Howard
Collins, Jackie
Jones, Old Man

Chapter 8
White, Randy
Paul, Billy
Walsh, John
Trelford, Stephen Edward
Weatherhead, Leslie
Lewis, C.S.
Pope, John Paul XXIII
Cowan, Max
Cowan, Margaret
Brown, Joy Lois
Mullinder, Wesley
Epstein, Brian
The Beatles
Caesar, Julius
Lord Harvey
Prince Faisal

Chapter 9
Judson, Doug
Martin, Bill
Hemingway, Ernest
Smith, Tedd
Beavan, Jerry
Evans, Robert
Bubeck, Mark
Ross, Autumn
Pocock, Maggie
Ross, Larry
Ellis, Robbie
Keon, Davey
Mahovolich, Frank
White, Margaret
Chambers, Irv

Chapter 10
Wallace, John
Wallace, Paula
Lindsey, Charles
Alou, Philippe
Waters, Ethel
Osborne, Dr.
Girvan, George
White, Hugh
White, Aileen
White, Brian
Wade, Wendy
Van Dyke, Vonda Kay
Kemple, Dick
Stam, Peter
Thomas, Edward
Frank, Vince
Ryan, Steve
Andersen, Paul
Bright, Bill
Jostlin, LaVonne
Jostlin, Eric
Cons, John
Wells, Russell
Wells, Lois
Wells, Grant
Wells, Jennifer
Wells, John
Wells, Margaret
Wells, Mark
Greene, Lorne
Graham, Billy
Barrows, Cliff
Shea, George Beverly
Wilson, T.W.
Johnson, Torrey
Pierce, Bob
Templeton, Chuck
Shuler, Jack
Cornell, Ted

Cornell, Zandra
Cornell, Ted Jr.
Cornell, Britney
Stewart, Nels
Bledsoe, Tom
Bledsoe, Terry
Presley, Elvis
Hall, Myrtle
Fasig, Bill
Wills, Stephanie
Leaning, Johnny
Leaning, Scott
Bell, Rhonda
Smith, Paul
Lastman, Mel
Thatcher, Ross
Robertson, Lloyd
Huston, Sterling

Chapter 11
Richard, Cliff
Tso, Peter
Roberts, Oral
Goodwin-Hudson, A.W.
McDonald, Jimmie
Peters, Frank
MacArthur, John
Southern, Dan
Musto, Steve
Goodall, Richard
Mitsuhashi, Mr. and Mrs.
Davies, Bob
Stephens, Bishop John
Carson, Johnny
Brady, Olga
President Marcos
Romeo
Gaugenzio
Boyzeo

323

Suddenly Silenced

Chapter 12
Kennedy, John F.
Kennedy, Robert
Luther, Martin
Monroe, Marilyn
Hendrix, Jimi
Joplin, Janis
Huxley, Aldous
Guevara, Che
Marx, Karl
Johnson, L.B
Leary, Timothy
Rubin, Jerry
Hoffman, Abbie
Manson, Charles
McKuen, Rod
Mai Tse Tung
Castro, Fidel
Mingh, Ho Chi
Marcuse, Herbert
Fabiano, Jerry
Spurgeon, Charles
Dylan, Bob
Zimmerman, Jack
McIntosh, Mike
Heitzig, Skip
Laurie, Greg
Colson, Charles
Watson, Merv
Watson, Merla
Foreman, George
Findley, Timothy
Trelford, Edward Lee
Hinn, Benny
Hinn, Costandi
Hinn, Clemence
McVety, Linda
McVety, Beverly
McVety, Douglas
White, Sheryl

Pointer, Jim
Kuhlman, Kathryn
Thomas, Rondo
Diefenbaker, John
Eisenhower, Dwight
Trudeau, Pierre Elliott
Clark, Joe
Nixon, Richard
McPherson, Aimee
Bell, Ralph
Nixon, Pat
Kennedy, Joseph
Kennedy, Bobby
Kennedy, Teddy
Winmill, Joan
Brown, Bill
Grier, Rosie
King, Larry
Shaw, George B.
Wallace, George
Smith, Anita
Armstrong, Neil
Salem, Beulah
Kopechne, Mary Jo
Blessit, Arthur
Rockefeller, Nelson
McGovern, George
Mulroney, Brian
Gustafson, Len
Reagan, Ronald
Ford, Gerald
Summers, Anthony
Horowitz, Michael
Bush, Barbara
Lynn, Dr.
Bush, Robin
Evans, Don
Evans, Susan
Bush, Laura
Bush, George H.W.

Kerry, John
Clemenger, Bruce
Martin, Paul
Harper, Stephen
Mackey, Lloyd
Manning, Preston
Quayle, Dan
Gore, Al
Trelford, Margaret
Whittall, John

Chapter 13
Tornquist, Evie
Tchividjian, Stephan
Dienert, Millie
Blanchard, Lewis
Hamilton, Sam
Hull, Bobby
Healey, Sid
James, Homer
Mainse, David
Mainse, Norma Jean
Wyrtzen, Jack
Dobbs, Gil
Jarvis, Doug
Reese, Jim
Cox, David
Haqq, Akbar
Bell, Ralph
Jones, Howard
Moore, Barry
Gzowski, Peter
Harpur, Tom
Alvi, Dr.
Shulman, Morton
Purling, Linus
Trott, Allan
Manson, Charles
Wood, Cathy
Fisher, Mike

Index of Names—By Chapter in Order of Appearance

Pollock, John
Schuller, Bob
Warkentin, Martha
Bloodgood, Jim
Wesley, Charles
Agajanian, Danny
Agajanian, Dennis
Ellerbie, Bruce
Ellerbie, Agnes
McQueen, Steve
McQueen, Barbara

Chapter 14
Wycliffe, John
Harvard, John
Mather, Cotton
Whitefield, George
Asbury, Francis
Dickinson, Jonathan
Edwards, Jonathan
Beecher, Lyman
Booth, William
Aberhart, William
Simpson, A.B.
Douglas, Tommy
Brown, John
Riley, W.B.
Maier, Walter A.
Fuller, Charles
Falwell, Jerry
Gifford, Kathie Lee
Robertson, Pat
Voskuyl, Roger
Thompson, Robert
Dinsdale, Walter
Reimer, Donald
Harrison, Rolland K.
Farquharson, Morris
Goheen, Allan
Judson, Douglas

Patterson, Marwood
Virgin, William
Zacharias, Ravi
Henderson, Paul
Onley, David
Flaherty, James
Hesburgh, Theodore
Grant, Amy
Reese, Allan
Jackson, Basil
Tchividjian, Gigi
Crouser, Harv
Armeding, Hudson
Ryan, Walter
Ryan, Jennifer
Osborne, Mark
Osborne, Madolyn
Emery, Cal
Spoelstra, Watson
Cosell, Howard
Howarth, Jerry
Howarth, Mary
Timlin, Mike
Carter, Joe
Burns, Britt
Hopp, Johnny
Thompson, Mychal
Johnson, Magic
McMahon, Mike Sr.
McMahon, Mike Jr.
McClintock, Joel
Johnson, Ben
Charest, Jean
Johnson, Dezrene
Khadafi, Momar

Chapter 15
Maughon, Grover
Maughon, Marcie
Maughon, Robert

Ceraula, Joe
Ceraula, Marlene
Greenwood, Glen
Majors, David
Cooper, Stephen
Livingstone, Jim
Graham, Jane
McGlassan, Billy Joe
Furman, Dick
Furman, Lowell
Pearson, Lester B.
Butters, Bill
Strum, Roseanne
Peltier, Bill
Plate, Leo
Coomes, Tommy
Beukema, Hank
Barnett, Sherman
Little, Danny
McCarthy, Herb
Marti, Bill
Newman, Paul
Cash, Johnny
Patti, Sandi
Gifford, Kathie Lee
Durrant, Peter
Duff, Sandra
Duff, Frank
Trudeau, Michel
Booth, Bonnie
Rubin, Bernard
Sobchak, Anatoly
Putin, Vladimir
James, Richard
Nesbitt, Lloyd
Rovenstine, Wendel
McCartney, Bill
Skaggs, Ricky
Graham, Mel Jr.
McElroy, Catherine

McCloy, Mr.
Adsett, Rob
Hollingworth, Peter
Van DeVenter, Judson W.
Patterson, Mark Sr.
Patterson, Mark Jr.
Rhoads, Ross
Rhoads, Carol
Barnhouse, D.G.
Smith, M.W.

Chapter 16
Durston, Fred
Gustafson, Roy
Merrill, Stephen
Allan, David
Davis, Linda
Hajik, Dr.
Hull, John
Hamilton, Doreen
Newman, Bill
Parrish, Preston
Fisher, David
Olerud, John
Huston, Todd
McLean, Elwood
Wetheral, Gordon
Molitor, Paul
Sprague, Ed
Parson, George
Holyfield, Evander
Cowper, William
Barker, Donna
Rees, Alf
Pauline, Ms.
Jacques, Mrs. Ike
Brooks, John
Shearer, Gary
Coren, Michael
Roddy, Bob

Boyes, David
Brown, Moira
Christensen, Marion
Cheatham, Melvin
Turner, John
Claremont, Patricia

Chapter 17
Hussein, Saddam
Bin Laden, Osama
Price, Charles Wesley
Price, Hannah
Price, Hilary
Price, Laura
Lotz, Anne Graham
Price, Matthew
Thomas, Major
Briscoe, Jill
Briscoe, Stuart
Taylor, Bentley Dr.
Knight, Lloyd
Knight, Stephen
Pope John Paul

Chapter 18
White, Grandmother
Manchester, William
Frist, Bill
White, Paula
White, William Sabastien
White, Izzy Peter
Rees, Bernadette

Index of Names

By Alphabetic Order

Abdul-Haqq, Akbar
Aberhart, William
Abraham, John
Adsett, Rob
Agajanian, Danny (Brother)
Agajanian, Dennis
Alderdice, David
Allan, David
Allan, Tom
Alou, Philippe
Alvi, Dr.
Andersen, Paul
Andrew, Sister
Apps, Syl
Armerding, Hudson
Armstrong, Neil
Asbury, Francis
Ayers, Lou

Baird, Clifford
Baird, Neville
Baird, Sam
Baird, Stephen
Baird, Trevor
Barker, Donna
Barnett, Sherman

Barnhouse, D.G.
Beatles, The
Beavan, Jerry
Beecher, Lyman
Bell, Ralph
Bell, Rhonda
Benjamin, Dwayne
Bentley-Taylor Dr.
Beukema, Hank
Bin Laden, Osama
Blair, Tony
Blanchard, Lewis
Bledsoe, Terry
Bledsoe, Tom
Blessit, Arthur
Blinco, Joe
Bloodgood, Jim
Booth, Bonnie
Booth, William
Boyes, David
Boyzeo
Brady, Olga
Briggs, James
Briggs, Mary
Bright, Bill
Briscoe, Jill
Briscoe, Stuart

Brooks, Joan
Brown, Bill
Brown, Joan
Brown, Joy Lois
Brown, Moira
Bubeck, Mark
Bullock, Bruce
Bullock, Jean
Burns, Britt
Busby, Russell
Bush, Barbara
Bush, George H.W.
Bush, George W.
Bush, Laura
Bush, Robin
Butler, Bill

Caesar, Julius
Cairns, Earle
Calderwood, Billy
Calderwood, Maidra
Calderwood, Mina Wilson
Calderwood, Ruth
Calderwood, William
Cantalon, Howard
Carpenter, Jerry
Carson, Johnny

Suddenly Silenced

Carter, Clarence
Carter, Joe
Cash, Johnny
Castro, Fidel
Ceraula, Joe
Ceraula, Marlene
Chambers, Irv
Chapman, Wilbur
Cheatham, Melvin
Christensen, Al
Christensen, Marion
Churchill, Winston
Clark, Joe
Claremount, Patricia
Clemenger, Bruce
Clews, Mrs. Charles
Clinton, Bill
Collins, Jackie
Colson, Charles
Cook, Bob
Coomes, Tommy
Cooper, Stephen
Coren, Michael
Cornell, Britney
Cornell, Ted
Cornell, Ted Jr.
Cornell, Zandra
Corts, John
Cosell, Howard
Cowan, Margaret
Cowan, Maxwell
Cowper, William
Cox, David
Cox, Harvey
Crawford, Percy
Criswell, W. A.
Crouser, Harv

Davies, Bob
Davis, Linda

DeBoer, Lester
Dickinson, Jonathan
Diefenbaker, John
Dienert, Millie
Dienert, Ted
Dillon, John
Dinsdale, Walter
Dobbie, Florence
Dobbie, Orde
Dobbie, William
Dodds, Gil
Drillon, Gordon
Duff, Frank
Duff, John
Duff, Sandra
Durrant, Peter
Durston, Fred
Dylan, Bob
Dynna, Dole
Dynna, Gilbert
Dynna, Harold
Dynna, Lillian

Edwards, Jonathan
Einstein, Albert
Eisenhower, Dwight
Elizabeth, Queen
Elizabeth, Queen Mother
Ellerbie, Agnes
Ellerbie, Bruce
Ellis, Perry
Ellis, Robbie
Emery, Cal
Epstein, Brian
Evans, Don
Evans, Robert
Evans, Susan
Everson, Hubert

Fabiano, Jerry

Faisal, Prince
Falwell, Jerry
Farquarson, Morris
Fasig, Bill
Findlay, John
Findley, Timothy
Finney, Charles
Fischer, Mike
Fisher, David
Flaherty, James
Ford, Gerald
Ford, Jean
Ford, Leighton
Foreman, George
Freeland, Gordon
Frist, Bill
Fuller, Charles
Furman, Dick
Furman, Lowell

Gaugenzio
George, King VI
Girvan, George
Goheen, Allen
Goodall, Richard
Goodwin-Hudson A.W.
Gore, Al
Graham, Billy
Graham, Franklin
Graham, Glenna
Graham, June
Graham, Mel
Graham, Mel Jr.
Graham, Ruth
Graham, Ruth Jr.
Graham, Will
Graham, William
   Franklin Sr.
Grant, Amy
Gray, James

Index of Names—By Alphabetic Order

Greene, Lorne
Greenwood, Glen
Gretzky, Wayne
Grier, Rosie
Gustafson, Len
Gustafson, Roy
Guevara, Che
Gzowski, Peter

Hajik, Dr.
Hall, Myrtle
Hamilton, Doreen
Hamilton, Sam
Harper, Stephen
Harpur, Tom
Harris, Trevor
Harrison, Rolland K.
Harvard, John
Harvey, Lord
Hawking, Stephen
Healey, Sid
Heitzig, Skip
Hemingway, Ernest
Henderson, Paul
Hendry, Gordon
Hendrix, Jimi
Hesburgh, Theodore Dr.
Hewitt, Foster
Hinn, Benny
Hinn, Clemence
Hinn, Constandi
Hitler, Adolf
Hoffman, Abbie
Hollands, Aunt Emma
Hollands, Fred
Hollands, Harold
Holliday, Don
Hollingworth, Peter
Holyfield, Evander
Hopp, Johnny

Horowitz, Michael
Howarth, Jerry
Howarth, Mary
Hull, Bobby
Hull, John
Humbard, Rex
Hussein, Saddam
Hustad, Don
Huston, Esther
Huston, Sterling
Hudson, Todd
Huxley, Aldous

Innis, John

Jackson, Basil
Jackson, Lowell
Jacques, Mrs. Ike
James, Homer
James, Richard
Janecek, Ed
Janecek, Janine
Janecek, Phil
Jarvis, Doug
Johnson, Ben
Johnson, Dezrene
Johnson, LB.
Johnson, Magic
Johnson, Torrey
Jones, Bob
Jones, Howard
Jones, Old Man
Joplin, Janis
Jostlin, Eric
Jostlin, LaVonne
Judson, Doug

Kathie, L.G.
Kemple, Dick
Kendall, Ron

Kennedy, Bobby
Kennedy, John F.
Kennedy, Joseph
Kennedy, Teddy
Keon, Davey
Kerry, John
Khadafi, Momar
King George
King, Larry
Kirk, Gordon
Kirk, John
Knight, Lloyd
Knight, Stephen
Kopechne, Mary Jo
Kuhlman, Kathryn

Landry, Tom
Lastman, Mel
Laurie, Greg
LaVonne, March
Layman, Eldon
Leary, Timothy
Lee, Robert
Lenning, Jerry
Lenning, Johnny
Lenning, Scott
Lenning, Tammy
Lewis, C.S.
Lindsey, Charles
Little, Danny
Livingstone, Jim
Lotz, Anne Graham
Lowry, Oscar
Luther, Martin
Lynn, Dr.

MacArthur, Douglas
MacArthur, John
Mahovolich, Frank
Maier, Walter A.

Suddenly Silenced

Mainse, David
Mainse, Norma Jean
Majors, David
Manchester, William
Manning, Ernest
Manning, Preston
Manson, Charles
Marcos, President
Marcuse, Herbert
Marti, Bill
Martin, Bill
Martin, Paul
Mather, Cotton
Marx Karl
Matier, Mina
Matier, Billy
Maughon, Grover
Maughon, Marcie
Maughon, Martha
Maughon, Robert
McCarthy, Herb
McCartney, Bill
McClintock, Mrs. Bill
McCloy, Mr.
McClung, Nellie
McCoy, Mike
McDonald, Jimmie
McDougall, Douglas
McElroy, Catherine
McGee, Vernon
McGlassan, Billy
McGovern, George
McIntosh, Mike
McKuen, Rod
McLean, Elwood
McLean, Glen
McPherson, Aimee
McQueen, Steve
McQueen, Barbara
McRae, William

McVety, Betty
McVety, Charles
McVety, Doug
McVety, Elmer
McVety, Hugh
McVety, Linda
Merrill, Stephen
Metz, Nick
Mingh, Ho Chi
Mitsuhashi, Mr. and Mrs.
Molitor, Paul
Monaghan, Rinty
Monroe, Marilyn
Moody, D. L.
Mooney, Nellie
Moore, Barry
Mosienko, Bill
Mullinder, Wesley
Mulroney, Brian
Munn, Allan
Musial, Stan
Musto, Steve

Nelsen, Frank
Nesbitt, Lloyd
Newman, Bill
Newman, Don
Newman, Paul
Nixon, Pat
Nixon, Richard
Nunn, Arthur

Olaf, King
Olerud, John
Onley, David
Osborne, Dr.
Osborne, Madolyn
Osborne, Mark

Paisley, Ian

Parrish, Preston
Parson, George
Paskett, Louis
Paskett, Shirley
Patterson, Mark
Patterson, Marwood
Patti, Sandi
Pattison, Jimmy
Paul, Billy
Pauline, Ms.
Pauling, Linus
Pearson, Lester B.
Peden, Sister
Peltier, Bill
Peters, Frank
Phillips, Randy
Pickering, John
Pickering, Olive
Pierce, Bob
Pilate, Pontius
Pocock, Maggie
Pollock, John
Pope, John Paul XXIII
Presley, Elvis
Price, Charles Wesley
Price, Hannah
Price, Hilary
Price, Laura
Price, Matthew
Pritchard, Lorne
Putin, Vladimir

Radar, Paul
Reagan, Ronald
Rees, Alf
Rees, Bernadette
Reese, Allan
Reese, Jim
Reimer, Donald
Rhoads, Carol

Index of Names—By Alphabetic Order

Rhoads, Ross
Richard, Cliff
Riley, W.B.
Robb, John
Roberts, Oral
Robertson, Lloyd
Robertson, Olga
Robertson, Pat
Rockefeller, Nelson
Roddy, Bob
Rogers, Adrian
Romeo
Roosevelt, Franklin D.
Rosell, Merv
Ross, Autumn
Ross, Larry
Rovenstine, Wendel
Rowlandson, Maurice
Rubin, Bernard
Rubin, Jerry
Ryan, Steve
Ryan, Walter

Salem, Beulah
Salem, Harold
Sargent, Jean
Schuller, Bob
Scriven, Joseph
Shakespeare, William
Shaw, George B.
Shea, George Beverly
Shea, Karlene
Shearer, Gary
Sheppard, Arthur
Sheppard, Harry
Sherrard, Sam
Shuler, Jack
Shulman, Morton
Simpson, A.B.
Skaggs, Ricky

Smith, Anita
Smith, Brent
Smith, M.W.
Smith, O.J.
Smith, Paul
Smith, Tedd
Sommerville, Albert
Sommerville, Dorothy
Sommerville, Kenneth
Sommerville, Roy
Southern, Dan
Spoelstra, Watson
Sprague, Ed
Spurgeon, Charles
Stam, Peter
Steinbeck, John
Stephens, Arthur
Stephens, Bishop John
Stewart, Nels
Stiller, Brian
Strand, Dr.
Strum, Roseanne
Stuart, Jimmy
Subchak, Anatoly
Summers, Anthony
Sweeting, George

Taylor, Mick
Tchividjian, Stephan
Templeton, Charles
Thatcher, Margaret
Thatcher, Ross
Thielman, Calvin
Thomas, Edward
Thomas, Major
Thompson, Mychal
Thompson, Robert
Timlin, Mike
Tornquist, Evie
Torrey, R.A.

Townsend, Colleen
Trelford, Edward Lee
Trelford, Margaret
Trelford, Sandy
Trelford, Stephen
Trott, Allan
Trudeau, Pierre Elliott
Trudeau, Michel
Tso, Peter
Tung Mai, Tse
Turner, John
Twist, Arlo

Upritchard, Harry

Van DeVenter, Judson W.
Van Dyke, Vonda Kay
Vince, Frank
Virgin, William
Voskyl, Roger

Wade, Wendy
Wagner, Linda
Walker, Hugh
Wallace, George
Wallace, John
Wallace, Paula
Walsh, John
Warkentin, Martha
Waters, Ethel
Watson, Merla
Watson, Merv
Weatherhead, Leslie
Wells, Jennifer
Wells, John
Wells, Lois
Wells, Margaret
Wells, Mark
Wells, Russell
Wesley, Charles

Wesley, John
Wetheral, Evelyn
Wetheral, Gordon
Wetheral, Jim
White, Aileen
White, Aunt Beryl
White, Betty
White, Brian
White, Charlton Bill
White, Clara
White, Elmore
White, Finnan
White, Frank
White, Grandmother
White, Hugh
White, Izzy
White, John Wesley
White, John Wesley Jr.
White, Kathleen Ellen
White, Lewis
White, Lorraine
White, Margaret
White, Martha Jean
White, Nok
White, Paul
White, Pearl
White, Paula
White, Randy
White, Richard
White, Roy
White, Sheryl
White, Timothy Randolf Dean
White, William
Whitefeather, Chief
Whitefield, George
Whittall, John
Williams, Garnett
Williams, Ted
Wills, Stephanie

Wilson, Grady
Wilson, T.W.
Wilson, Woodrow
Winmill, Joan
Winstone, Howard
Wood, Cathy
Wycliffe, John
Wyrtzen, Jack

Zacharias, Ravi
Zimmerman, Jack